Implementing a global health programme

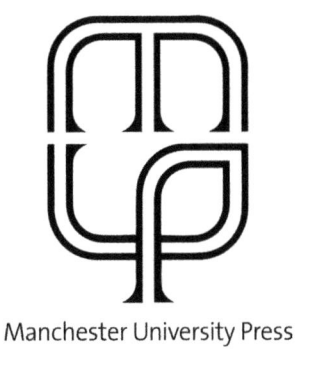

Manchester University Press

SSHM

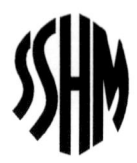

SOCIAL HISTORIES OF MEDICINE

Series Editors
David Cantor, Anne Hanley and Elaine Leong

Editorial Board
Diego Armus, Swarthmore College, PA, USA
Rana Hogarth, University of Illinois, Urbana-Champaign, USA
Angela Ki Che Leung, University of Hong Kong, China
Ian Miller, Ulster University, Northern Ireland

Social Histories of Medicine is concerned with all aspects of health, illness and medicine, from prehistory to the present, in every part of the world. The series covers the circumstances that promote health or illness, the ways in which people experience and explain such conditions, and what, practically, they do about them. Practitioners of all approaches to health and healing come within its scope, as do their ideas, beliefs, and practices, and the social, economic and cultural contexts in which they operate. Methodologically, the series welcomes relevant studies in social, economic, cultural and intellectual history, as well as approaches derived from other disciplines in the arts, sciences, social sciences and humanities. The series is a collaboration between Manchester University Press and the Society for the Social History of Medicine.

To buy or to find out more about the books currently available in this series, please go to: https://manchesteruniversitypress.co.uk/series/social-histories-of-medicine/

Implementing a global health programme

Smallpox and Nepal

Susan Heydon

MANCHESTER UNIVERSITY PRESS

Copyright © Susan Heydon 2025

The right of Susan Heydon to be identified as the author of this work has been asserted in accordance with the Copyright, Designs and Patents Act 1988.

Published by Manchester University Press
Oxford Road, Manchester, M13 9PL

www.manchesteruniversitypress.co.uk

British Library Cataloguing-in-Publication Data
A catalogue record for this book is available from the British Library

ISBN 978 1 5261 7666 0 hardback

First published 2025

The publisher has no responsibility for the persistence or accuracy of URLs for any external or third-party internet websites referred to in this book, and does not guarantee that any content on such websites is, or will remain, accurate or appropriate.

Typeset by Newgen Publishing UK

Contents

Figures, maps and tables	vii
Acknowledgements	viii
Abbreviations	xi
Notes on spelling and terminology	xiii
Key events	xiv
Maps	xvii
Introduction	1
1 Writing Nepal into global smallpox history	24
2 Smallpox in Nepal	45
3 Nepal – a nation state	67
4 1963–64 – epidemic smallpox	93
5 Engaging global policy – from control to eradication	118
6 Vaccination and global strategies	143
7 A time of transition	168
8 Expanding nationwide	193
9 Success	218
Conclusion: Implementing a global health programme – and making it work	252
Appendices	
1 Smallpox cases reported by year, 1961–75	268
2 Selected health and socio-economic indicators, 1951–76	269
3 Financial inputs by the Government of Nepal and WHO, 1962–76 (US$)	271
4 Vaccinations carried out through the HMG/WHO smallpox programme	272

Glossary 273
Bibliography 275
Index 291

Figures, maps and tables

Figures

0.1	Child with smallpox	2
5.1	A vaccination team near Boudhanath Stupa, Kathmandu Valley	132
6.1	Bridge under construction over the Parajuli river, Dailekh district, Bheri zone	150

Maps

1	Nepal – districts and zones	xviii
2	Nepal – elevation and rivers	xx

Tables

4.1	Notified smallpox cases and deaths, Kathmandu, April 1963–January 1964	100
7.1	'Modern' health services in the sample villages of the Nepal Health Survey	175
7.2	Preparatory, attack and maintenance phases in Nepal's plan to eradicate smallpox	185

Acknowledgements

I could not have completed this book without the help of many people and organisations over many years and in many countries. You have all made this book and I thank you very much. Email and Zoom do not replace in-person communication, but these enabled me to keep in contact and work around the challenges from another communicable disease, COVID-19, that helps make this history of implementing a global health programme relevant and topical for today's ongoing health challenges.

People's stories are at the heart of the book – they enrich and they disrupt. My journey with Nepal's smallpox story began with the 1963 smallpox epidemic in the Mt Everest region where we had lived for two years – people told me about it even if it was absent from the official written record. Later, Professor Sanjoy Bhattacharya showed me a copy of the account about Nepal in the global programme's official history and thought I might like to do some research! At the time I did not know this was the only published account of the project in Nepal. Nor did I appreciate its significance. Importantly, Sanjoy also funded me to give a talk at WHO in Geneva, which enabled me to visit the library and archives. Reynald Erard and Tomas Allen have given me much help. A few months later I was in Kathmandu where Dr Pratyoush Onta and the Martin Chautari research centre had invited me to give an exploratory talk about my proposed research. I had precious little to contribute about Nepal and smallpox at that point, but shortly before leaving and just a week before the massive 2015 earthquake my pharmacist colleague Kiran Bajracharya asked if I would like to talk with a friend of his father who had smallpox as a child. We

Acknowledgements

also went to the temple at Swayambhunath. My smallpox in Nepal journey shifted focus to my thinking about a devastating disease that was part of people's lives and from which many people died. Like so many people from countries where smallpox had disappeared, I had only thought about prevention and vaccination. Two years later I was able to return to Kathmandu, and we went and talked with people in the nearby small town of Kirtipur.

Information about the Kathmandu area tends to dominate writings about Nepal but following up on a magazine article I was introduced to former Peace Corps volunteers Don Messerschmidt and Bruce Morrison who carried out vaccinations in the Lamjung area of central Nepal as part of responses to the 1963–64 epidemic. Bruce died in August 2023 but was pleased to know that I would be telling their smallpox story, which is not mentioned in the Peace Corps publication about the organisation's contribution to the global smallpox programme. Don introduced me to Doug Hall and the wonderful collection of photos about Nepal of the Peace Corps photo project. He also met up with Dr Edward Crippen's family at a reunion, visited and was given papers about smallpox to pass on to me. Jay Friedman, WHO Technical Officer in the later years of Nepal's smallpox programme, has also been very generous with his time, although I was disappointed that we were not able to locate his old car, which he had tracked to New Zealand!

In Nepal, I continue to owe much to the valuable conversations and insights from Dr Kami Temba Sherpa and Dr Lhakpa Norbu Sherpa. Professor Hemang Dixit has provided me with much help over the years introducing me to people who might be able to help, finding literature and translating, checking information and answering my many questions. Through an email to his public health colleagues, I met with Dr Benu Karki and Dr Rita Thapa. Dr Karki also explained much about how the public service works.

Nepal is a special place to many New Zealanders. My book begins with the Mt Everest region as does my own introduction to Nepal with our family's involvement with the Himalayan Trust and the ongoing work of Sir Edmund Hillary. More recently, I would like to thank Peter and Sarah Hillary for permission to access and use their father's papers and photos. Mike Gill has given me permission to use the emotive image of a child with smallpox. In 1963 New Zealand's only medical school was at the University of Otago in Dunedin. The head of the Department of Preventive and Social Medicine was international smallpox expert Professor Cyril Dixon. The University has a considerable collection of WHO publications, including a hard copy of the Big Red Book. The unstinting help of Health Sciences library staff throughout is very much appreciated. I would also like to thank Chris Garden from the School of Geography for assistance with maps and the School of Pharmacy for enabling me to carry out this research.

Finally, I have had wonderful support from my family who have now 'lived' with smallpox for many years. This book is a very big thank you to them and to all who have helped me.

Abbreviations

AMEE	American Mount Everest Expedition
ANZ	Archives New Zealand
BCG	Bacille Calmette-Guérin (vaccine against tuberculosis/TB)
CDC	1946: Communicable Disease Center; 1970: Center for Disease Control; 1992: Centers for Disease Control and Prevention
DDT	Dichloro-diphenyl-trichloroethane
DPT	Diptheria–pertussis–tetanus (vaccine)
EPI	Expanded Programme on Immunization
FP/MCI I	Family Planning and Maternal Child Health
HMG	His Majesty's Government
IOR	India Office Records (UK)
JNMA	*Journal of Nepal Medical Association*
KH	Khunde Hospital
NMA	Nepal Medical Association
NMEO	Nepal Malaria Eradication Organization
NMEP	National Malaria Eradication Programme
PDW	Panchayat development worker
PRC	People's Republic of China
SEARO	South-East Asia Regional Office (WHO)
SEP	Smallpox Eradication Programme. In Nepal, SEP or NESP denotes Nepal's Smallpox Eradication Project/Programme
TAR	Tibet Autonomous Region (of China)
TNA	The National Archives (UK)
UMN	United Mission to Nepal

Abbreviations

UN	United Nations
UNESCO	United Nations Educational, Scientific and Cultural Organization
UNICEF	United Nations Children's Fund
USAID	United States Agency for International Development
USOM	United States Operations Mission
WER	*Weekly Epidemiological Record*
WHA	World Health Assembly
WHO	World Health Organization; WHO HQ: Headquarters in Geneva
WPC&R	WHO Programme Coordinator and Representative; also WR: WHO country representative

Notes on spelling and terminology

Many versions of names and places in Nepal exist. Where used in quotes, the spelling will be according to the source. Nepali words and terms used in the main text are italicised and explained on first use.

Following practice in Nepali discourse I use Nepali and Nepalis throughout, rather than Nepalese to denote nationality and Nepali the language. Gurkha, however, is used to refer to Nepali troops in the British Army. Sherpa or Sherpas denote the ethnic group and not an occupational category in expeditions.

Many Nepalis use their ethnicity or caste name as their surname. Names such as Shrestha or Sherpa, therefore, denote the family or wider group rather than a person's given name. Full names are given. Some names are common in this book – such as Shrestha – and where there is the potential for confusion in subsequent references initials are added for clarity.

I use the Gregorian calendar. The Bikram Sambat is the official calendar of Nepal and started fifty-seven years earlier.

In Nepal, the term 'modern medicine' is used commonly, as is 'allopathic', to refer to what is variously called in the literature western medicine, modern medicine, biomedicine, scientific medicine, cosmopolitan medicine or allopathic medicine. Multiple terms reflect multiple views.

Public health and epidemiological terms are used throughout the book. They are defined in the text but also key terms regarding the smallpox programme are listed in a glossary.

Key events

1743	Prithvi Narayan Shah crowned king of Gorkha
1814–16	Anglo-Gorkha War; Treaty of Sagauli leads to the permanent establishment of a British Resident in Kathmandu; British East India Company starts recruiting Gurkha soldiers
1816	Death of King Girvan Yuddha Bikram Shah from smallpox
1846	Kot Massacre; Jang Bahadur becomes prime minister and in 1849 assumes the name of Rana; control of the government is held by the Rana family as hereditary prime ministers until 1951; 1850 Jang Bahadur visits Europe
1889	Opening of Bir Hospital in Kathmandu
1914–18	About 100,000 Nepali troops support Britain in the First World War
1923	Britain in a treaty with Nepal formally recognises Nepal's independence
1934	January: massive earthquake causes widespread destruction
1939–45	Nepal supports Britain in the Second World War
1947	Following India's independence from Britain, India receives twelve and Britain eight of the existing Gurkha battalions; the USA recognises Nepal as an independent state and signs an Agreement of Commerce and Friendship

Key events

1948	World Health Organization (WHO) established; November: the WHO Regional Office for South-East Asia established in New Delhi with the first members being Afghanistan, India, Burma (Myanmar), Ceylon (Sri Lanka) and Thailand
1950	Treaty of Peace and Friendship between India and Nepal, November: King Tribhuvan's flight to the Indian Embassy
1951	General Agreement for Technical Cooperation with the USA; February: formal end of Rana regime and establishment of government coalition under King Tribhuvan; coalition collapses – sets pattern for several years of political instability and changes of government
1953	First ascent of Mt Everest by New Zealander Edmund Hillary and Tenzing Norgay from Nepal with the British Mount Everest expedition; Nepal becomes a member of WHO
1955	Nepal becomes a member of the United Nations
1958	Epidemics of smallpox and cholera in Nepal
1959	Promulgation of constitution; general election; World Health Assembly (WHA) adopts goal of worldwide smallpox eradication; China intensified its presence in Tibet
1960	King Mahendra imposes direct royal rule; Treaty of Peace and Friendship between China and Nepal
1962	Start of joint Government of Nepal (HMG)/WHO Smallpox Control Pilot Project; war between India and China; promulgation of new constitution in Nepal setting up the panchayat system of government
1963	New Civil Code (Muluki Ain); widespread smallpox epidemic
1965	Administrative reorganisation creating 14 zones and 75 districts

1966	Revised plan signed between HMG and WHO to eradicate smallpox and control communicable diseases
1967	Plan solely concerned with smallpox eradication (SEP); start of global intensified smallpox eradication programme
1971	War in East Pakistan leads to the establishment of the independent nation state of Bangladesh
1973	Nepal classified as non-endemic for smallpox
1974	Major epidemic of smallpox in north-east India
1975	Last case of smallpox in Nepal; emergency rule declared in India; last case of smallpox in India; world's last case of endemic variola major, in Bangladesh
1977	Smallpox declared eradicated from Nepal following visit of International Commission; world's last case of endemic smallpox, variola minor, in Somalia
1979	Global Commission certifies eradication of the disease of smallpox
1980	Thirty-third World Health Assembly formally declares smallpox eradicated globally

Maps

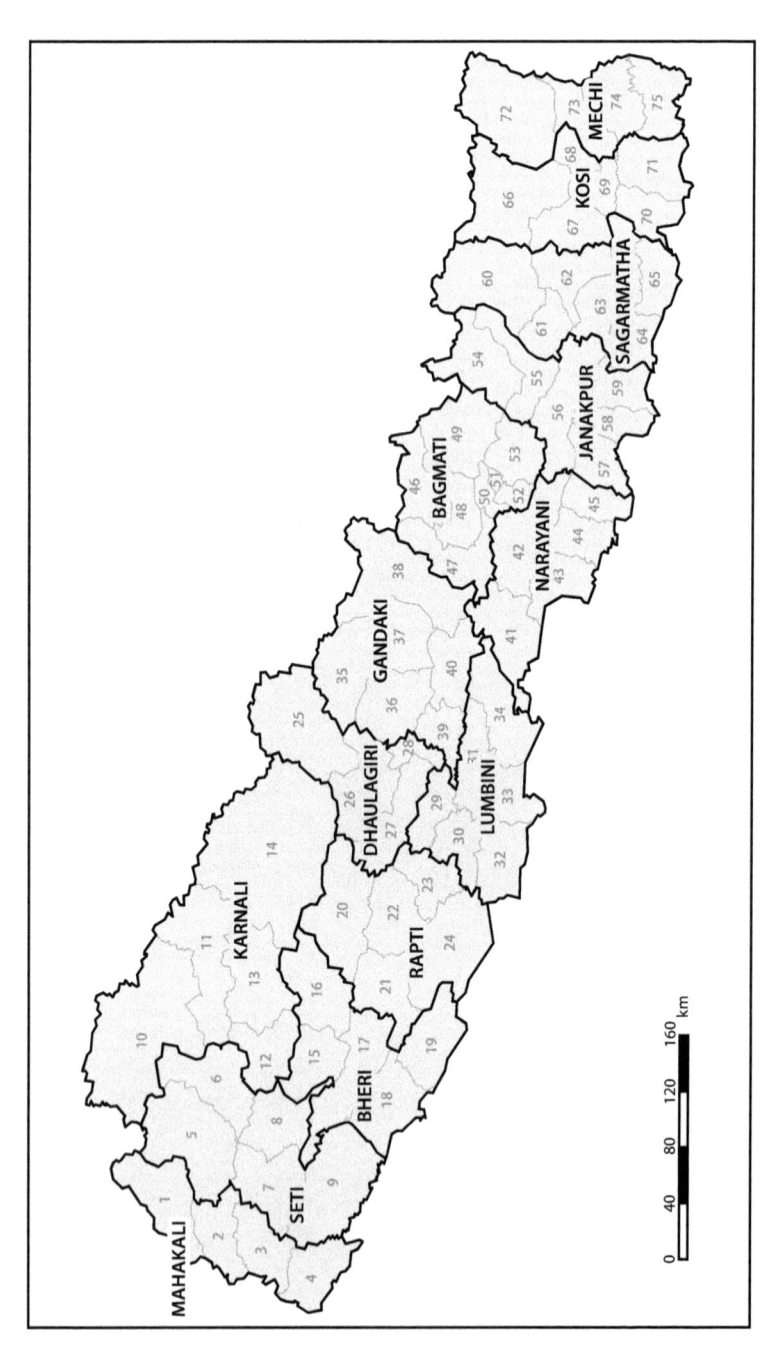

Map 1 Nepal – districts and zones

1	Darchula	39	Syangja
2	Baitadi	40	Tanahun
3	Dadeldhura	41	Chitwan
4	Kanchanpur	42	Makwanpur
5	Bajhang	43	Parsa
6	Bajura	44	Bara
7	Doti	45	Rautahat
8	Achham	46	Rasuwa
9	Kailali	47	Dhading
10	Humla	48	Nuwakot
11	Mugu	49	Sindhupalchok
12	Kalikot	50	Kathmandu
13	Jumla	51	Bhaktapur
14	Dolpa	52	Laltipur (Patan)
15	Dailekh	53	Kabhrepalanchok
16	Jajarkot	54	Dolakha
17	Surkhet	55	Ramechhap
18	Bardiya	56	Sindhuli
19	Banke	57	Sarlahi
20	Rukum	58	Mahottari
21	Salyan	59	Dhanusha
22	Rolpa	60	Solukhumbu
23	Pyuthan	61	Okhaldhunga
24	Dang	62	Khotang
25	Mustang	63	Udayapur
26	Myagdi	64	Siraha
27	Baglung	65	Saptari
28	Parbat	66	Sankhuwasabha
29	Gulmi	67	Bhojpur
30	Arghakhanchi	68	Terhathum
31	Palpa	69	Dhankuta
32	Kapilvastu	70	Sunsari
33	Rupandehi	71	Morang
34	Nawalparasi	72	Taplejung
35	Manang	73	Panchthar
36	Kaski	74	Ilam
37	Lamjung	75	Jhapa
38	Gorkha		

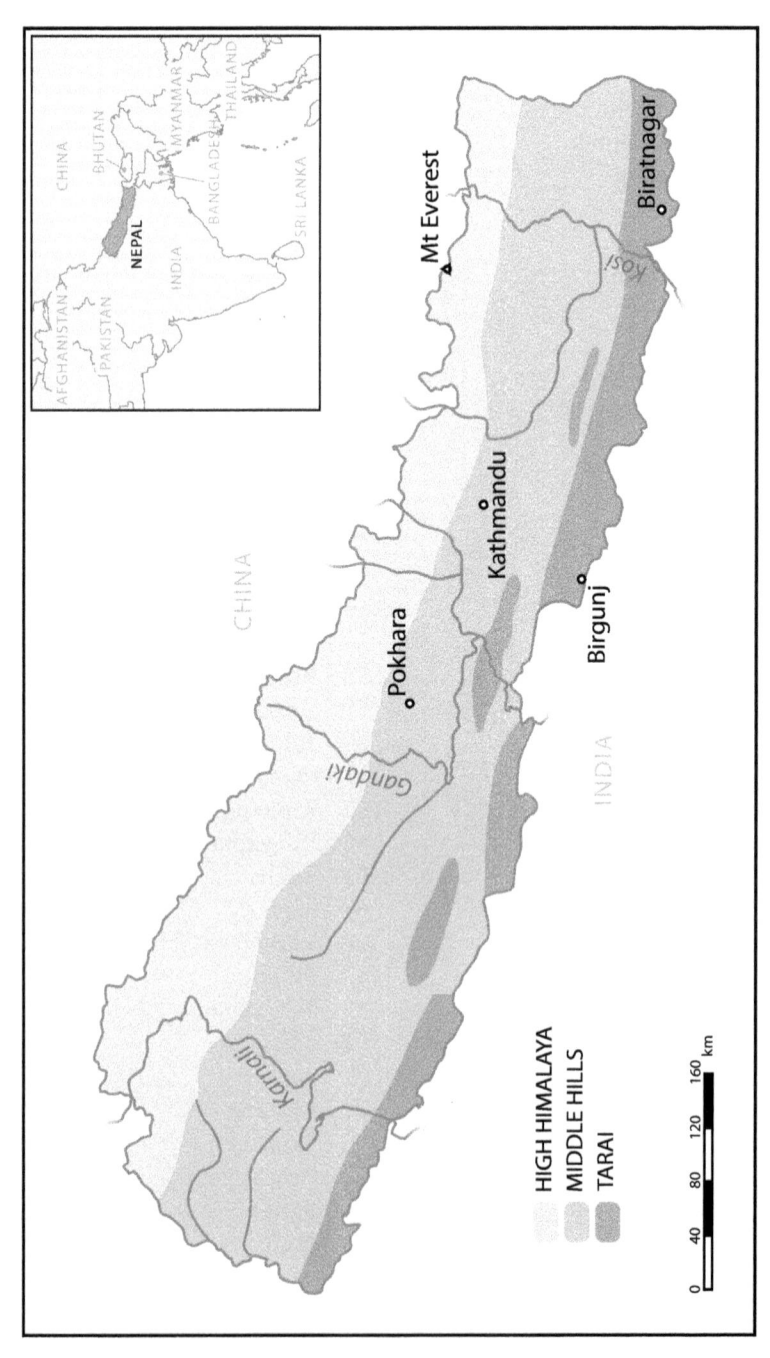

Map 2 Nepal – elevation and rivers

Introduction

The first cases of an outbreak of smallpox in the remote Mt Everest area appeared in early March 1963. Few government services of the small Himalayan kingdom of Nepal reached the high mountains near its northern border with the Tibet Autonomous Region (TAR) of China. Dr Lhakpa Norbu Sherpa from Thangte (Upper Thame) village was not yet a teenager in 1963 as he talked about his vivid memories of the epidemic and what he had learned about his family's experiences.[1] For most people in the area the vaccination they received was their first experience of the 'modern' medicine that they had only heard about.[2] His village was one of the most badly affected and some of his relatives died. His house became a vaccination centre, but his parents were worried by the number of people crowding into their home who might spread the infection. Furthermore, the men vaccinating were not local, or government health workers or from elsewhere in Nepal, but were foreigners from a small New Zealand aid expedition.[3]

Epidemics in crowded urban areas such as the capital Kathmandu were not uncommon, but they were in a sparsely populated region such as Khumbu, the local Sherpa name for the Mt Everest area. There are no roads in Khumbu; a young Sherpa man had walked for several days from his village to Kathmandu to look for employment. He wanted to find work as a porter carrying supplies and equipment for one of the foreign expeditions that were becoming regular visitors to Nepal.[4] While he was in Kathmandu he was infected with the smallpox (variola) virus, but it was only during the long two-week walk back into the mountains with the American Mount Everest Expedition (AMEE) that he became sick. This large expedition had over 900 porters. He continued his journey, but his condition worsened. Although other porters knew he had smallpox and shunned him on the trail, friends and family helped with his load so that he would not lose his wages. He stopped at houses along the way, coming into contact with villagers and other travellers, and later died. The walking track was a highway and steep-sided valleys concentrated people together whether they were local or strangers passing through. With high mountains on either side there was nowhere else for people to go. The disease began to spread.

On another occasion and in a different part of the country a grandmother asked me what I was going to do with her story.[5] I said I was going to tell it in a book. Four of her children had smallpox; she said that everyone along her street had someone who had died of smallpox. Like others, she looked after her sick children at home. We were in the hill town of Kirtipur on the edge of the Kathmandu Valley. Most of its inhabitants are Newar, who are often mentioned in accounts as being opposed to vaccination.

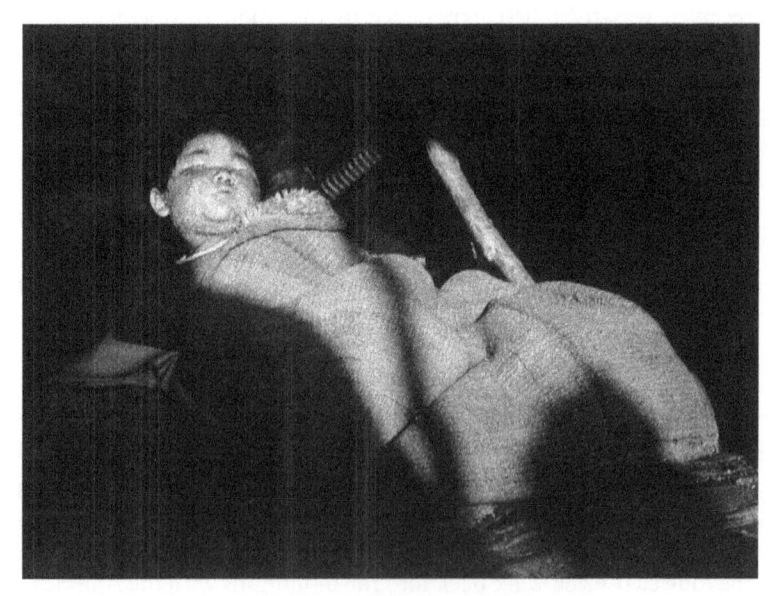

Figure 0.1 Child with smallpox.
Source: Mike Gill.

Not surprisingly, as I listened, people's stories about the disease and vaccination were complex. Some people were in favour, others less so and some changed their mind. Different factors influenced people's decisions. My colleague, pharmacist Kiran Bajracharya, who is Newar and from Kirtipur, helped me as interpreter. He told me that families talked together, but his friend had never heard his mother talk in such a way about the anguish she felt of seeing her child suffer with smallpox. Two years earlier we had talked with a man in Kathmandu city who had smallpox as a child.[6] His brother and sister had been vaccinated but had died. He did not know the cause of their deaths, but his mother had not wanted him – her only other child – to be vaccinated.

I not only wanted to tell these and other stories in a book but had in mind another audience for whom the smallpox narrative of the 1960s and 1970s usually culminates in the worldwide 'eradication' of the disease. Such stories as I was hearing are absent. This other narrative focuses on the successful implementation of a global health programme led and co-ordinated by the World Health Organization (WHO) with a goal of ridding the world of the disease of smallpox. Historically, eradication has had different meanings with different diseases and was often used to describe what today in health programmes for the wider population (public health) is considered as 'control' or 'elimination'.[7] Elimination was the achievement of smallpox-free status by individual countries – eradication was used for continents. The proposed global programme to eradicate smallpox meant the permanent reduction to zero of the incidence (number of new cases) of infection worldwide caused by a specific agent as a result of deliberate efforts.[8] Eradication was and remains controversial; the debates and literature about eradication and its benefits and drawbacks are wide-ranging and ongoing.[9] Success with the eradication programme, however, would mean that intervention measures were no longer needed in any country and money saved could be spent on other health issues.

The focus of this book is not on the concept of eradication or of making an *eradication* programme work. The stories I was hearing were not about this. This book is about the broader theme of implementing a global health programme and using Nepal's experiences to help understand vaccination and public health interventions more generally. Based initially on mass vaccination which involved delivering vaccinations to large numbers of people in various locations in a limited time, people's experiences are largely absent from the smallpox programme narrative, yet for the people I talked to, their ideas, practices and experiences of smallpox the disease were integral to how they approached being vaccinated.[10] For most Nepalis, vaccination meant smallpox and most Nepali people believed in its efficacy, but many factors influenced their decisions. The 'local' and the 'global', therefore, were deeply connected.

Although I had read about the 1963 epidemic in Sir Edmund Hillary's diary and book and in the AMEE expedition account, I had found few other references to the epidemic or to smallpox in Nepal. Talking with people brought to light people's experiences and the impact that the disease of smallpox had on their lives. Smallpox was experienced and looked after in the home and therefore away from the historical record of health services. Like most other people from countries which did not have the disease, I had only thought about vaccination. Unlike Nepal, much of the world in 1963 was already free of the disease but fear was aroused when a case occurred, imported from overseas. The worldwide spread of disease had long concerned international health authorities; quarantine was a key public health 'tool' but was to be balanced against disrupted international trade and increased political tension.[11] The aeroplane now enabled both people and the variola virus to travel more quickly and further afield. Smallpox had no cure, but it could be prevented through vaccination and revaccination since one dose did not give lifelong protection.

Smallpox was widespread in Nepal in 1963. To older Nepalis I talked with, it was a disease of their childhood, and many still carried the scars. My mentioning smallpox led to people talking about a disease that affected them, their family and their community. They were the survivors. Many people died, although the number of cases and deaths are unknown because there were no statistics. Elsewhere, mortality was known to be around 30 per cent.[12] A person with smallpox went through several stages as the disease progressed. Typically, smallpox had an incubation period of seven to seventeen days after exposure, but a person only became infectious once early symptoms such as fever and fatigue developed. Two to three days later, a characteristic rash appeared and could cover the whole body. The bumps were full of a clear liquid that later filled with pus. A crust then formed that dried and eventually fell off. Almost without exception, people either died or acquired long-lasting immunity, although accompanied by varying degrees of disfigurement. Despite its severity, smallpox was just one of many serious diseases facing Nepali people. Malaria, tuberculosis and cholera were major problems. Nepal was a poor country and the country's health infrastructure was extremely limited. Some vaccination was provided; smallpox was much feared, but its control was not a priority – neither for the government nor the people.

Vaccination had spread rapidly around much of the world since its introduction in Britain at the end of the eighteenth century, reaching India in 1802 and Nepal in 1816.[13] Although Nepal was defeated militarily by the East India Company in 1816, it did not become a British colony. Much has been written about smallpox vaccination as a 'site of conflict' between western medicine and the spread of empire, although other scholars have shown that the situation was complex.[14] In the case of Nepal, its government approached the newly imposed British Resident who organised for vaccine to be brought in from India. Many people were vaccinated in and around Kathmandu, although the practice did not spread.[15] The government did not consider a service such as vaccination to be part of its role. Towards the end of the nineteenth century the government began to provide some health services, but most of Nepal's overwhelmingly rural population was unable to access these.[16] Not until after 1951, when the monarchy returned to power after a century in the shadows and promised change, did vaccination begin to become more widespread. Education and health services expanded, but Nepal remained one of the world's most under-developed nation states. Being located strategically between the growing post-World War regional powers of India and China, it was beginning to attract considerable outside interest and foreign aid. The big new player was the United States of America (USA).

The twentieth century had brought the formation of a number of new institutions and organisations that focused on health issues. Following the destruction of the Second World War, the WHO with its headquarters in Geneva (Switzerland) was one of these. Established as an agency of the United Nations (UN) in 1948, the WHO grew out of past international organisation and cooperation taking over the notification responsibilities of its predecessor. The politics of the Cold War, however, had a considerable impact on the workings of WHO. The US and its allies were able to exert a dominating influence when in 1949 the Soviet Union (USSR) and other communist countries walked out of the UN system and therefore WHO. With their return in 1956 the balance of power in the World Health Assembly (WHA) – the governing forum and policy-setting body for the WHO – shifted. At a meeting in Minneapolis (USA), the member states of the WHA voted in 1958 in favour of a proposal put forward by the USSR representative, Viktor Zhdanov who was Deputy Minister of Health of the USSR, to go further than controlling smallpox and to support a policy of eradicating the disease worldwide based on mass vaccination.[17] In 1959, the WHA committed to undertaking a smallpox eradication programme.[18] Technological solutions characterised WHO's approach in these early years.[19] The yaws campaign in the early 1950s used the new penicillin. By the end of the decade, the WHO's principal activity was an increasingly expensive malaria eradication programme employing pesticides.

The WHO worked with nation states. Nepal became a member in 1953 functioning through the organisation's South-East Asia Region based in New Delhi, India.[20] Although its headquarters was in Geneva, the WHO had a decentralised structure and way of working with six regional offices. Following WHA policy to move towards worldwide smallpox eradication, the South-East Asia Regional Committee passed a Resolution at its meeting in September 1958 to support the initiative.[21] By 1960, Afghanistan, Burma (Myanmar), India, Indonesia and Thailand had started plans for eradication while Ceylon (Sri Lanka) had reported no cases for the previous two years.[22] That only left Nepal.[23] In 1959 the proposed regional budget for 1961 included funding to start a WHO-assisted pilot control project in the Kathmandu Valley. The aim was to build up a core of expertise and then expand to other parts of the country.

Over the next few years, smallpox was eliminated from other states in Asia, Africa and South America but progress was considered insufficient.[24] In 1966 the WHA voted to intensify its smallpox programme in 1967 and target the countries where the disease remained endemic (regularly present among the population). These included Nepal. Mass vaccination remained the global programme's initial strategy; increasingly, this shifted towards surveillance and containment operations as smallpox spread more slowly than was thought and not everyone needed to be vaccinated. One benefit of such knowledge was that less vaccine would be required for the programme. Surveillance and containment involved active searching to find cases, rigorous isolation of patients, and vaccination and surveillance of close contacts to contain outbreaks.[25]

In 1967 Nepal became part of the intensified global programme. With a story that the official history regarded as an 'impressive achievement', Nepal became free of smallpox.[26] It faced enormous geographical and infrastructural challenges, but central to its success were the local district smallpox supervisors, who were responsible for running the programme in their area, and after 1971 to a change in vaccination strategy to a time-limited annual programme that aligned with people's views as to when vaccination should be carried out. Despite the shorter period, vaccination numbers increased. Nepal was one of the last countries in the world to achieve success, but in 1973 it was no longer classified by WHO as an endemic country and in 1975 it recorded its last case. In 1977 an international commission certified that Nepal no longer had smallpox. In December 1979 the final report of the Global Commission for the Certification of Smallpox Eradication concluded that eradication had been achieved throughout the world and that there was no evidence that smallpox would return as an endemic disease. On 8 May 1980 the Thirty-third WHA proclaimed officially that the disease of smallpox had been eradicated from the globe.[27]

Over the decades, different anniversaries have been marked. In Geneva, on the fortieth anniversary, a plaque was unveiled in the room where on 9 December 1979 Dr Purushottam Narayan Shrestha from Nepal and the other members of the Global Commission had certified that the world was free of the disease of smallpox. Shrestha had led Nepal's programme from 1969 to 1977. The WHO Director-General, Dr Tedros Adhanom Ghebreyesus, spoke of 'what we can achieve when all nations work together'. 'When it comes to epidemic disease, we have a shared responsibility and a shared destiny.'[28] He reminded people how the successful smallpox eradication programme 'yielded vital knowledge and tools for … fighting diseases'. The diseases the Director-General used as examples were poliomyelitis (polio) and the Ebola virus, but a few months later on the fortieth anniversary of the official declaration by the WHA of smallpox eradication, the world was in the grip of a pandemic from the disease caused by the SARS-CoV-2 virus known as COVID-19. With heightened urgency, Tedros spoke of the need for the world to work together 'now more than ever'.[29]

Nation states around the world were facing a 'common threat', but their responses were very different. Tedros emphasised the importance of 'basic public health' tools used successfully against smallpox: disease surveillance, case reporting, contact tracing and mass communication campaigns to inform affected populations. Unlike smallpox, in May 2020 no vaccine existed for COVID-19. The tools mentioned by the Director-General, however, are one part of what is required. They do not exist in a vacuum.[30] To enable these to work, more is involved. The WHO is not the centre of this book but learning from Nepal's experience with eradicating smallpox can add to the 'basic public health' toolbox needed today. Nepal was successful because it found a way to adapt the global programme to the Nepali context. Its programme was also one of the least expensive to implement. As historian Agnieszka Sobocinska has reminded us, historians need 'to go beyond plans and track how projects were actually delivered, to capture the complex and often fraught negotiations taking place at ground level'.[31] Leading medical anthropologist Mark Nichter takes this further. We need to appreciate how the different groups involved conceptualise the problems 'if we are to develop culturally sensitive and socially responsible health programs and policies'.[32]

In the subsequent drawing together of lessons, benefits and legacy for public health, Nepal's contribution to the global programme has dropped out of people's consideration. Nepal's experiences, however, can be used to highlight the complexities of a global programme when faced with realities on the ground in any location. International cooperation, organisation and support are needed but the roots to success will differ. More than the tools – it is how and how well they are used, by whom and the context in which they are used. Nepal achieved success by moving away from the top-down and centre-led structure and effectively decentralised its operations to deal with the tremendous challenges it faced. It had to. Epidemiology takes into consideration social, political, economic, and environmental factors but these need to be thought of as equally important tools for public health interventions. Barriers need to be overcome or worked around and enablers need to be taken advantage of. Nepal's story with smallpox shows what can be achieved, although like elsewhere it also needs to be remembered that at the time it was 'anything but clear and straightforward'.[33]

The authors of the official history of the eradication programme published in 1988 wrote about the disease in the past tense. Although the clinical disease no longer exists, the long history of smallpox and its prevention remains a popular topic in the literature.[34] Smallpox is also referred to in discussions about globalisation with the success of the eradication programme feeding into and helping sustain the focus on 'global' in history generally and health history more specifically.[35] The variola virus, however, has not been destroyed. Cold War politics and threats of bioterrorism have entered the historiography.[36] Research continues into a better vaccine and some countries hold stocks of smallpox vaccine. This vaccine has been used to help against the spread of the closely related disease of mpox (monkeypox) as cases began to appear unexpectedly around the world. Nevertheless, with the passage of time since 1980, the achievement of the smallpox campaign is being reduced to a phase of an ongoing history.[37] The wealth of unpublished, published and online detail vital to understanding the implementation of a global health programme in different local settings and still valuable today is lost from brief summaries or lessons learned.

Why this book?

This book is about smallpox and Nepal and how a global health programme was adapted and decentralised to make it work on the ground. The book shifts the focus from the WHO to the nation state and to the individual being vaccinated. By exploring Nepal's experiences with smallpox, it brings the local into the global narrative. Nepal's story disrupts. As such, it is important not only for smallpox but also for other diseases. The many issues raised, the challenges faced and the solutions devised are important in how we think about and deal with communicable disease more generally.

At the forefront of this book are people's experiences of the disease and vaccination. A successful vaccination programme needs people to be vaccinated. People's experiences remind us of the awfulness of smallpox and that experiences as well as beliefs influence vaccination behaviour.[38] Vaccination remains a popular topic in a wide variety of literature. Being vaccinated has long been viewed as an individual behaviour that helps protect not only the body of an individual person but also the 'social body', the community.[39] A third dimension has been added – the global, where the benefits of vaccination cross national borders. People encountered and responded to smallpox as individuals, families and members of local communities, but a global effort introduced measures that in the case of smallpox moved ongoing national or regional efforts beyond prevention and control to worldwide eradication.[40] In practice, these many levels are more blurred and less stable.[41] Although the global smallpox programme was a response to a health issue, mass vaccination campaigns are political projects. National governments, however, occupy a middle space, since they might be seen as distant by individuals or small communities but local or regional by a global organisation such as the WHO.[42]

Along with India, Bangladesh, Pakistan and Afghanistan in the Himalayan and South Asian region, Nepal was one of the last small group of countries to eliminate the disease. A study of Nepal offers us a longer lens to view smallpox activities in one setting from early initiatives through to the programme's final stages. Unlike much of the South and South-East Asian region Nepal was not colonised, and through the lens of vaccination provides an opportunity to investigate colonial and post-colonial narratives.[43] The book brings to the fore a small country's experiences and shows local agency but also highlights the practice in public health to operate through the framework of nation states.[44] As historian Sanjoy Bhattacharya has urged, using a case study of Nepal and smallpox can 'show how the regional, national, and local components of this multifaceted programme were important and consistently active sites of negotiation and adaptation'.[45]

A central theme is the many challenges facing Nepal in the mid-twentieth century that affected not just smallpox but almost everything. The underlying question this book asks is why was smallpox eradication successful in Nepal?[46] This question may seem pointless when the programme succeeded everywhere, but that assumption brings in the benefit of hindsight and was not evident for most of the global programme. The enormous difficulties in Nepal that are described in the official history are usually offered as reasons why a programme does not work or takes too long. Why something worked is unusual.[47] Initially from the global perspective Nepal was not a high priority.[48] The global community knew little about Nepal since much of their attention was on Nepal's much larger neighbour India. In 1967, 83,943 (63.9 per cent) of the world's 131,418 reported cases were in India.[49] Nepal reported 110 cases (Appendix 1). As the number of countries with smallpox decreased, Nepal's visibility increased. In answering the question of why Nepal's Smallpox Eradication Project (SEP) succeeded it becomes possible to question the ongoing top-down narrative of the global programme and to identify what mattered on the ground if this or another programme was to succeed. It is in the implementation of the smallpox programme in Nepal that we can see it being made to work to overcome the many problems presented by the country's physical and human environment.

In their history of the WHO, Marcos Cueto, Theodore Brown and Elizabeth Fee firmly locate the success of the smallpox eradication programme in US support from 1965 and the Cold War détente.[50] The reduction of tension between the USA and the USSR in the later 1960s was significant if a global programme was to be based on cooperation.[51] Bhattacharya and Carlos Campani offer a different viewpoint and reassess the 'foundations' provided by previous multi-level and multi-sited negotiations, initiatives and activities worldwide.[52] In so doing, the programme's history adopts a wider geographical focus and longer timeframe than recent smallpox historiography suggests.[53] The later success, as Bhattacharya and Campani argue and Nepal also demonstrates, took time to develop and was built on what was created and learned from earlier successes and failures and the involvement of multiple actors to provide a richer history and alternative narrative timeline.

The official history of the global smallpox programme was written to record what happened but also to identify what was learned that might be useful for other programmes. Bhattacharya, whose earlier study of the eradication of smallpox from India was built on detailed local research, has done much to encourage historians to interrogate the common narrative of the success of the smallpox eradication programme being due to a set of definite ideas and the actions of a relatively small number of people.[54] 'The regional, national, and local chapters of the global smallpox eradication programme … never took the predetermined paths that some senior WHO and government officials hoped they would.'[55] That eradication in Nepal was achieved differently does not at all undermine the value of having an organisation such as the WHO, but it does question some of the messages implied in the ongoing smallpox narrative.

In Nepal, the 'outstanding international public leaders' that Cueto, Brown and Fee are thinking about were not the reason for its success.[56] Writing about the principles and lessons of the WHO-led programme, global project leader Dr Donald Henderson from the USA, considered that 'each national programme must have an administrative structure and pattern of operations compatible with its own health structure and socio-cultural environment'.[57] Nepal was divided administratively into seventy-five districts and the authors of the global programme's official history identified the 'vital' role of the Nepali district supervisors.[58] With most travel of necessity on foot and with very few health services, national programme leaders had to come up with a viable alternative strategy; this led them to rely on district staff. Nowhere else in the official history in the conclusions drawn from different national programmes is such a decentralised strategy referred to as a reason for success.[59] It is also absent from the wider literature.

In his introduction to *A Global History of Medicine*, Mark Jackson highlights the need for historians to find ways to research and write histories 'that are sensitive to promiscuous linkages between global, regional, and local dimensions of health and disease'.[60] This detailed case study of a small country provides, as American social scientist Robert K. Yin argues, the opportunity to look in-depth at a complex topic in a 'real-world' context and in so doing explore these linkages and local dimensions.[61] In the field of health, however, in the hierarchy or levels of evidence, which enable different research methods to be ranked according to the validity of their findings, case studies usually rank low and are seen as 'soft'. This perception should be questioned.[62]

Wanting to write a book that reflected many viewpoints requires a wide range of primary sources. These have been collected over several years from people and institutions in Nepal, Switzerland, the United Kingdom (UK), the USA and New Zealand. I also lived in Nepal for just over two years in the Sherpa community of the Mt Everest region where our family were volunteers for Sir Edmund Hillary and the Himalayan Trust at the small hospital in Khunde built in 1966, partly in response to the 1963 smallpox epidemic.[63] From sitting in the winter sunshine in a stone-walled field talking to a man from Thame village to the WHO Library and archives in Geneva underscores my own local–global journey.

Smallpox had been present in Nepal for centuries, but despite its visibility little has been recorded about the disease. Many people in Nepal today, however, remember smallpox. This book makes extensive use throughout of people's oral and written accounts of their experiences, whether having the disease themselves or caring for others. As the start of this introduction illustrates, their stories are about the lived experiences and heartaches that as time passes will get forgotten, yet these were integral to their acceptance of vaccination. Other perspectives come from health practitioners, people providing vaccination or those involved with the smallpox programme, before and after 1967. Many have helped me on numerous occasions and over several years with information, replying to questions or helping trace people and whether they were still alive or in good health.[64]

Unlike many other countries in the region, Nepal does not have the written records of a colonial past. Documents from the British Residency established in 1816 are limited.[65] There were no health statistics to inform either national or foreign staff.[66] Adding to the challenge, in 1973 a devastating fire gutted most of Nepal's main government building and record repository, the Singha Durbar. Communications from WHO passed through the Ministry of Foreign Affairs, but after 1960 its archives are not publicly available even to Nepali citizens.[67] Another difficulty is obtaining countrywide information rather than just for the Kathmandu Valley which tends to predominate in the literature.[68] Where possible, this book draws on material from other parts of the country. Even in the 1960s, newspaper coverage was extremely limited, but overseas visitors liked to write about Nepal and their experiences, and many of the scattered references to smallpox from the late 1940s onwards come from such sources.

As one of the last countries from which smallpox was eradicated, Nepal was involved in the final stages of the global programme. Detailed reporting was central to its success; even for a small country such as Nepal much information exists in the WHO headquarters (HQ) and South-East Asia regional office (SEARO) files – especially from 1971.[69] The surveillance–containment strategy of the later years of the programme depended on good quality reporting. At all levels, information was needed to evaluate progress and problems. Policymakers and planners required evidence. Officials charged with implementing the global programme needed data about what was being done in small communities, large towns, districts, nation states, and at regional and global levels. This was the kind of information that the authors of the official history also wanted and regarded as the most reliable and authoritative. Importantly, however, in the files are unpublished letters and other documents that can interpret and provide different perspectives, as can the accounts and talking with those involved with the programme.

Each chapter in the book has an individual focus and significance, but several themes run throughout and are pulled together in the conclusion. The book begins by discussing the writing of the global smallpox story, arguing that this is important because of the programme's ongoing influence in global health policy and practice. It thus has important implications for implementing programmes more generally. The chapter's emphasis is on the programme rather than eradication as a concept. The writing is also important because the only published account of Nepal's involvement with the global smallpox programme is in the massive official history published in 1988. This account highlights that Nepal's project leaders decentralised in response to the many challenges they faced and established an effective programme based on Nepal's seventy-five districts (Map 1). Later historiography of smallpox and global health, which inform people today, promote the success of smallpox eradication as a top-down and centre-led programme. Local detail is lost and Nepal's contribution to the global story has become invisible.

Chapters 2 and 3 set the scene prior to 1960 and provide a longer and wider lens for considering smallpox in Nepal. These contextual aspects are essential to understanding what happens and the eventual success. Chapter 2 focuses on the disease, which was widespread and looked after mainly in the home, but which was just one of many serious diseases people faced. At an international level the global eradication of smallpox was seen as a triumph for the epidemiological or population-based approach to health, but for people with the disease and their families the experience was intensely personal and one they might not survive. The control and later eradication of smallpox was for them not just about prevention – their own experiences and the presence of the disease in the community influenced their ideas and actions, including vaccination. Chapter 3 explores the nation state of Nepal and how this influenced and shaped its responses to the worldwide smallpox programme. Responding to contagious and epidemic diseases and their prevention had long been viewed as a major task for governments – but not in Nepal. Political changes in Nepal after 1950 brought the promise and hopes of modernisation, including providing education and expanding the very limited health services. The chapter also discusses Nepal's external relations and early involvement with the WHO. Development was difficult, slow and patchy as new systems were also being built on the roots of an older social and political fabric. The smallpox programme in Nepal was ultimately successful because it learned to work with both.

The next two chapters investigate the early 1960s. Chapter 4 provides 'snapshots' of responses to epidemic smallpox in 1963–64 from three very different geographical areas of Nepal. They illustrate the many and fragmented responses that collectively tell us about Nepal and smallpox prior to the intensification of the global programme but separately highlight the need for local adaptation and the importance of local people's beliefs which influenced their practices. The official history noted 1958 as the last smallpox epidemic and suggested that the disease's transmission could not be sustained for long in most of the country.[70] This chapter shows the limitations of this approach and what could happen. Mostly written from the perspectives of local people and foreigners caught up in helping, it makes visible Nepal's last major epidemic. The outsiders in this chapter did not come to Nepal as smallpox experts – their involvement with the disease was chance and temporary – but in each setting they exerted influence, operating independently or in conjunction with the government or local officials.

Chapter 5 examines how Nepal was becoming caught up in an uneasy world of foreign aid and donors. Little financial support was provided for the global smallpox programme meaning that after 1959 the disease was still a problem for nation states to control and fund. For smallpox, the key external relationship for Nepal's central government was at a regional level with WHO SEARO. I argue that the joint Government of Nepal/WHO Smallpox Control Pilot Project (Nepal 9), which started in three districts of the Kathmandu Valley in early 1962, provided the foundation for Nepal's implementation of the intensified global programme after 1967. Both WHO and the government drew different conclusions from the project, reiterating the need to consider the smallpox programme from multiple perspectives. I also suggest that a local initiative in 1965 in part of the southern Tarai region better demonstrated that improved results could be achieved using local vaccinators who people trusted.

Vaccination lay at the centre of the global smallpox programme and global policies are discussed in Chapter 6. Although the goal changed from control to eradication and the strategy later shifted away from mass vaccination to surveillance and containment, vaccination throughout remained the available tool. Globally, logistics was considered critical to the success of the programme after 1967. In Nepal logistics was important before 1967 and influenced plans for developing the project after 1967. From this perspective, a successful vaccination programme required an appropriate vaccine, an adequate supply, and an ability to store and distribute to where it was needed. Nepal relied on outside sources for smallpox vaccine and the country had few refrigerators. A successful programme also relied on people being vaccinated. The chapter argues that issues concerning vaccine, vaccination and vaccination behaviour could be both separate and linked and need to be considered as such. Understanding the specific vaccine and the context is crucial if a vaccination programme is to work. Faulty vaccine was related to technical aspects of the vaccine and problems of storage and distribution in Nepal, but these issues also influenced people's responses to vaccination. Most Nepali people supported vaccination, but individual vaccination behaviour was complex and influenced by many factors.

Building on the foundations of the earlier chapters, the final three chapters of the book examine Nepal's Smallpox Eradication Project (SEP) and how it became Nepal's first nationwide healthcare programme. Although this was carried out through the auspices of a global programme, how this was implemented and adapted was deeply embedded in the local context. The chapters highlight the interplay, networks and relationships operating at all levels and how these evolved over time in response to a range of issues.

Chapter 7 argues that the mid-1960s was a period of transition as global and national policies began to come together in intent and practice. A joint revised plan of operation for the eradication of smallpox and control of other communicable diseases was agreed and signed by the government and WHO in November 1966 but was followed by a modified implementation plan in 1967 solely concerned with smallpox. Both built on earlier experiences with the pilot project in the Kathmandu Valley and local initiative in the Tarai. Nepal's first national health survey (1965–66) showed to a wider audience that smallpox was still widespread; it also demonstrated the country's very limited health infrastructure and low level of vaccination. The chapter highlights the limited foreign involvement with the programme, examining how Nepal's officials engaged with global smallpox policy and vice versa of how the new and small WHO smallpox unit in Geneva and the regional office in New Delhi interacted with nation states.

Chapters 8 and 9 explore how the plan's goal was achieved in Nepal. The first few years were characterised by continuing outsider references to the problems and need for improvement, but progress was being made. Chapter 8 focuses on the programme's gradual but planned nationwide expansion and decentralisation, zone by zone and district by district. Each year further areas were added until the SEP became operational in all districts in 1972–73. Vaccine was secured, stored and distributed; staff were recruited and trained; reporting increased, and information began to appear that could be used within the country, and in New Delhi and Geneva. A structure and way of operating was established that is key to understanding how Nepal was able to transition to a surveillance–containment strategy. This is examined in Chapter 9. A change in strategy in mid-1971 to time-limited annual mass vaccination undertaken around Nepali people's preference for vaccination during the winter months remained an important and complementary component. This freed staff to concentrate on surveillance and containment for the rest of the year. External factors, however, could threaten a programme's progress. The dominating concern became the importation of cases from outside Nepal, especially during an epidemic over the border with India in Bihar. Nepal's last case of smallpox was in 1975 and was followed by two years of externally driven monitoring before the visit of an international commission to certify that smallpox was no longer present in the country. Celebration speeches highlighted many of the themes discussed throughout this book, but the final speech returned to the theme of where this book starts – the anguish that smallpox had caused in people's lives.

Notes

1 Dr Lhakpa Norbu Sherpa, conversation, 50th Everest anniversary celebrations, Kathmandu, May 2003, and written communication to author, July 2017. Lhakpa was the first Sherpa to gain a PhD and today is a respected Sherpa cultural authority.
2 In Nepal, the term 'modern medicine' is commonly used. See notes on spelling and terminology.
3 The 1963 Himalayan Schoolhouse Expedition was led by New Zealander Sir Edmund Hillary. Hillary and Tenzing Norgay were the first to climb Mt Everest on 29 May 1953.
4 Sir Edmund Hillary, *Schoolhouse in the Clouds* (London: Hodder and Stoughton, 1964), chapter 3; James Ramsey Ullman, *Americans on Everest* (Philadelphia, PA: J. B. Lippincott, 1964), pp. 81–2.
5 Interview with author, Kirtipur, May 2017.
6 Interview with author, Kathmandu, 16 April 2015.
7 F. Fenner, A. J. Hall and W. R. Dowdle, 'What is eradication?', in W. R. Dowdle and D. R. Hopkins (eds), *The Eradication of Infectious Diseases* (Chichester: John Wiley & Sons, 1998), pp. 3–17.
8 Walter R. Dowdle, 'The principles of disease elimination and eradication', *Bulletin of the World Health Organization*, 76:Suppl. 2 (1998), 22–5.
9 See Nancy Stepan, *Eradication: Ridding the World of Diseases Forever?* (Ithaca, NY: Cornell University Press, 2011).
10 Mass vaccination with new vaccines was being used to combat an international rise in epidemics of poliomyelitis (polio). Despite the

Cold War, Eastern Europe was important in laying the foundations for the later global polio eradication programme. Dora Vargha, 'Vaccination and the communist state: Polio in Eastern Europe', in Christine Holmberg, Stuart Blume and Paul Greenough (eds), *The Politics of Vaccination: A Global History* (Manchester: Manchester University Press, 2017), p. 77.
11 Stuart Blume, *Immunization: How Vaccines Became Controversial* (London: Reaktion Books, 2017), p. 63.
12 Alfred W. Crosby, 'Smallpox', in Kenneth F. Kiple (ed.), *The Cambridge World History of Human Disease* (Cambridge: Cambridge University Press, 1993), pp. 1008–13 http://dx.doi.org/10.1017/CHOL9780521332866.190 (accessed 22 June 2016). For public health practice in the early 1970s, see Abram S. Benenson (ed.), *Control of Communicable Diseases in Man*, 12th edn (Washington: American Public Health Association, 1975).
13 Michael Bennett, *War Against Smallpox: Edward Jenner and the Global Spread of Vaccination* (Cambridge: Cambridge University Press, 2020); Susan Heydon, 'Death of the king: The introduction of vaccination into Nepal in 1816', *Medical History*, 63:1 (2019), 24–43. For its later introduction into Japan, see Ann Jannetta, *The Vaccinators: Smallpox, Medical Knowledge, and the 'Opening' of Japan* (Stanford, CA: Stanford University Press, 2007).
14 David Arnold, *Colonizing the Body: State Medicine and Epidemic Disease in Nineteenth-Century India* (Berkeley, CA, and London: University of California Press, 1993), p. 144. For complexity, see, for example, Sanjoy Bhattacharya, Mark Harrison and Michael Worboys, *Fractured States: Smallpox, Public Health and Vaccination Policy in British India 1800–1947* (New Delhi: Orient Longman, 2005); Niels Brimnes, 'Variolation, vaccination and popular resistance in early Colonial South India', *Medical History*, 48:2 (2004), 199–228. For an introduction to public health and colonialism see Alison Bashford, 'The history of public health during colonialism', in Harald Kristian (Kris) Heggenhougen and Stella Quah (eds), *International Encyclopedia of Public Health* (ebook, Academic, 2008), pp. 398–404; see also Alison Bashford, *Imperial Hygiene: A Critical History of Colonialism, Nationalism and Public Health* (Basingstoke: Palgrave Macmillan, 2004).
15 Heydon, 'Death of the king'.
16 Babu Ram Marasini, 'Health and hospital development in Nepal: Past and present', *Journal of Nepal Medical Association* (JNMA), 42:149 (2003), 306–11.
17 Resolution WHA11.54.

18 Resolution WHA12.54.
19 For a wider discussion see Marcos Cueto, Theodore M. Brown and Elizabeth Fee, *The World Health Organization: A History* (Cambridge: Cambridge University Press, 2019).
20 World Health Organization, *The First Ten Years of the World Health Organization* (Geneva: WHO, 1958), p. 474.
21 SEA/RC11/R6. In World Health Organization, Regional Office for South-East Asia, *Twenty Years in South-East Asia 1948–1967* (New Delhi: WHO Regional Office for South-East Asia, 1967), p. 174. www.who.int/iris/handle/10665/126401.
22 *Ibid*.
23 Other parts of geographical South-East Asia became part of WHO's Western Pacific Region established in 1951 with its headquarters in Manila in the Philippines.
24 For the official history, see F. Fenner, D. A. Henderson, I. Arita, Z. Jezek and I. D. Ladnyi, *Smallpox and Its Eradication* (Geneva: WHO, 1988).
25 World Health Organization, SE/69.1, 'Surveillance-containment operations: principles and operational procedures' https://apps.who.int/iris/handle/10665/67974 (accessed 19 June 2023).
26 Fenner et al., *Smallpox and Its Eradication*, p. 804.
27 Resolution WHA33.3. The last naturally occurring case of smallpox worldwide was in Africa in Somalia in 1977.
28 WHO, 'WHO commemorates the 40th anniversary of smallpox eradication' www.who.int/news/item/13-12-2019-who-commemorates-the-40th-anniversary-of-smallpox-eradication (accessed 13 May 2021).
29 WHO, 'WHO Director-General's opening remarks at the media briefing on COVID-19–8 May 2020' www.who.int/director-general/speeches/detail/who-director-general-s-opening-remarks-at-the-media-briefing-on-covid-19---8-may-2020 (accessed 3 July 2020).
30 See Akihito Suzuki, 'Smallpox and the epidemiological heritage of modern Japan: Towards a total history', *Medical History*, 55:3 (2011), 313–18. For how basic differences in political and administrative systems have shaped how individual states responded to epidemic disease in Europe, see Peter Baldwin, *Contagion and the State in Europe, 1830–1930* (Cambridge: Cambridge University Press, 1999).
31 Agnieszka Sobocinska, 'New histories of foreign aid', *History Australia*, 17:4 (2020), 595–610. For a multi-level ethnography of the polio eradication programme in Pakistan see Svea Closser, *Chasing Polio in Pakistan: Why the World's Largest Public Health Initiative May Fail* (Nashville, TN: Vanderbilt University Press, 2010). As Closser mentions (p. 8), the 'classic' in the genre of the anthropology of global health, is a study on Nepal by Judith Justice, *Policies, Plans &*

People: Foreign Aid and Health Development (Kathmandu: Mandala, in association with University of California Press, 1989).
32 Mark Nichter, *Global Health: Why Cultural Perceptions, Social Representations, and Biopolitics Matter* (Tucson, AZ: University of Arizona Press, 2008), p. 3.
33 Cueto, Brown and Fee, *The World Health Organization*, p. 144.
34 See, for example, Donald R. Hopkins, *Princes and Peasants: Smallpox in History* (Chicago, IL: University of Chicago Press, 1983) with a second edition in 2002 titled *The Greatest Killer: Smallpox in History*; S. L. Kotar and J. E. Gessler, *Smallpox: A History* (Jefferson, NC, and London: McFarland & Co., 2013); Jonathan B. Tucker, *Scourge: The Once and Future Threat of Smallpox* (New York: Grove Press, 2001); Gareth Williams, *Angel of Death: The Story of Smallpox* (Basingstoke: Palgrave Macmillan, 2010). A recent addition to the literature is Jennifer D. Penschow, *Battling Smallpox before Vaccination: Inoculation in Eighteenth-Century Germany*, Clio Medica Series (Leiden: Brill, 2022), which examines the rejection and adoption of inoculation by different social groups.
35 Mark Harrison, 'A global perspective: Reframing the history of health, medicine, and disease', *Bulletin of the History of Medicine*, 89:4 (2015), 639–89; Randall M. Packard, *A History of Global Health: Interventions into the Lives of Other Peoples* (Baltimore, MD: Johns Hopkins University Press, 2016); Erez Manela, 'Smallpox and the globalization of development', in Stephen J. Macekura and Erez Manela (eds), *The Development Century: A Global History* (Cambridge: Cambridge University Press, 2018), 83–103; Sarah Hodges, 'The global menace', *Social History of Medicine*, 25:3 (2012), 719–28; J. P. Koplan, T. C. Bond, M. H. Merson, K. S. Reddy, M. H. Rodriguez, N. K. Sewankambo, J. N. Wasserheit and Consortium of Universities for Global Health Executive Board, 'Towards a common definition of global health', *The Lancet*, 373:9679 (2009), 1993–5.
36 As well as Bob R. Reinhardt, *The End of a Global Pox: America and the Eradication of Smallpox in the Cold War Era* (Chapel Hill, NC: University of North Carolina Press, 2015), see particularly Erez Manela, 'A pox on your narrative: Writing disease control into Cold War history', *Diplomatic History*, 34:2 (2010), 299–323.
37 See, for example, Williams, *Angel of Death*, chapter 15.
38 World Health Organization, 'Report of the SAGE Working Group on Vaccine Hesitancy, 12 November 2014' www.asset-scienceinsociety. eu/sites/default/files/sage_working_group_revised_report_vaccine_ hesitancy.pdf (accessed 9 January 2023).
39 Blume, *Immunization*, p. 19.

40 J. N. Hays, *The Burdens of Disease: Epidemics and Human Response in Western History*, rev. edn (New Brunswick, NJ, and London: Rutgers University Press, 2009).

41 Sidsel Roalkvam, Desmond McNeill and Stuart Blume (eds), *Protecting the World's Children: Immunisation Policies and Practices* (Oxford: Oxford University Press, 2013), p. 41.

42 Holmberg, Blume and Greenough (eds), *The Politics of Vaccination*. Compared with other scales of historical analysis, a region is more fluid and less easily defined than local, national or global. Paul A. Kramer, 'Region in global history', in Douglas Northrop (ed.), *A Companion to World History*, 1st edn (Oxford: Blackwell, 2012), pp. 201–12. For a discussion that considers international organisations as mechanisms to foster unity in a divided world, see Akira Iriye, *Global Community: The Role of International Organizations in the Making of the Contemporary World* (Berkeley, CA: University of California Press, 2002).

43 See Chapter 3. For how Nepal's political status influenced the introduction of vaccination see Heydon, 'Death of the king'.

44 Sanjoy Bhattacharya, 'International health and the limits of its global influence: Bhutan and the worldwide Smallpox Eradication Programme', *Medical History*, 57:4 (2013), 461–86; Peter Baldwin, *Contagion and the State in Europe, 1830–1930* (Cambridge: Cambridge University Press, 1999).

45 Sanjoy Bhattacharya, 'Global and local histories of medicine: Interpretative challenges and future possibilities', in Mark Jackson (ed.), *A Global History of Medicine* (Oxford: Oxford University Press, 2018), p. 255.

46 For understandings of success, see Anne-Emanuelle Birn, 'The stages of international (global) health: histories of success or successes of history?', *Global Public Health*, 4:1 (2009), 50–68.

47 Likewise, see Mark Liechty, *What Went Right: Sustainability versus Dependence in Nepal's Hydropower Development* (Cambridge: Cambridge University Press, 2022).

48 Fenner et al., *Smallpox and Its Eradication*, p. 792.

49 Sanjoy Bhattacharya, *Expunging Variola: The Control and Eradication of Smallpox in India 1947–1977* (New Delhi: Orient Longman, 2006), p. 6.

50 Cueto, Brown and Fee, *The World Health Organization*, chapter 5.

51 *Ibid.*, p. 115. In 1956 the Soviet Union returned to active participation in the WHO.

52 Sanjoy Bhattacharya and Carlos Eduardo D'Avila Pereira Campani, 'Re-assessing the foundations: Worldwide smallpox eradication, 1957–67', *Medical History*, 64:1 (2020), 71–93.

Introduction 23

53 See, for example, Reinhardt, *The End of a Global Pox*.
54 Bhattacharya, *Expunging Variola*.
55 Bhattacharya, 'Global and local histories of medicine', p. 256.
56 Cueto, Brown and Fee, *The World Health Organization*, p. 145.
57 D. A. Henderson, 'Principles and lessons from the smallpox eradication programme', *Bulletin of the World Health Organization*, 65:4 (1987), 535–46.
58 Fenner et al., *Smallpox and Its Eradication*, p. 804.
59 For a later global eradication programme that focused on primary healthcare and community participation, see Jonathan David Roberts, 'Participating in eradication: How Guinea worm redefined eradication, and eradication redefined Guinea work, 1985–2022', *Medical History*, 67:2 (2023), 148–71.
60 Mark Jackson, 'One world, one health? Towards a global history of medicine', in Jackson (ed.), *A Global History of Medicine* (Oxford: Oxford University Press, 2018), p. 4.
61 Robert K. Yin, *Case Study Research and Applications: Design and Methods*, 6th edn (Thousand Oaks, CA: SAGE Publications, 2018), p. 5.
62 Yin, *Case Study Research and Applications*, p. 6; Zina O'Leary, *Researching Real-World Problems: A Guide to Methods of Inquiry* (London: SAGE Publications, 2005), p. 80.
63 Susan Heydon, *Modern Medicine and International Aid: Khunde Hospital, Nepal, 1966–1998* (New Delhi: Orient BlackSwan, 2009).
64 I have acknowledged this valuable help throughout the book, particularly in the chapter endnotes.
65 They are held in the British Library, London. The next formal presence was the USA which recognised Nepal in 1947 and established diplomatic relations in 1948.
66 For a review of the situation in 1960 see WHO, SEA/PHA/15, Dr D. P. Nath, Assignment Report on Assistance to Central Health Directorate, Nepal, WHO Project: Nepal 4, August 1957–October 1960, 2 December 1960.
67 Bandana Gyawali, email communication, 19 July 2020.
68 John Whelpton, *A History of Nepal* (Cambridge: Cambridge University Press, 2005), p. 2.
69 Unfortunately, some of the earlier files have been destroyed.
70 Fenner et al., *Smallpox and Its Eradication*, p. 792.

1

Writing Nepal into global smallpox history

In their anthropology of biomedicine, Margaret Lock and Vinh-Kim Nguyen write that the successful eradication of the disease of smallpox 'is still celebrated as a triumph of international cooperation and of the ability of biomedicine to bring nations together'.[1] Indeed, it is the 'most consistently cited success by global health decision-makers' says Anne-Emanuelle Birn.[2] Cueto, Brown and Fee call the eradication of smallpox a 'landmark historical event' with the WHO acting as a 'supranational organization and a leader of global affairs'.[3] Writing about its history, therefore, is of more than a general academic interest. Increasing amounts of documentation arose from the global programme and the intention of the authors of the vast official history was not only that it would record and interpret the what, when, where and why of what happened but that it would also act as a reference for subsequent policies and practices for other diseases.[4] Bhattacharya and Campani have called the official history a 'diplomatic exercise' and that it 'does not present us with value-free sets of information'.[5] Nevertheless, anyone wanting to find out about Nepal's experiences during this period has to start with the official history because it still contains the only published account, located in a chapter about India and the Himalayan area.[6] Its conclusion acknowledges Nepal's exceptionalism.

Geographically, the nation state of Nepal is sandwiched between the large regional powers of India and China. It is rectangular in shape, approximately 800 km long by 200 km wide, and is divided into three broadly horizontal areas – the lowland Tarai to the south, the middle hills, and the mountains to the north (Map 2). The three major river systems of the Karnali, Gandaki and Kosi drain much of the country. Standing on the narrow walking track above Namche Bazar, the administrative centre of the Mt Everest area, the view is of steep-sided river valleys and ridge after ridge that disappear into a hazy distance that leads from the mountains, through the hills and on to the Tarai and Nepal's southern border with India. On the other side of this porous frontier are the densely populated Indian states of Bihar and Uttar Pradesh. To Nepal's east lies Sikkim, which until 1975 was an independent state although externally controlled by India from 1947; beyond is the small kingdom of Bhutan. In the north are the mountains of the high Himalaya that form most of the country's border with the TAR. On the visit of King Mahendra to China in 1961 the two states signed a boundary treaty which placed the summit of Mt Everest on the border.[7] The People's Republic of China (PRC), which controlled mainland China after 1949, was not recognised by the UN until 1971.[8]

This chapter is in two parts. The first section examines how the global smallpox programme's history has been written. Drawing on WHO archives, it begins with the official record published by the WHO in 1988, *Smallpox and Its Eradication*, popularly known as the 'Big Red Book' because of the colour of its leather-bound cover. This vast book of 1,460 pages sets out to 'properly record' the 'unique accomplishment'.[9] It contains a wealth of information, but not surprisingly the book's focus is the successful 'intensified' global eradication programme after 1967. The second section writes Nepal into global smallpox history. In the later years of the global programme – as more information became available and was disseminated widely – Nepal became visible in the narrative. Every case of smallpox and everywhere worldwide now mattered. It also became visible because its success was built on developing and adapting the global programme to meet and overcome the considerable local challenges that existed in its implementation.

The Big Red Book and global smallpox history

In December 1979 the Global Commission for the Certification of Smallpox Eradication released its final report, concluding that eradication had been achieved throughout the world and that there was no evidence that smallpox would return as an endemic disease.[10]

Its chair was Australian virologist Professor Frank Fenner, from the Australian National University in Canberra, who initially became involved with the smallpox programme to help provide 'greater certainty' to the belief that the smallpox virus only affected humans.[11] As author of one of the principal textbooks on virology, he was a member of the WHO group convened in 1969 to investigate a new virus that caused a smallpox-like disease in monkeys. Fenner demonstrated 'scientific confidence' but was also 'the voice of calm and reason'.[12] Among the twenty-one members of the Global Commission was Dr Purushottam Shrestha, Chief of the Planning Division of the Institute of Medicine, Maharajgunja, Kathmandu. Shrestha was Nepal's national project chief throughout most of the intensified smallpox programme (1969–77) and a member of the International Commissions for the Certification of Smallpox Eradication for Burma (1977), Bangladesh (1977) and Somalia (1979), and chairman for Afghanistan (1976).[13]

The Global Commission made a series of recommendations as 'policy for the post-eradication era', including two that related to the programme's documentation. It was 'essential for future historians' that the programme be 'fully documented'.[14] The Commission considered it important that experiences of the programme that were applicable to other health programmes should be 'defined and elaborated, in order to help public health officials develop strategies and tactics for the conduct of other programmes'. This applied particularly to infectious diseases but acknowledged that this was a complex area 'since the lessons learnt from the smallpox eradication programme need to be evaluated in each instance by the health programme to which they may be applied'. Under recommendation 16, 'WHO should ensure that appropriate publications are produced describing smallpox and its eradication and the principles and methods that are applicable to other programmes.' Under recommendation 17, 'All relevant scientific, operational and administrative data should be catalogued and retained for archival purposes in WHO headquarters and perhaps also in several centres interested in the history of medicine.'[15] In May 1980 the WHA formally accepted the report and its recommendations. Historians, practitioners and policymakers would be provided with a wealth of data that was evidence of what had occurred and how this programme could be drawn on to develop and assist others.

The authors of the official history were keen to promote the Big Red Book as 'a truly collaborative effort', but Fenner was responsible for the overall organisation, the reference lists and indexes.[16] He wrote the early chapters and edited the drafts prepared by Dr Isao Arita, who took over as Chief of the Smallpox Eradication Unit after Henderson left Geneva in 1977 to return to the USA and become Dean of the Johns Hopkins School of Public Health.[17] In his book about his own and his father's lives, Fenner clearly saw himself as the lead author of the official history and devoted a whole chapter and a considerable part of another to his involvement with smallpox, certification and the book.[18] Australian law required that he retire from his paid university position at the age of sixty-five years at the end of 1979, but in March 1978 he had written to Arita that 'he would like to make the production of the smallpox book my principal post-retirement activity'.[19]

Henderson, previously chief of the epidemiology intelligence service at the Communicable Disease Center (CDC), was the main author for the chapters about the implementation of the programme after 1967. This included Nepal. Although he visited many countries, Henderson never visited Nepal; in the programme's archives he appeared at times to struggle with comprehending Nepal's situation on the ground. He also wrote chapter 31 Lessons and benefits. Key to the programme's success for Henderson was the 'extraordinary achievement which was possible when countries throughout the world collaborated in the pursuit of a common aim, making use of the structures of an international organization and acting under its auspices'.[20] The WHA provided 'the necessary and, indeed, the only forum in which global health policies can be agreed upon', while the WHO 'alone has the requisite channels of communication with the national authorities through which their several programmes can be coordinated, with the support of the international scientific expertise upon which the Organization can draw'.[21] A 'network of professional WHO staff, although small in number compared to the tens of thousands of national staff', were central as they 'facilitated the rapid communication of new information throughout the world and assisted in adapting and applying it to national programmes'.[22] 'In brief, it was clear that comparatively few, strongly motivated and knowledgeable professionals could organize and effectively mobilize large numbers of persons and that in most countries they could count on the eager support of the health staff and the general population alike.'[23] In Nepal, Dr Benu Bahadur Karki, who worked with Nepal's programme from December 1972 to October 1975 and at times was the medical officer in charge when Shrestha was away, said that they did not like the Big Red Book because it only mentioned 'the big people'.[24]

While each chapter draft for the official history was reviewed widely, commented on and revised, drafts about the programme at a country level were sent by the Director-General, Dr Halfdan Mahler, to the directors of the various regional offices for final comment.[25] Opinions varied. In South-East Asia, the Regional Office intended to review the relevant drafts but also contacted the WHO Programme Coordinator and Representatives (WPC&R) to share the draft 'with any national officials you deem appropriate for their comments'.[26] Comments were wanted at SEARO by 3 December 1984 for return to Geneva by 21 December. On 29 November, Dr P. Micovic, the acting WPC&R for Nepal, replied attaching comments from Shrestha. These were the first to be received from any country in any of the WHO Regions. Overall, Shrestha considered it 'well-written' and 'clear and concise' but listed twenty-two detailed points 'to present an accurate picture'.[27]

The monumental *Smallpox and Its Eradication* was not the first attempt at writing a record of the smallpox eradication programme. Drafts from 1976 and 1978 of an earlier manuscript exist in five binders in the programme archive in Geneva.[28] While Henderson planned a 'technical reference volume', writer David Preston (also from the USA) was contracted for extended periods between 1975 and the end of 1978 to assist in the preparation and revision of a book *The Eradication of Smallpox* about the 'background and execution of the Programme'.[29] In Preston's draft Nepal appeared before India because eradication in Nepal was achieved first.[30] Fenner made no mention of any earlier activity and in his own book traced the genesis of the Big Red Book to his own involvement as Chair of the Global Commission and his impending retirement.[31]

Preston also commented that the 'basic modern work on the disease' was the book written by Professor Cyril Dixon, an epidemiologist from the UK who in 1959 became Head of the Department of Preventive and Social Medicine at the University of Otago in New Zealand.[32] Dixon's book, published twenty-six years earlier than the official history, was about a disease that still existed and was devastating in many parts of the world. It was full of practical suggestions for the health practitioner being confronted with smallpox or the possibility of the disease whether in hospital or the community. Dixon was an internationally recognised smallpox expert, but his contribution to the smallpox story was scarcely acknowledged in the official history. The caption to his photo did not even mention that he was a member of the First WHO Expert Committee on Smallpox in 1964.[33] More glaring was the omission that Dixon had published an article on the effective use of the strategy that would become known as surveillance and containment. Dixon had used this strategy of 'ring vaccination' during an outbreak of smallpox in Tripolitania (Tripoli) in 1946.[34] Henderson credited Dr William Foege with being the first to implement the new strategy in Eastern Nigeria in 1967.[35] Dixon now has been acknowledged in smallpox historiography.[36]

Other publications also were produced. In 1979 SEARO published the detailed account of the eradication of smallpox from India which had been recommended by the International Commission that had certified India free from the disease.[37] This conveyed a strong sense of triumph and highlighted cooperation, but as Bhattacharya has demonstrated downplayed the complexity and disunity, and the many people and agencies involved in the everyday implementation of the programme.[38] Publications also appeared about the programmes in Bangladesh (1980), Somalia (1981) and Ethiopia (1984).[39] Numerous articles, written by WHO staff and others connected with the programme, appeared in a range of publications. Some published accounts of their own involvement and with the increasing passage of time their memoirs.[40] Use of the English language predominated, but Dr Ivan Ladyni was the author of a book in Russian in 1985, *Smallpox Eradication and Prevention of Its Return*.[41] A simple search using Google elicited no mention of this, unlike writings for Fenner or Henderson. Arita's recent book, *The Smallpox Eradication Saga: An Insider's View*, is based on an earlier account *Smallpox Eradication: Target Zero* written in Japanese.[42]

Countries and organisations also produced publications to highlight their role in the successful campaign. The CDC's (renamed Centers for Disease Control) book appeared in 1987 to mark the tenth anniversary of the world's last naturally occurring case of smallpox. If other accounts promoted themes of 'worldwide' and 'cooperation', this narrative was about the involvement of the CDC and its operatives. In their foreword, CDC directors, David Sencer, William Foege and James Mason, acknowledged the 'different and even conflicting priorities' of US health authorities and African governments in the Smallpox Eradication/Measles Control Program in West and Central Africa, which began in 1967 and was funded by the United States Agency for International Development (USAID) and largely executed by the CDC.[43] The central role of the USA is also the theme of the more recent Peace Corps report on the activities of their volunteers.[44] Dedicated to smallpox eradication's thirtieth anniversary, is Professor Svetlana Marennikova's edited collection about Russian participation. While West Africa is central to the US narrative, Marennikova's volume directs the reader to the Global Smallpox Eradication Program, launched by the WHA in 1959 from the initiative of the Soviet Union.[45]

Outside the programme, historians have also collaborated with WHO to publicise and discuss the programme, its achievement, and challenges.[46] Such joint endeavours offer opportunities to revisit and to reinforce themes but also to present different perspectives. Alan Schnur was a mid-level fieldworker for WHO operating for part of the time in Uttar Pradesh near the border with Nepal. Despite the top-down narrative of the official history, Schnur's account highlights 'the culture of empowerment and innovation' at the province and district level that was essential to the eradication effort and that also indicated a two-way flow of information and ideas.[47]

With the rise of the internet and the digitisation of archives, many documents and publications are now widely available. The programme archives are held at WHO headquarters in Geneva and have been digitised, but other repositories have also been established.[48] In 2016 WHO nominated the records of the Smallpox Eradication Programme for inclusion in the United Nations Educational, Scientific and Cultural Organization's (UNESCO) Memory of the World programme, which promotes the preservation of and access to the world's significant documentary heritage.[49] In 2017 this was accepted.

Both the book on India and the official history of the global programme generally ignored the wider context in which this public health project was carried out. The smallpox programme was a response to a health issue, but such programmes do not take place in a vacuum from what else is happening at the time whether locally, nationally or internationally, and that they have had a major impact on public health activities in any given location and at any given time. Much later historiography, for example, situates the global smallpox programme in an environment of international Cold War politics, biosecurity and support from the USA. Cueto, Brown and Fee even title their chapter on smallpox eradication 'Overcoming the warming of the Cold War'.[50] For Cueto, Brown and Fee, the Soviet Union is their focus, but in South and South-East Asia the threat was seen as China.[51] This focus on the Cold War, unfortunately, also has the effect of obscuring other factors. Regionally, Asia after the end of the Second World War was complex, changing and affected by conflicts between and within countries. This war had already brought an upsurge in the number of smallpox cases and re-established the disease as endemic in Indonesia, Malaysia and the Philippines. Regional administrative challenges also occurred. The last case of smallpox in Asia was in Bangladesh, which has a separate chapter in the Big Red Book, but from 1947 until December 1971 was East Pakistan. Bangladesh became a member of WHO's South-East Asia Region while Pakistan continued as part of the Eastern Mediterranean Region. Nepal was not part of any conflict but was affected by the movement of people across its border. Internally, however, Nepal was experiencing major political and social changes in the 1950s and 1960s that impacted on individual Nepali people's lives and organisations working in Nepal, such as the WHO which had its tentative first involvement in the early 1950s.

Writing Nepal into global smallpox history

Limited literature and references are available about Nepal and smallpox. Speaking in 1965 at the annual meeting of the American Public Health Association in Chicago, Scottish epidemiologist Dr W. Charles Cockburn, Chief Medical Officer Virus Diseases, Division of Communicable Diseases, WHO, compared the global smallpox situation in 1964 with 1944 and commented on the absence of reporting from Nepal in 1944.[52] What is presented and how, therefore, becomes central to how people view the programme in Nepal and what they might seek to learn from it.

In writing about Nepal's history, historian John Whelpton identifies two key themes that are also relevant to writing about the history of smallpox and the country's involvement with the global programme. First, the relationship between the people and their environment is complex.[53] Nepal's population in 1961 was 9,412,999, of which an overwhelming 96.4 per cent were classified in the census as rural.[54] This was an increase of 14 per cent since the 1952–54 census, although human pressure on the environment began well before wider changes in the 1950s. Settlements with a population of 5,000 were classified as urban and increased in number from just ten to sixteen in 1961.The climate ranges from the heat of the jungle and plains to the icy Himalayan peaks of the highest mountains in the world. The often rugged, if spectacular, landscape influenced people's way of life as well as where they lived. Two seasons predominate, although there are marked variations between the different regions: a hot season from April to September and a cold season from October to March. People escaped to the hills from the summer heat and disease, but successful malaria eradication activities in the 1950s increased the availability of land for settlement in areas formerly prone to the disease.[55] Much of the Tarai region was opened up. A second theme is that Nepal, which lies on the edge of the Indian and Chinese cultural worlds, is also a cultural contact zone. Hinduism was the state religion while the Sherpa of the Mt Everest area, for example, are Buddhist, but Whelpton cautions not to oversimplify Nepal's complex cultural and ethnic diversity by focusing too much on the southern Hindu and northern Buddhist dichotomy.[56] WHO officials' understanding of the relationship between religion and people's response to vaccination suffered at times from thinking this way.

Although smallpox was an important disease in Nepal with a long history, little has been written about it. The history of disease and public health has been portrayed largely from development and anthropological perspectives, such as through the work over several years of Nepali scholar Madhusudan Subedi and Ian Harper.[57] Neither write about smallpox. Dr Hemang Dixit's valuable account of the development of health services in Nepal provides brief mentions of the disease.[58] Dixit has produced four editions of his book published between 1995 and 2014. In the first edition smallpox appeared in a chapter on 'Diseases that matter in Nepal'.[59] He noted the death of King Girvan from smallpox in 1816 and the vaccination of Prime Minister Jang Bahadur Rana's eldest son in 1850. Public awareness of the need for vaccination existed but little activity occurred until after 'the ushering of democracy in 1951'. The later editions add a little more detail with an earlier royal death and mention of the 1963–64 epidemic, which Dixit refers to as Nepal's 'last big epidemic'.[60] Dixit's strategy with his book has been to see it as an evolving work with each edition responding to knowledge learned or a new focus.[61] With smallpox, Nepalis 'have had over the years plenty of experience with this disease'.[62]

During the implementation of the global programme a small number of publications appeared. Coinciding with the government's agreement with 'international agencies' in 1966 to launch a smallpox eradication programme, the *Journal of Nepal Medical Association* (JNMA) published an article about smallpox, international control and eradication, and activities in Nepal.[63] The authors, Dr B. N. Vaidya and H. V. Gurubacharya who worked in the Department of Health Services, linked the new programme to the experiences and limits of the previous joint government and WHO pilot project, which started in 1962. Beginning their article with the global situation in 1963 and the large number of cases, they also commented that many countries in Europe had few cases but that 'One sick man in a hospital is news to the world.'[64] Nepal's limited health infrastructure made 'a national public health programme such as smallpox eradication' 'difficult to envisage and to start'.[65] The key to success would be 'active community participation'. Nepal's programme was intending to use 'local man power at the village panchayat [local authority] level' as vaccinators, which had been shown to work in 1965 in a community-initiated scheme (see Chapter 5). As the programme expanded, WHO epidemiologist Dr Satnam Singh published in the *Indian Journal of Public Health* in 1970 an article about the epidemiology of the disease in Nepal. Singh was in Nepal to advise on smallpox and the control of other communicable diseases. Henderson assisted with the drafts and considered this particular journal would reach an appropriate audience as part of the article related to smallpox in the border region of the Tarai and cases entering Nepal from India.[66] In 1972, national project chief Shrestha published an article about the history of smallpox, although it was mostly a general history of the disease with a few scattered references to Nepal such as the death of the king in 1816 and people's belief in the goddess Sitala.[67]

While such articles might reach a targeted but limited audience in Nepal or India, also appearing in 1972 was an article in the October edition of the WHO's magazine *World Health* featuring 'Smallpox Target Zero', the final phase of the campaign. Henderson wrote about the global strategy, but articles about the campaigns in Ethiopia and Nepal where smallpox was still endemic highlighted that

> the success of the programme relies ultimately on the persistence and dedication of a comparatively small band of workers who, in these and other endemic countries, have to contend not only with smallpox but with mountains and uncharted desert wastes, with storms and floods, with abject poverty, with superstition and unreasoning hostility.[68]

The article on Nepal, entitled 'The anger of a goddess', was written by Nedd Willard, a US author and artist who spent six years as chief of public information for WHO in India and South-East Asia.[69] In setting the scene, Willard captured the romantic outsider view of the country but then grounded it in an appreciation of the reality.

> The popular image of Nepal remains that of a land of Sherpas and hippies, with Mount Everest at one end and the enchanted valley of Kathmandu at the other. To many people the very word Kathmandu suggests a faraway place of strange temples, friendly people, mystic lore and cheap drugs.
>
> Like all legends, this one contains both truth and fantasy.[70]

Willard was well-informed about smallpox and the programme in Nepal, again linking it to the pilot project started in 1962.

These few references emphasise the importance of the account in the official history of Nepal's programme and experiences. The first point to note is that it was viewed and written about in the context of India and India's programme. From the perspective of WHO programme planners, the assumption was that epidemiologically Nepal was a 'mountainous extension' of the neighbouring Indian states of

Bihar and central and eastern Uttar Pradesh.[71] Nepal was not a priority, and it was thought that eradication in Nepal would depend on progress in India. Sharing a common border, the histories of smallpox in India and Nepal were linked, although in the end success came to Nepal first. India regarded much of its northern border with the Himalayan region as remote and difficult to access, but for Nepal the open border with the states of Bihar and Uttar Pradesh was seen primarily as the route for importing smallpox cases into Nepal.[72] High case numbers in these two states were closely associated with the incidence of smallpox in Nepal. More cases entered Nepal than vice versa. In his review of the draft account of Nepal's programme for the official history, Shrestha commented that while such a view was true for the 1970s, earlier the disease was known to be endemic without importation.[73] As malaria came under control in the Tarai the population had increased rapidly, with the area of the eastern Tarai bordering Bihar being more densely populated than the western Tarai. In another comment, Shrestha gave a lower population figure for the western Tarai. While his comments overall were recorded as being accepted, they did not always appear in the final printed version of the official history.[74]

The planners also considered that 'the mainly mountainous terrain, the predominantly rural population and the poor communications between villages in Nepal suggested that smallpox transmission could not be long sustained in most of the country'.[75] The occurrence of smallpox in Nepal in 1963 is mentioned in terms of the limited reporting of the disease which began that year, but the cases enumerated were only from the three districts of the joint government and WHO pilot project in the Kathmandu Valley. None are included from elsewhere. Epidemics were noted to occur, like India, about every five years with the last epidemic said to have been in 1958. No mention is made of the epidemic in 1963 or of one in the mountains. Yet if the reader looks at the numbers of cases officially reported from Nepal for 1963 the total is much higher compared with subsequent years.[76]

Unsurprisingly, the chapter's primary focus was India, but unlike the few paragraphs for Sikkim and Bhutan, the account for Nepal was nine pages.[77] The authors wanted to record 'the closely related and ultimately well-executed Nepalese programme, of which there is no published description' and were able to draw on an unpublished detailed description and analysis that was prepared in 1977 for the certification process.[78] The account is divided into an introduction; the country – geographical and socio-cultural considerations where it was noted that 'socio-economic and demographic factors played unusually important roles in the development of the programme and in the pattern of occurrence of the disease';[79] the smallpox control pilot project beginning in 1962 which it deemed 'ineffective';[80] and extension of the project beyond the Kathmandu Valley in 1968. Over half of the account of Nepal was about the programme strategy changes introduced from 1971. The start of this section, however, is inaccurate in that American WHO Technical Officer David Bassett only arrived in Nepal in 1974 while Briton Royston (Roy) Mason (1970–74) was not mentioned.[81] Also, district supervisors were part of the project's staffing structure before 1971. A final paragraph noted the low cost of the programme for the government and the WHO compared to outlay on other programmes such as malaria control. The overall chapter conclusion, however, identified the 'vital role' played by Nepal's district supervisors in extending the programme throughout the country and developing the first national disease reporting system.[82] Not mentioned was that because of the enormous communication challenges these district smallpox supervisors were entrusted with decision-making responsibilities. Nepal's programme was 'an impressive achievement' given the low staff to population ratio and 'no less remarkable' than India's success.[83]

Few foreigners were involved with the programme in Nepal and therefore the potential for foreigners to write or talk about the programme and their experiences was limited. Nepal features little in the later smallpox literature. The senior WHO staff member was Dr Manickavasagar Sathianathan (1970–76) from Ceylon (Sri Lanka). He worked alongside Shrestha, but despite the respect with which he was held and his length of time in Nepal, his voice is absent.[84] The second WHO technical officer, Jay Friedman (1972–77), a 'CDC veteran of the campaign in West Africa' was interviewed for the *Global Health Chronicles* and is briefly mentioned in Horace Ogden's book about CDC involvement with the smallpox campaign.[85] Two points are of interest. The example of 'Friedman and his helicopter' is used in trying to reach a remote settlement, but in practice helicopters were not widely used in Nepal, especially not early on, except to investigate some later outbreaks in the roadless western hills. In the official history, a photo caption noted that roads at times were almost impassable, but a more appropriate comment to add could have been to note that no roads existed in most of the country.[86] Ogden went on to write that on one helicopter trip Friedman was 'hopelessly lost' and he was faced with a 'no less than a five-day trek' – a not unusual occurrence in Nepal. A 'young [Nepali] man' was asked to come in the helicopter as a passenger and point out to the pilot the correct village, prompting the comment that 'Not all the heroes of global smallpox eradication were formally enrolled in the campaign.' They are also often nameless in such accounts and so remain invisible. Although attributing success to the 'national program', Ogden was promoting CDC involvement and at the end of the section mentioned that in response to epidemics in Bihar and cases being imported into Nepal Friedman was involved in devising an 'informal system of cross-notification … that bypassed the cumbersome official reported process via Katmandu and New Delhi'.[87] Friedman was also a former Peace Corps Volunteer and is mentioned in the Peace Corps report.[88]

Most significantly, Nepal appears in Henderson's memoirs as a one-page box inset at the end of the chapter about India.[89] Henderson acknowledged that the programme's main concern was India, but he highlighted Nepal's 'unique program' after 1971 and the introduction of mass vaccination for one month each year. 'It was a new and surprisingly effective tactic in the eradication program.' He praised smallpox eradication for being the 'first national program in Nepal, the first to extend to all parts of the country, and the first to establish a national disease-reporting system'. These were 'remarkable accomplishments' and 'further highlighted the pathetic performance of the two adjacent Indian states of Bihar and Uttar Pradesh'. Nepal's story with smallpox had become part of the global history of smallpox.

Conclusion

Despite the absence of any case of the disease of smallpox for more than forty years, smallpox remains topical in the literature and the success of the global programme continues to be celebrated.

Participants then and later wrote about their involvement and organisations promoted their contribution. Documenting the programme's achievement and learning from its experiences were major recommendations of the Global Commission's Final Report in 1979 and resulted in the vast official history published in 1988. Although identifying the need to consider local context, the authors emphasised the important role of an organisation such as the WHO, which could work with the various nation state members, and international scientific expertise as key factors in the programme's success. This narrative is important because of the programme's ongoing influence in global health policy and practice and therefore has important implications for implementing programmes more generally.

The official history is also important because it contains the only published account of Nepal's involvement with the global smallpox programme. Nepal was not a priority, whether before or after 1967. Its programme was viewed as an extension of that of India which had the highest number of cases worldwide, but chapter 15 in its conclusion acknowledged Nepal's different strategy as did Henderson more recently in his memoirs. Nepal's project leaders decentralised in response to the many challenges they faced and established an effective programme based on Nepal's seventy-five districts. District smallpox supervisors were key. The account particularly referred to the period after a change in strategy in 1971. Surveillance and containment became the focus but included a time-limited period of mass vaccination each year timed to take advantage of people's preferences about when best to vaccinate. This later success, however, was built on knowledge and experiences, positive and negative, from earlier activities that are either dismissed or not mentioned.

In the subsequent drawing together of lessons and benefits and legacy for public health, Nepal's contribution to the global programme has dropped out of people's consideration. Later historiography of smallpox and global health, which inform people today, promote the success of smallpox eradication as a top-down and centre-led programme. Local detail is lost and Nepal's part in the global story has become invisible. Yet Nepal's experiences highlight the complexities of a global programme when faced with realities on the ground in any location and provide evidence that these could be overcome by moving away from the top-down model. The next chapter begins this endeavour by examining the longer history of smallpox in Nepal prior to WHO involvement.

Notes

1 Margaret Lock and Vinh-Kim Nguyen, *An Anthropology of Biomedicine* (Chichester: Blackwell, 2010), p. 155. Their revised second edition contains the same sentence except that 'biomedicine' becomes 'biomedical endeavours' (Hoboken, NJ: Wiley, 2018), p. 87.
2 Birn, 'The stages of international (global) health', 50.
3 Cueto, Brown and Fee, *The World Health Organization*, p. 115.
4 Fenner et al., *Smallpox and Its Eradication*, p. ix.
5 Bhattacharya and Campani, 'Re-assessing the foundations', 74.
6 Fenner et al., *Smallpox and Its Eradication*, pp. 792–801.
7 5 October. Ram Rahul, *The Himalaya as a Frontier* (New Delhi: Vikas Publishing House, 1978), p. 73. Nepal formally recognised the TAR as part of China.
8 For the history of smallpox eradication in China and relations with WHO see Lu Chen, 'China in the worldwide eradication of smallpox, 1900–1985: Recovering and democratizing histories of international health' (PhD dissertation, University of York, 2021). After certification, new information was received indicating that the last outbreak was 1963–65 in Shanxi Province and Inner Mongolia rather than Yunnan in 1961, pp. 259–60.
9 Fenner et al., *Smallpox and Its Eradication*, p. vii.
10 WHO, 'The global eradication of smallpox: Final report of the Global Commission for the Certification of Smallpox Eradication, Geneva, December 1979' (Geneva: WHO, 1980) www.who.int/iris/handle/10665/39253 (accessed 1 June 2019).
11 Donald A. Henderson, 'Frank Fenner (1914–2010): A guiding light of the campaign to eradicate smallpox', obituary, *Nature*, 469:7328 (2011), 35.
12 *Ibid.*
13 Fenner et al., *Smallpox and Its Eradication*, pp. 1140–6. Fenner also served on a number of the International Commissions, including India (1977). Burma became Myanmar in 1989.
14 WHO, 'Final report of the Global Commission for the Certification of Smallpox Eradication', p. 14.
15 *Ibid.*, p. 15.

16 Fenner et al., *Smallpox and Its Eradication*, p. ix. The official history initially had four designated authors: Fenner, Henderson, Dr Isao Arita and Dr Ivan D. Ladnyi, an epidemiologist from the Soviet Union who from 1965 to 1971 was a WHO Intercountry Adviser on smallpox eradication in Africa and in 1976 was appointed WHO Deputy Director-General responsible for the control of infectious diseases. S. S. Marennikova (ed.), *How It Was: The Global Smallpox Eradication Program in Reminiscences of Its Participants* (Novosibirsk: CERIS, 2018), p. 253. Dr Zdenek Ježek, a medical officer with the Smallpox Eradication Unit in Geneva, was added.

17 Smallpox Eradication Archives, World Health Organization, Geneva, Switzerland (hereafter SEA/WHO), File 1242, Box 667, Correspondence with D. A. Henderson and F. Fenner 'Smallpox and Its Eradication' 1981–83.

18 Frank Fenner, *Nature, Nurture and Chance: The Lives of Frank and Charles Fenner* (Canberra: ANU E Press, 2006).

19 *Ibid.*, p. 164.

20 Fenner et al., *Smallpox and Its Eradication*, p. 1346.

21 *Ibid.*, p. 1349.

22 *Ibid.*, p. 1351.

23 *Ibid.*, p. 1358.

24 Interview with author, Kathmandu, 25 May 2017. The only Nepali mentioned by name is Shrestha (p. 796).

25 See: SEA/WHO, File 1239, Box 666, Comments from Regions on 'Smallpox and Its Eradication' and Progress Review/Status; File 1242, Box 667, Correspondence with D. A. Henderson and F. Fenner 'Smallpox and Its Eradication' 1981–83.

26 SEA/WHO, File 1239, Box 666, 9 October 1984.

27 *Ibid.*, 26 November 1984 and 15 November 1985; for his comments, see the next section in this chapter.

28 SEA/WHO, Files SMEPRESTON1–5, Box 723, The eradication of Smallpox by David Preston – binders 1–5.

29 WHO Library, Geneva: Catalogue, vol. 1, Publications and Records, pp. 313–14; email to author from Reynald Erard, WHO Records and Archives, 22 July 2020.

30 Nepal 13 April 1977; India and Bhutan 23 April 1977.

31 Fenner, *Nature, Nurture and Chance*, p. 159.

32 SEA/WHO, Files SMEPRESTON1, Box 723, The eradication of smallpox by David Preston – binder 1 (pages unnumbered); C. W. Dixon, *Smallpox* (London: J & A Churchill, 1962).

33 Fenner et al., *Smallpox and Its Eradication*, pp. 194, 402–3.

34 C. W. Dixon, 'Smallpox in Tripolitania, 1946: An epidemiological and clinical study of 500 cases, including trials of penicillin treatment',

Journal of Hygiene, 46:4 (1948), 351–77. The article is often cited but is referenced in the official history for a different point. Fenner et al., *Smallpox and Its Eradication*, p. 196. Professor Viktor Zhdanov's plan to the WHA in 1958 also used surveillance and containment. Kotar and Gessler, *Smallpox: A History*, p. 357. The strategy of 'ring vaccination' was already known. It had first been used in Leicester in England a century earlier where there was considerable opposition to vaccination. Stuart M. F. Fraser, 'Leicester and smallpox: The Leicester method', *Medical History*, 24:3 (1980), 315–32.

35 D. A. Henderson, *Smallpox: The Death of a Disease: The Inside Story of Eradicating a Worldwide Killer* (New York: Prometheus Books, 2009), p. 91.

36 Reinhardt, *The End of a Global Pox*, p. 110.

37 R. N. Basu, Z. Jezek and N. A. Ward, *The Eradication of Smallpox from India* (New Delhi: WHO, 1979), p. vi. See also L. B. Brilliant, *The Management of Smallpox Eradication in India* (Ann Arbor, MI: University of Michigan Press, 1985). This account targeted a broader audience and engaged with wider debate about different types of programmes.

38 Bhattacharya, *Expunging Variola*, pp. 8–9.

39 Fenner et al., *Smallpox and Its Eradication*, p. 1284.

40 See, for example: Henderson, *Smallpox: The Death of a Disease*; Isao Arita, *The Smallpox Eradication Saga: An Insider's View* (Hyderabad: Orient Blackswan, 2010); William H. Foege, *House on Fire: The Fight to Eradicate Smallpox* (Berkeley, CA: University of California Press and Milbank Memorial Fund, 2011).

41 Marennikova, *How It Was: The Global Smallpox Eradication Program in Reminiscences of Its Participants.*

42 Isao Arita, *Smallpox Eradication: Target Zero* (Japan: Mainichi Press, 1979).

43 Horace G. Ogden, *CDC and the Smallpox Crusade* (Washington, DC: US Department of Health and Human Services, Center for Disease Control, 1987), pp. ix–x.

44 Peace Corps, *The Peace Corps' Contributions to the Global Smallpox Eradication Program* (Office of Strategic Information, Research, and Planning, 2016).

45 Marennikova, *How It Was: The Global Smallpox Eradication Program in Reminiscences of Its Participants.* Marennikova was the head of the National Smallpox Center in Moscow which supported the eradication programme throughout.

46 Bhattacharya has been at the forefront of this initiative. See Sanjoy Bhattacharya and Sharon Messenger (eds), *The Global Eradication of Smallpox* (New Delhi: Orient BlackSwan, 2010).

47 Alan Schnur, 'Innovation as an integral part of smallpox eradication: A fieldworker's perspective', in Sanjoy Bhattacharya and Sharon Messenger (eds), *The Global Eradication of Smallpox* (New Delhi: Orient BlackSwan, 2010), p. 107.

48 For example, Target Zero: Smallpox Eradication Archive www.zeropox.info/index.htm. As well as the WHO programme, this US-based archive now includes the CDC Smallpox Eradication/Measles Control Program in West and Central Africa.

49 Email from Donna Kynaston, Head, Records and Archives, WHO, Geneva, to author, 12 May 2016. Registered for inclusion on the Memory of the World Register 2017.

50 Cueto, Brown and Fee, *The World Health Organization*, p. 115.

51 For Nepal and Cold War politics see Thomas Robertson, '"Front line of the Cold War": The US and Point Four development programs in Cold War Nepal 1950–1953', *Studies in Nepali History and Society*, 24:1 (2019), 41–72.

52 W. Charles Cockburn, 'Progress in international smallpox eradication', *American Journal of Public Health*, 56:10 (1966), 1628–33.

53 Whelpton, *A History of Nepal*, p. 2.

54 Economic and Social Commission for Asia and the Pacific (ESCAP), *Population of Nepal*, Country Monograph Series No. 6 (Bangkok: United Nations, 1980), pp. 13, 21.

55 For an environmental history approach see Thomas B. Robertson, 'DDT and the Cold War jungle: American environmental and social engineering in the Rapti valley of Nepal', *Journal of American History*, 104:4 (2018), 904–30.

56 Whelpton, *A History of Nepal*, p. 3.

57 See, for example, Madhusudan Subedi, *State, Society and Health in Nepal* (Abingdon: Routledge, 2018) and Ian Harper, *Development and Public Health in the Himalaya: Reflections on Healing in Contemporary Nepal* (Abingdon: Routledge, 2014).

58 For brief mentions see also Marasini, 'Health and hospital development in Nepal'.

59 Hemang Dixit, *The Quest for Health: The Health Services of Nepal*, 1st edn (Kathmandu: Educational Publishing House, 1995), pp. 99–100.

60 Hemang Dixit, Nepal's Quest for Health: The Health Services of Nepal, 4th edn (Kathmandu: Educational Publishing House, 2014), p. 24.

61 Personal communication with the author.

62 Hemang Dixit, *The Quest for Health: The Health Services of Nepal*, 2nd edn (Kathmandu: Educational Enterprise, 1999), p. 113.

63 B. N. Vaidya and H. V. Gurubacharya, 'On smallpox', *JNMA*, 4:4 (1966), 339–43.

64 *Ibid.*, p. 339.

65 *Ibid.*, p. 343.
66 Satnam Singh, 'Some aspects of the epidemiology of smallpox in Nepal', *Indian Journal of Public Health*, 14:4 (1970), 129–35. In the official history, the reference WHO/SE/69.10 was used.
67 P. N. Shrestha, 'History of smallpox', *JNMA*, 10:2 (1972), 107–11. See also B. B. Karki, 'A review of global smallpox eradication', *JNMA*, 13:1–2 (1975), 18–24.
68 'Smallpox Target Zero', *World Health* (October 1972), 3. Nepal had two WHO employees involved with smallpox at the time.
69 Nedd Willard, 'The anger of a goddess', *World Health* (October 1972), 18–21. Willard became chief editor for *World Health*.
70 *Ibid.*, 18.
71 Fenner et al., *Smallpox and Its Eradication*, p. 792. This is stated in the first line.
72 Basu, Jezek and Ward, *The Eradication of Smallpox from India*.
73 WHO/SEP, File 1239, Box 666, Attached comments, Acting WPCR Nepal to Regional Director, SEARO, 29 November 1984.
74 *Ibid.*
75 Fenner et al., *Smallpox and Its Eradication*, p. 792.
76 *Ibid.*, p. 796.
77 For Bhutan, see Bhattacharya, 'International health and the limits of its global influence'.
78 Fenner et al., *Smallpox and Its Eradication*, p. 715; P. N. Shrestha, D. A. Robinson, J. Friedman and WHO, *The Nepal Smallpox Eradication Programme: Description and Analysis* (Geneva: WHO, 1977) www.who.int/iris/handle/10665/68287. In the official history, the reference SME/77.1 was used.
79 Fenner et al., *Smallpox and Its Eradication*, p. 793. Shrestha commented that it was only some sections of Newars who resisted vaccination, and this was added, p. 794.
80 *Ibid.*, p. 795.
81 *Ibid.*, p. 796.
82 *Ibid.*, p. 804.
83 *Ibid.*, pp. 804–5.
84 Although independent from Britain since 1948, Ceylon in 1972 on becoming a republic changed its name to Sri Lanka. In the official history, Sathianathan is described as 'an experienced smallpox adviser' (p. 796) but is one of the few people in the Index of Names to only be given an initial (p. 1417). Known to those he worked with as 'Sathi', I am very grateful for the assistance of present and former WHO staff, Hemanthi and Hema Dassanayake, and Shiv Kumar Varma, in enabling me to identify his given name.
85 Ogden, *CDC and the Smallpox Crusade*, p. 98.

86 Fenner et al., *Smallpox and Its Eradication*, p. 794.
87 Ogden, *CDC and the Smallpox Crusade*, p. 98.
88 Peace Corps, *The Peace Corps' Contributions to the Global Smallpox Eradication Program*, pp. 84–5.
89 Henderson, *Smallpox: The Death of a Disease*, p. 185.

2

Smallpox in Nepal

Smallpox was widespread throughout much of Nepal which had the variola major form of the virus that was prevalent throughout Asia and much of Africa. It was particularly common in childhood and people with acute variola major were usually very sick. During the first half of the twentieth century, a variola minor variant became endemic in North and South America and parts of Europe and Africa but not in South Asia.[1] The only difference was in the 'spectrum of severity' and a case fatality rate (total number of deaths as a proportion of reported smallpox cases) of less than 1 per cent.[2] Today many older Nepalis retain vivid and often painful memories of their encounters with smallpox and so for them smallpox was about much more than prevention or vaccination. Their own experiences and the disease's presence in the community influenced their ideas and actions, including vaccination which few were able to access.[3] Much that emerged during the global campaign reflected Nepali people's long-held ideas and practices.

This chapter is in two parts. Using oral and written sources about different areas of the country, the first part places individual people's beliefs and experiences at the forefront but also incorporates the framework used in the official history to provide a population-based (epidemiological) perspective. From this latter viewpoint much information is considered 'anecdotal' and less reliable, but with few other sources available this nevertheless provides missing but valuable context.[4] The second section discusses the practice of variolation and the very limited provision of vaccination until expansion in the 1950s. Vaccination was introduced in 1816 at the request of Nepal's government and demonstrates the existence of boundaries and limits to colonial authority and influence and that governments may adopt and use technologies on their own terms and for their own purposes.

Smallpox

The boy was barely five years old when he contracted smallpox.[5] The family lived in the town of Biratnagar in the Tarai where his father worked for the district administration. When bullets flew in 1950 at the start of the revolution that brought down the national government, the family moved out of their house into a bunker before taking up an offer to move into a neighbour's house.[6] Although the family had their own separate rooms in the compound, the child played with other boys. When his mother learned that there was smallpox in the area, she would not let him go out, but it was already too late. Of the approximately fifteen other small boys, half died.

People with smallpox were looked after at home. Indeed, in countries where the health infrastructure was poor they often did better at home.[7] When the boy began to show signs of the disease, he was isolated in a small room on the top floor and kept away from others. His mother was with him all the time – he was her only son still alive. When the vesicles on the boy's body burst his mother wiped away the fluid. She worried that if he scratched more fluid would come. She soothed him with a peacock feather – it gave him relief even if it tickled. Another man recalled sleeping on banana leaves with a cradle placed over him so that nothing could touch him.[8] In many parts of South Asia the leaves of the neem tree (*Azadirachta indica*), which in Nepal grew in the foothills, were used widely for a variety of healing purposes including smallpox. When his mother went out of the room, he would scratch the soft skin of his lips until they were raw. She put sheep's ghee on his lip, which had a 'horrible' smell, and told him 'Don't lick!' Itchiness was not mentioned in the official history, and Dixon also thought it was 'not a serious problem, except when the eruption is drying up and there is much scaling and scabbing'.[9] Mothers talked about the itching and trying to stop their children from scratching.[10] The boy's mother made a rice paste. Very few girls in Nepal went to school at this time, and what she knew about smallpox she had learned from her family. Although many types of healers were present in communities, most people with smallpox never saw a health practitioner.[11] Of the people I talked with, one man recalled how he had a fever, and then developed a rash which affected his eyes. A 'healer' came to the house in the morning and the evening, 'blowing' his eyes with black pepper grains and afterwards it cleared up.[12]

Rituals and religious practices were an integral part of how people responded to the disease. The Hindu deity Sitala held a central place in many people's beliefs and practices, although these varied among the different groups and location. Most of the literature focuses on India.[13] Belief in Sitala and vaccination were not mutually exclusive. Lauren Minsky discusses how people in colonial Punjab actively sought safe and effective protection from smallpox and that it is a mistake to focus only on the 'religiosity'.[14] This point is important; it is discussed further in Chapter 6 about global vaccination strategies in the 1960s. In later accounts, including the official history of the global programme, non-acceptance of vaccination became conflated with the idea of 'cultural resistance' and was particularly associated with belief in and worship of the goddess Sitala rather than any other beliefs or concerns. Minsky noted how because of vaccination's side effects affecting people's ability to work, parents from the agrarian lower classes preferred to have their children vaccinated before the spring harvest and only when smallpox was present.[15]

In the Kathmandu Valley, many Newar practise a mixture of Hinduism and Buddhism. The major Buddhist temple complex of Swayambhunath contains a square, two-storey temple devoted to the worship of Sitala.[16] It was rebuilt following major damage in 1800 by order of the ex-king Rana Bahadur.[17] His beloved Brahmin mistress Kantavati, who was a widow and so could not remarry, had died by suicide after losing her beauty through being disfigured by the scars from an attack of smallpox. Rana Bahadur had abdicated a few months earlier to ensure their infant son, Girvan, became king. The ex-king's grief, his actions and his forbidding people to worship the goddess illustrate royal power but also how strong and widespread belief was in Sitala and supports the view that Sitala was more than a village/folk deity.[18] A genealogical history, the

Vansāvalī, blamed King Girvan's death from smallpox on the fury of the goddess Sitala.[19] The reason for the goddess being angry was not given, but Brahmin astrologers had reflected many people's unhappiness with the socially unacceptable relationship between Girvan's parents and spread a rumour that their child would die of smallpox.[20] Despite such reaction and people's fear of smallpox, responses to Sitala should be understood more in terms of worship and healing.[21] In the mid-nineteenth century the temple was visited annually by 'thousands' of Buddhists as well as Hindus.[22] Included among the Buddhists were groups of Tibetans, 'numbers of whom annually visit Nipal, and who suffer fearfully from the ravages of small-pox'.[23] To Buddhist Newar, the temple at Swayambu is for Hariti or Ajima and is devoted to a mother (*ma*) figure and protector of children rather than the 'dreaded goddess of smallpox'.[24] The goddess was believed to 'afford the necessary protection to all those who sought her aid'.

Ceremonies were carried out in other parts of the country. In 1954, David Snellgrove, a lecturer in Tibetan studies in London, visited Jiwong monastery in the hill region of Solu in eastern Nepal. He noted that the monks gathered together for general ceremonies not only on set feast days but also

> at the request of one of their members or of any layman, who has some private objective in view. ... and several parents came to ask for the after-death ceremony to be performed on behalf of children who had died of small-pox, of which there happened to be an epidemic.[25]

For such private ceremonies the cost was the responsibility of the instigator, 'which is normally between 200 and 300 rupees. This is a large sum in a simple agricultural economy, but no attempt is made to limit it, for much of the efficacy of the rite consists in unregretted giving.'

Individually, Nepali people's beliefs and practices differed, but collectively many understood that smallpox was contagious and affected not just the person with the disease but could spread to those around them and the wider population. The official history's account of Nepal's programme focuses on the situation in the 1960s and gives little historical context. While sources agree that Nepal had a long history of smallpox, how long is unclear. Statistical data on the morbidity and mortality from smallpox do not exist and as the state did not collect vital statistics such as births and deaths, it would have been impossible to calculate any rates for incidence (number of new cases) and prevalence (number of cases of a disease present in a particular population at a given time or over a period of time).

Smallpox had distinctive clinical features; facial pockmarks were a visible reminder of the disease's presence in a community. People belonging to Nepal's many different ethnic groups had long recognised smallpox as a disease entity and gave it a name. Sherpa called it *blendum*. Other examples can be found in earlier written sources. While William Kirkpatrick did not discuss smallpox, he listed it in his vocabulary that he compiled for two of the main vernacular languages following his visit in 1793. Each had a specific word for smallpox, the only disease to be listed.[26] Other words about illnesses were more about signs and symptoms such as 'A cough', 'A fever' or 'The venereal disease'. The existence of a word for smallpox did not mean necessarily that the disease was present, but it suggested that sometime in the past there had been an encounter. During his fieldwork in the Gurung village of Thak in central Nepal (north of Pokhara) from the late 1960s, British anthropologist Alan Macfarlane found no evidence of epidemics in Thak records or evidence of smallpox scars, but the Gurung people had a word – *pro*.[27]

Children were particularly prone to getting smallpox, but in the literature the most commonly referred to or widely known information was when royalty or those around them died from the disease. King Mahindra Malla of Lalitpur died in 1715, the mistress of King Rana Bahadur Shah in 1800 and King Girvan in 1816. Sources also suggest that smallpox affected society widely. A royal order in 1805 recorded an outbreak of smallpox among the *jhara* (bonded) labourers at Chisapani in the hills around the Kathmandu Valley.[28] Nepali society was hierarchical and based on caste. The young boy from Biratnagar in the initial story came from a Brahmin family, the highest caste.

References to smallpox indicate that the disease was severe and that the case-fatality rate was high. British residency surgeon Daniel Wright mentioned in an introductory sketch to his *History of Nepal* the epidemic in 1816 and that 'Soon after the British arrived in the country, smallpox broke out, and committed great ravages among the people.'[29] Indian explorer Hari Ram travelled through the Mt Everest region in 1885 and secretly gathered information for the

Survey of India, reporting an outbreak of 'virulent small-pox ... which carried off a large number of the inhabitants of Khumbu'.[30] Given the vast under-reporting and under-estimation of the disease, such brief glimpses convey their message vividly. The official history noted that the worldwide history of smallpox before the twentieth century was full of 'epidemic years' against a background of endemicity.[31] This fitted the evidence from Nepal. During the 1940s and 1950s epidemics were noted to have occurred regularly in Nepal – 1946, 1950, 1954 and 1958.[32] On this timeline, the next epidemic was expected around 1962 or 1963.[33]

The Kathmandu Valley was the most densely populated part of Nepal which aided the spread of a range of infectious diseases. In 1856, Prime Minister Jang Bahadur instigated the first population census of Nepal. Data collected for urban and rural Kathmandu, Patan and Bhadgaun (Bhaktapur), referred to houses depopulated as a result of epidemics. Urban Patan had 22,000 'old Newar houses', but this total was 'exclusive of 2,000 houses depopulated as a result of a pox epidemic' and urban Bhadgaun had 11,500 'old Newar houses', a total 'exclusive of 500 houses depopulated as a result of a smallpox epidemic'.[34] Such information illustrates that accurate statistical data could be gathered when wanted. Depopulation also occurred in rural areas as Hari Ram noted in his travels.[35]

Most infectious diseases show characteristic seasonal variations in incidence. Smallpox in temperate climates was similar to measles and chickenpox being a winter/spring disease; the variola virus survived most easily in cool and dry conditions and so was most infectious in the winter and spring. In tropical climates this could be blurred. In Nepal it varied; it was generally more frequent in the low-lying Tarai in January and February, the Kathmandu Valley in March and April, and higher altitude areas in May and June.[36]

While the clinical picture of smallpox is concerned with how the virus spread within the body of an individual and how the body responded (pathogenesis), the epidemiological perspective is concerned with how the virus particles moved between human beings. The only source of the variola virus was human and there were no long-term carriers. As a person was infectious from the onset of fever, the most likely source of infection was contact with someone with the disease. The mode of transmission was usually direct through implantation of infective droplets from the respiratory tract. Indirect was less common. Mobility, family size and composition, occupation and 'dangerous situations' such as an undiagnosed case in an institution influenced transmission.[37]

A common response, when a person was thought to have the disease, was isolation. In 1816 this occurred when King Girvan was separated from his family after his two sons developed the disease. In an earlier epidemic, his father 'ordered that all children be sent elsewhere. The order had been issued with the aim of saving them from death, but it imposed severe hardships on the people.'[38] The event is remembered through the well-known and very sad Newar song, 'Sitala Maju', which dates from the early nineteenth century and captures the anguish and hardship of the parents with their young children being forced 'out of the country' (the Kathmandu Valley) and across the river Tamakoshi: 'There was nothing to eat. There was nothing to wear. There was no place for me to rest. It was not with a whip, it was not with a cane, it was with a bundle of stinging nettles that they were beaten. They were surrounded by soldiers.'[39] Many of the Newar towns outside the Kathmandu Valley can be traced to this expulsion in 1793.[40] A later unforced example is the hill-top settlement of Bandipur (Tanahun district) situated between Kathmandu and Pokhara, which was founded in the 1850s when a group of Newar fled an epidemic.[41]

In small houses isolation was difficult, but Newar houses in the urban areas of the Kathmandu Valley were multi-storeyed. Since people with smallpox stayed at home, those most at risk were other members of the household and especially those involved in the caring. Mothers looked after their children, irrespective of whether they had had the disease or had been variolated or vaccinated. While in the late nineteenth century controversy existed in other countries over the siting of hospitals and airborne spread, Nepal in the 1950s had few schools or hospitals even in the capital and so smallpox had limited opportunity for institutional spread of the virus.[42] After the smallpox victim (whether alive or dead), the next most important source of infection was the person's clothing and bedding. Normal washing and airing were insufficient to prevent transmission of the virus, but a poor family could not afford to destroy such items as Hillary and his team found in the Mt Everest area in 1963. 'But what will my daughter wear – what will she sleep in? We have nothing else and I have no money.'[43]

Various factors such as the viability of the virus, changes in host susceptibility or the wider political, social and economic environment affected the spread of smallpox, which did not have the associated stigma of a disease such as leprosy and 'lessened the tendency to conceal cases'.[44] Smallpox spread, however, varied in different settings. Even where it was 'essentially uncontrolled', such as Nepal, 'it was never uniformly distributed within a country'.[45] When populations were first exposed to the smallpox virus, people of all ages and both sexes were affected; after it became endemic it was mainly a disease of childhood. Rural areas and small villages often escaped infection for several years.

In Nepal, the movement of people was central to understanding how smallpox spread among different groups. Activities such as visiting family and other social, religious or public events which brought people together could affect the transmission of the disease. Among the Tharu of the Tarai it was customary to grant the wish of someone who had smallpox; this might involve visiting family in a nearby village and so encouraged short-distance spread.[46] Although fighting did not occur in Nepal during its war (1814–16) with the British East India Company or the later World Wars, military activities involved the movement of large numbers of people – not just soldiers but others associated with their support.[47] Natural disasters, the need for work or the shortage of food also led to the movement of people and the spread of disease.[48] A 1958 survey of 908 villages in central Nepal, carried out by the Nepal–America Cooperative Service for Industrial Development, revealed that 86.7 per cent of the men left their homes and went looking for seasonal employment.[49] The incubation period of the virus of around two weeks meant that people could travel long distances before the disease became apparent.

During the 1950s, political changes in Nepal brought both instability and opportunities; it also brought new groups of foreigners into the country. Dr Michael Ward was with the 1951 British Mount Everest reconnaissance expedition and spent three weeks walking from Jogbani on the Indian border through the hills of eastern Nepal. Smallpox and cholera were noted in Dhankuta (Kosi zone).[50] While the number of foreign climbers might only be small, large numbers of local people were employed to assist and carry supplies through the country. These porters had to look after themselves with food and accommodation. 'Hundreds of foraging porters' travelling from village to village could spread not just smallpox but also other diseases.[51]

Vaccination

Controlling smallpox by deliberate intervention began long before such measures were adopted for other infectious diseases. Part of the landscape of responses to smallpox in Nepal prior to 1959 was the practice of variolation, which if successful was considered to achieve the desired immunity. Since variolation used live smallpox matter, cases of the disease might result and lead to further spread, although fewer people died than from naturally occurring smallpox.[52] David Arnold has suggested that the practice of variolation was 'virtually unknown' in Nepal but Shrestha, although giving no source or any other information, considered that variolation was well known during the eighteenth century.[53] It continued to be used at the highest social level after the introduction of vaccination. In 1830 'Dhirja Vaidya, who had conducted variolation on a royal prince' was granted exemption from various forced-labour and tax obligations.[54] This was a significant payment given the extreme burden under which most Nepalis lived. Atsuko Nano suggests that in colonial Burma, variolation or inoculation was a popular and widely diffused practice rather than a profession.[55] An outline of Newar castes, however, listed the *kaussa* who were 'inoculators for small-pox'.[56] They were regarded as inferior in status to some Buddhists although were still a clean caste.

In his autobiography, Professor Dr Bhisma Raj Prasai describes the practice of variolation around 1938 in his village of Nirudadin in Jhapa, the easternmost district in Nepal (Map 1). People were 'frightened' as an epidemic spread towards their village; they believed that an outbreak of smallpox was a 'visitation' of the goddess and responded with rituals. On hearing news of an epidemic, the local baidya (Ayurvedic practitioner) went to the village.

> They would break the vesicle on the body of the infected person and collect the material from it in a small container. Any child who was not infected would then have a small incision on the ventral aspect of the forearm with a knife or any sharp pointed object. Once a little

blood started flowing from the site of the incision, they would then put a drop of the material from the vesicle of the infected child and rub it on the site of the incision. The crying child would be firmly held by the parents whilst the baidya applied the material from the smallpox vesicles and carried on rubbing it. This was known as putting on the 'Kholi'. The baidya would receive money or some rice grains as remuneration for his services.[57]

A few days later the child's arm became swollen and the child feverish. Vesicles began to develop and then cover the body. Those who survived developed increased immunity and people believed they had 'won over' the disease. Unfortunately, a cousin and some of his friends died.

In 1950, in another district in eastern Nepal, villagers invited a variolator to come and inoculate their children after a young boy developed the disease.[58] A 'camp' was set up that operated under the healer's strict rules surrounding neatness, cleanliness and ritual purity. The children 'nicely cleaned' were brought together and variolated at the same time. They were kept in a room and provided with food from a separate kitchen. No meat or eggs were allowed. Each child was looked after by a family member, usually the mother, who likewise had to follow strict rules about dress and cleanliness.[59] Visitors were allowed but also had to be 'neat and clean' and could not touch the children. Although variolation was a source for the spread of smallpox as it used live smallpox matter, people recognised this and kept those being variolated separated. The children had to stay until 'it was all over', which could be three to four weeks; the healer also stayed throughout. All survived. Afterwards a 'big' *puja* (religious ceremony) was held, and the camp closed. Although people thought of smallpox as a children's disease, two adults died in the small community at this time.

By far the most important factor influencing transmission of the virus was immunity provided by vaccination, but vaccination in Nepal was extremely limited when the global campaign commenced. At times it may not have been successful. The boy in Biratnagar was puzzled that he got smallpox because he understood from his mother that although his parents were not vaccinated, and his sister underwent variolation, he had been vaccinated. He did not know where this was done or by whom. Nepal did not produce its own vaccine, which needed bringing into the country from India.[60] It was quite possible that the heat of the Tarai and lack of cold storage for the liquid vaccine in use at the time had rendered it ineffective.[61] Considering people's mixed experiences with vaccination, that the more common variolation was mostly effective and that practitioners used both variola or vaccine which they bought from India,[62] vaccination's benefit was not obvious to the majority of the population.

Vaccination was introduced into Nepal in 1816, appeared widely accepted but was not expanded further into the country. It arrived in South Asia at a time of growing British power in the region, and India became a hub for the spread of vaccination further afield. Within a few years of its introduction into India in 1802 vaccination had become well established in British India and Ceylon (Sri Lanka), but local populations throughout South Asia were less enthusiastic.[63] In Nepal, government officials requested vaccination from the new British representative or 'resident' in response to a smallpox epidemic in the capital.[64] This newcomer to Nepal was part of the terms of the Treaty of Sagauli imposed in 1816 after Nepal's military defeat by the British. It was highly unpopular with the Nepali government, but it is through the Resident's letters that we know about the events that brought vaccination into the Kathmandu Valley and that the initiative came from Nepal.[65] One of the principal functions of a resident was to provide a regular flow of information to the East India Company's headquarters in India and then on to London.[66] The Honourable Edward Gardner, a Company civil servant with an empathy for India, reached Kathmandu in July. Over the next six months, the Government of Nepal and the Governor-General in Fort William, through the channel of the Resident, commenced negotiations which included the return of parts of the Tarai to Nepal. In a private letter to John Adam, acting Chief Secretary, Gardner wrote that the senior Nepali officials he was meeting with had requested the 'introduction of Vaccination'.[67] Their concern was that smallpox was 'raging' in the country 'and the Raja [king] has never had the disease'.

Gardner arrived in India in 1802 and so had several years of experience in the region. He clearly saw the political opportunity that was being presented. 'It would not only be an act of humanity to introduce the Vaccination, but be a desirable object, perhaps to have the Raja and the Officers of the Court inoculated by us' and asked Assistant Surgeon Charles Everest to obtain some 'Matter' (vaccine).[68] Gardner was unsure if Everest would be successful and wrote to Adam privately that it was important that he obtain 'the necessary quantity and of a wholesome quality from Calcutta, or wherever it can best be procured'.[69] By early September 'several packets of the vaccine matter' had been received at the residency in Kathmandu.[70]

This early correspondence demonstrated Gardner's awareness of two key aspects about smallpox vaccination if this diplomatic strategy was to be successful: a sufficient and reliable supply of vaccine; and vaccine of appropriate quality. In the early nineteenth century, the viability and efficacy of the vaccine was uncertain, a problem heightened by the effects of distance and travel time. The journey from northern India to Kathmandu took several weeks and was through difficult terrain. It was also the monsoon. Arm-to-arm vaccination using children was widely considered to be the most effective way of maintaining a source of the virus, but Gardner's letter referred to 'packets'.[71] Although the hot, wet and humid weather and the dangers of malaria in the Tarai were conditions found elsewhere in India and did not prevent the use of human-to-human transmission, it is unlikely that this method would have been used to get the vaccine to Nepal because the travel route was little used at that time of year.[72] The contents of the packets most likely were preserved vaccinia crusts.

Vaccinating began on 13 September 1816 at Banepa to the south-east of the Kathmandu Valley and was the preferred location of Nepal's powerful *mukhtiyar* (executive head of administration) Bhimsen Thapa. Everest vaccinated 'numerous patients' – although no numbers were recorded.[73] Gardner kept a close watch on what was happening. His letters conveyed the optimism that many felt about vaccination and the superiority of 'western' 'scientific' medicine and indicated that he was keen to introduce what he referred to as the 'benefit' of vaccination.[74] The King and his immediate family were said to be showing 'reluctance', although vaccination was being taken up by 'the families of the immediate members of the Court and of the Principal Chiefs and People of the Country'. Religious objection, therefore, was unlikely to be the reason. Political intrigue was rife at court, but also there could be a valid

Smallpox in Nepal 57

reason concerning the procedure. The content of vaccinia crusts was known to be unreliable and was considered inferior to variolation in the production of effective immunity against smallpox. In early November, Gardner wrote that he had received a proposal in person from Bhimsen Thapa 'for the immediate vaccination of the Raja and his family' but that it would be delayed until 'a living subject' could be used.[75]

We are not told why such concerns appeared only in connection with the royal family and Gardner was not allowed to communicate directly with the King. It may have been too late. On 18 November Gardner received a visit from another senior official, Gajraj Misra, 'to communicate to me that the Raja had unfortunately taken the smallpox'.[76] Two days later, Gardner conveyed the news of the King's death from smallpox.[77] It was apparently very quick and, as was Hindu custom, preparations were soon underway for his funeral. Soon afterwards the junior queen, Gorakshya Rajya Laxmi, was said to have died from smallpox. This surprised Gardner as 'it was always understood that she had had the smallpox in her youth' and would therefore be immune to the disease.[78] Speculation of foul play circulated among different groups at the court after the King's death, although Gardner believed both deaths were due to natural causes.

This episode was over thirty years before the more familiar reference by the residency's Surgeon Henry Oldfield to support for vaccination in Nepal from the Prime Minister Jang Bahadur Rana who visited Britain in 1850.[79] Oldfield also mentioned that Jang Bahadur carried out a few vaccinations himself. Gardner had hoped that vaccination would begin in the Kathmandu Valley and then extend to other parts of the country, but this had not occurred. Vaccination was available at the small residency hospital and Tibetans, wrote Surgeon George Gimlette, 'are among our cold weather clients; they principally come to be vaccinated, and seem to fully appreciate the efficacy of the operation'.[80] The residency surgeons at times were called on to provide medical services and vaccination for high-ranking families.[81] In 1885, Gimlette mentioned that he examined Gurkha recruits for the British Army, but made no note of smallpox, vaccination or scars.

In the early twentieth century vaccination appeared to be increasing as government health services began to develop, although neither Dixit nor Babu Ram Marasini mention vaccination during this period. While some early hospital archives exist, they are relatively unstudied.[82] Who carried out vaccination and where is not known, or how much was being done. We also learn nothing about what was happening in other parts of the country. The resident's annual report of the medical work from the residency mentioned that in 1912–13 the 'Darbar' (central government) was 'energetically' pursuing vaccination. The Residency had assisted in obtaining a supply of lymph from the Lahore Vaccine Department.[83] It was also believed 'that orders making it compulsory in the Nepal valley, if not beyond, have frequently been issued'. Nepal was one of several areas outside India receiving vaccine, but as the reports of the newly established Vaccine Institute combined these into an 'Out of Punjab' category, individual totals were not listed.[84] The calf lymph vaccine was despatched in small glass tubes carefully packed in wooden boxes. The tubes contained one gram of vaccine, which was found to be more tolerant of heat and exposure than smaller quantities.[85]

Despite assisting the government with obtaining vaccine, residency medical staff had little or no interaction with government staff. Some people from the town went to the residency hospital as did 'a large number of wandering people from the hills. The practice of inoculation [variolation] has not yet fallen into disuse here.'[86] The Residency had a military escort of about eighty and in the report for 1919–20 it was noted that 'All non-commissioned officers and men are well protected against small pox by recent vaccination.'[87] Outlining medical developments under Prime Minister Chandra Shamsher (1901–29), English writer Perceval Landon wrote that 'Vaccination is not compulsory, but it is free to those who choose to avail themselves of this protection against a disease.'[88] Although free, the rich were more likely to be able to access any that was available.[89] A later reference suggested that the vaidya (baidya) when using vaccine rather than variola, charged 'about one rupee, plus a small quantity of rice'.[90]

Variolation continued to be practised and vaccination only became available more widely throughout the country during the 1950s. The Directorate of Health Services obtained lymph vaccine from India from the Vaccine Institute at Patwadangar in Uttar Pradesh and in 1957 vaccinated 40,101 people at 'collecting points'.

Acceptance of vaccination was considered 'good'. The number of vaccinations had increased to 74,421 in 1959 but given the size of Nepal's population was still very low.[91] People only received one vaccination and were not revaccinated. A young boy at the time in Kathmandu recalled being vaccinated at school, although remembered a cholera vaccine more as they were given a holiday.[92] Indeed at 122,007, the number of vaccinations against cholera in 1959 was higher.[93] Nevertheless, smallpox vaccinators had reached even Namche Bazar in the Mt Everest region, as a man from Thame recalled being taken there to be vaccinated.[94] He also believed that this had prevented him from getting smallpox in 1963. Community leaders and religious personnel could also be influential in people being vaccinated. In the Mt Everest region, vaccination had been given the seal of approval when in the early 1940s, the new five-year old *rinpoche* (reincarnate head lama) at the Buddhist monastery at Tengboche was taken to Kathmandu to be vaccinated, although we do not know where the procedure was done or by whom.[95]

Another source of evidence referring to expanding, if limited, vaccination services can be found in accounts written by visitors. Dr Frederick Dunn travelled in the high-altitude remote Kali Gandaki valley in central Nepal. He commented that smallpox vaccination 'was limited to those few villagers whose travels south and east had brought them in contact with vaccinators'.[96] That the vaccinators went to certain places but did not go further afield tallies with the information of vaccination in the Mt Everest area. While some visitor accounts tended to associate belief in the goddess Sitala with resistance to vaccination, Dr George Moore with the United States Operations Mission (USOM) presented a different view.[97] He conferred with Hindu and Buddhist priests

> about using Sitala, the goddess of smallpox, in our campaign to induce people to be vaccinated. They readily agreed, and we quickly produced large campaign posters showing Sitala in full regalia with her four hands holding syringes and other medical items. The inscriptions in Nepali exhorted the people to be immunized for her sake. Runners delivered the posters to the village priests and lamas who plastered them on their homes and temples for all to see. Most of the people were illiterate, but the religious leaders (always the first to be vaccinated) read the message to them and announced the arrival of the team. Villagers greeted us festively.[98]

Moore spent two years in Nepal. He was able to acquire freeze-dried vaccine from the USA, but his practices were not part of the slowly developing government vaccination services and illustrate the fractured responses to smallpox at this time and the activities of foreigners which are the focus of Chapter 4.

Conclusion

Talking with people about smallpox, drawing on a wide range of sources and considering different perspectives confirms that smallpox was both endemic and epidemic but that it was one of many major diseases that confronted Nepali people prior to 1959. Although very little has been written about smallpox in Nepal from an epidemiological perspective, it is possible to build up a broader societal picture prior to the country's involvement in the global smallpox programme. Few Nepali people would have been surprised to know that smallpox had long been present in Nepal and was widespread throughout the country; it was severe and had a high mortality; all society was at risk; it was seasonal; and epidemics occurred every few years. Only newcomers in the 1950s expressed concern at the potential of smallpox to spread into remote areas.

People's various experiences, beliefs and practices influenced and shaped their responses to smallpox. Nepali people were familiar with the course of the disease and how to look after someone. Smallpox was managed in the home, particularly by mothers. Today many older people retain vivid and often painful memories, either of having the disease or of caring for their children. Rituals and worship were an important and integral part of people's varying responses to the presence of the disease, but they could believe both in the powers of deities and be variolated or vaccinated. Isolation of cases of smallpox in the home or in variolation camps helped contain the spread of the disease.

Vaccination, with vaccine from India, was introduced into the Kathmandu Valley in 1816 at the request of senior Nepali government officials during an epidemic in which the King later died from smallpox. Many people were vaccinated; resistance was not mentioned in the British Resident's correspondence. Despite his hopes and although some vaccine continued to be brought in from India, vaccination did not spread widely. Although vaccination expanded during the 1950s, it still did not reach many parts of the country and especially not most remote areas. Variolation remained popular, especially in rural Nepal. The WHO worked with governments, but Nepal had little history of providing services as understood by international organisations. The next chapter explores the development of Nepal as a nation state to provide the background and framework to the introduction and implementation of the global smallpox programme in Nepal.

Notes

1 Fenner et al., *Smallpox and Its Eradication*, p. 3.
2 Dixon, *Smallpox*, p. 57.
3 Highlighting the importance of social conceptions of smallpox and how the disease shaped society and worldviews, see Oluwatoyin Babatunde Oduntan, 'Culture and colonial medicine: Smallpox in Abeokuta, Western Nigeria', *Social History of Medicine*, 30:1 (2017), 48–70.
4 The topic continues to be an active debate in the literature. On the complementary value of anecdotal information, see, for example, M. W. Enkin and A. R. Jadad, 'Using anecdotal information in evidence-based health care: Heresy or necessity?', *Annals of Oncology*, 9 (1998), 963–6; on its flexible position on the boundary between science and its publics, see Alfred Moore and Jack Stilgoe, 'Experts and anecdotes: The role of "anecdotal evidence" in public scientific controversies', *Science, Technology, & Human Values*, 34:5 (2009), 654–77. See also Mathilde Frèrot, Annick Lefebvre, Simon Aho, Patrick Callier, Karine Astruc and Ludwig Serge Aho Glèlè, 'What is epidemiology? Changing definitions of epidemiology 1978–2017', *PLoSONE*, 13:12 (2018), e0208442.
5 Interview with author, Kathmandu, 19 May 2017.
6 Leo E. Rose, *Nepal: Strategy for Survival* (Berkeley, CA: University of California Press/Kathmandu: Mandala Book Point, 1971), p. 190.
7 Fenner et al., *Smallpox and Its Eradication*, p. 8.
8 Bhisma Raj Prasai, *Afu Lai Farkera Hereko* (Looking Back at Oneself) (Kathmandu: Ghost Writing Nepal, 2017). I am very grateful to Professor Hemang Dixit for this reference and for his translation (with permission from Dr Prasai).
9 Dixon, *Smallpox*, p. 101.
10 Interviews with author, Kirtipur, May 2017.

11 Madhusudan Sharma Subedi, *Medical Anthropology of Nepal* (Kathmandu: Udaya Books, 2001).
12 Interview with author, Kathmandu, 25 May 2017.
13 Ralph W. Nicholas, 'The goddess Sitala and epidemic smallpox in Bengal', *Journal of Asian Studies*, 41:1 (1981), 21–44; Susan S. Wadley, 'Sitala: The cool one', *Asian Folklore Studies*, 39:1 (1980), 33–62. In Sichuan, China, in the early twentieth century people worshipped the smallpox goddess, praying first for a good variolation and then later for a good vaccination. Chieng-Ling Liu, 'Relocating Pastorian medicine: Accommodation and acclimatization of Pastorian practices against smallpox at the Pasteur Institute of Chengdu, China, 1908–1927', *Science in Context*, 30:1 (2017), 51.
14 Lauren Minsky, 'Pursuing protection from disease: The making of smallpox prophylactic practice in colonial Punjab', *Bulletin of the History of Medicine*, 83:1 (2009), 17; see also Bhattacharya, *Fractured States*, pp. 220–1.
15 Minsky, 'Pursuing protection from disease', 185.
16 Among Newar the story of Sitala has been passed down through traditional songs. Interview with composer, Kathmandu, 16 April 2015. I am very grateful to Kiran Bajracharya for taking me to Swayambhunath and talking to me about current Newar beliefs and practices. His father was a community priest.
17 Henry Ambrose Oldfield, *Sketches from Nipal* (London: W. H. Allen, 1880), vol. 2, pp. 35–6. Oldfield was a member of the Indian Medical Service and was residency surgeon in Kathmandu 1850–63.
18 Fabrizio M. Ferrari, *Religion, Devotion and Medicine in North India: The Healing Power of Śītalā* (London: Bloomsbury, 2015), p. xx.
19 Daniel Wright, *History of Nepal* (New Delhi: Rupa, 2007 [1877]), pp. 53, 267. Wright became residency surgeon in 1863. In Kathmandu he collected documents and took many to the UK. See also John Whelpton, 'A reading guide to Nepalese history', *Himalaya*, 25:1 (2005): Article 5.
20 Chittaranjan Nepali, 'Reign and abdication of King Rana Bahadur Shah', Regmi Research Series (Kathmandu) (hereafter RRS), 3:1 (1971), p. 8.
21 Ferrari, *Religion, Devotion and Medicine in North India*.
22 Oldfield, *Sketches from Nipal*, vol. 1, p. 236.
23 *Ibid.*, p. 237.
24 Perceval Landon, *Nepal* (New Delhi: Asian Educational Services, 1993 [1928]), vol. 1, p. 202. The temple remains popular.
25 D. L. Snellgrove, *Buddhist Himalaya: Travels and Studies in Quest of the Origins and Nature of Tibetan Religion* (Oxford: Bruno Cassirer, 1957), p. 220.

26 Colonel Kirkpatrick, *An Account of the Kingdom of Nepaul Being the Substance of Observations Made during a Mission to That Country in the Year 1793* (New Delhi: Manjusri Publishing House, 1969 [1811]), p. 238.
27 Alan Macfarlane, 'Death, disease and curing in a Himalayan village', in Christoph von Fürer-Haimendorf (ed.), *Asian Highland Societies in Anthropological Perspective* (New Delhi: Sterling, 1981), pp. 99–100.
28 Smallpox Epidemic in Chisapani, royal order to Subedar Antya Khawzas and Subedar Niranja, RRS, 20:11 (1988), p. 160. Chisapani was a communication point.
29 Wright, *History of Nepal*, p. 53.
30 'Report on routes by explorer Hari Ram', *Records of the Survey of India* 8 (Dehra Dun: Survey of India, 1915), part 2, p. 386.
31 Fenner et al., *Smallpox and Its Eradication*, p. 178.
32 WHO library, SEA/CD/8 21 August 1961, Dr M. Radovanovic, Regional Adviser on Communicable Diseases, Report on field visit to Nepal, 1–4 August 1961, p. 1.
33 Interval length between epidemics was related to whether an epidemic was followed by greatly increased vaccination rates. Fenner et al., *Smallpox and Its Eradication*, p. 179. The phenomenon was analysed in detail for measles. M. S. Bartlett, 'Measles periodicity and community size', *Journal of the Royal Statistical Society. Series A (General)*, 120:1 (1957), 48–70.
34 Population of Kathmandu Valley, 1856, RRS, 2:5 (1970), pp. 117–18.
35 'Report on routes by Explorer Hari Ram', p. 386.
36 SEA/CD/8, Radovanovic, Report on field visit to Nepal 1961, p. 1.
37 C. W. Dixon and WHO, Expert Committee on Smallpox, Meeting (1964: Geneva, Switzerland), C.W. Dixon, 'Factors involved in transmission of smallpox and duration of immunity', pp. 1–4 https://apps.who.int/iris/handle/10665/67697.
38 Dr Shiva Prasad Dabaral 'Charan', 'The Yamuna to the Sutlej', *RRS*, 19:4 (1987), p. 53.
39 Siegfried Lienhard, *Songs of Nepal: An Anthology of Nevar Folksongs and Hymns* (Delhi: Motilal Banarsidass, 1992), p. 100.
40 Mary Slusser, 'Nepali sculptures: New discoveries', in P. Lal (ed.), *Aspects of Indian Art: Papers Presented in a Symposium at the Los Angeles County Museum of Art, October, 1970* (Leiden: Brill, 1972), p. 98.
41 Sagar S. J. B. Rana, *Singha Durbar: Rise and Fall of the Rana Regime of Nepal* (New Delhi: Rupa Publications, 2017), p. 172. By road this is 146 km from Kathmandu.
42 Subsequent research undertaken elsewhere was to show that the rate of hospital infections was low.
43 Hillary, *Schoolhouse in the Clouds*, p. 41.

44 Fenner et al., *Smallpox and Its Eradication*, p. 196.
45 *Ibid.*, p. 199.
46 SME/77.1, Shrestha, Robinson and Friedman, *The Nepal Smallpox Eradication Programme*, p. 11.
47 An article on Gurkha recruitment in the mid-1950s makes no mention of smallpox or the vaccination status of the recruits. W. S. Millar, 'Some aspects, mainly medical, of the Gurkha recruiting season, 1955', *Journal of the Royal Army Medical Corps*, 103:3 (1957), 147–54.
48 See, for example, David Arnold, 'Social crisis and epidemic disease in the famines of nineteenth-century India', *Social History of Medicine*, 6:3 (1993), 385–404.
49 Eugene Bramer Mihaly, *Foreign Aid and Politics in Nepal: A Case Study*, 2nd edn (Lalitpur: Himal Books, 2002 [1965]), p. 12.
50 Michael Ward, 'In Eastern Nepal', *The Lancet*, 263:2 (1952), 238–9.
51 Ralph Izzard, *An Innocent on Everest* (New York: E. P. Dutton, 1954), p. 111.
52 Fenner et al., *Smallpox and Its Eradication*, pp. 246–8.
53 Arnold, *Colonizing the Body*, p. 130; Shrestha, 'History of smallpox', 109. For discussion of a complex continuum of practice around smallpox prevention see Christiana Bastos, 'Borrowing, adapting, and learning the practices of smallpox: Notes from Colonial Goa', *Bulletin of the History of Medicine*, 83:1 (2009), 141–63.
54 Tax Exemption (Ashadh Badi 9, 1887) [1830], RRS, 7:2 (1975), p. 26. The name Vaidya suggests he was a practitioner of Ayurvedic medicine.
55 Atsuko Nano, 'Inoculators, the indigenous obstacle to vaccination in Colonial Burma', *Journal of Burma Studies*, 14 (2010), 91–114.
56 Oldfield, *Sketches from Nipal*, vol. 1, p. 186.
57 Prasai, *Afu Lai Farkera Hereko* (Looking Back at Oneself), pp. 10–11.
58 Interview with author, Kathmandu, 25 May 2017 and email communication, September 2021.
59 A menstruating mother was not allowed to look after her child.
60 For vaccine production in India see Sanjoy Bhattacharya, 'Re-devising Jennerian vaccines? European technologies, Indian innovation and the control of smallpox in South Asia, 1850–1950', *Social Scientist*, 26:11/12 (1998), 27–66.
61 When I explained this to him, he realised he could continue to believe he had been vaccinated and that he and his mother were not wrong. This was important to him.
62 WHO library, SEA/CD/14 14 February 1968, Dr B. Ignjatovic, Regional Adviser in Communicable Diseases, Report on a visit to Nepal, 12–17 November 1967, p. 2.
63 Bennett, *War Against Smallpox*, pp. 256–8; Niels Brimnes, 'Fallacy, sacrilege, betrayal and conspiracy: the cultural construction of

opposition to immunization in India', in Holmberg, Blume and Greenough (eds), *The Politics of Vaccination*, pp. 51–76.
64 For a more detailed account of vaccination's introduction see Heydon, 'Death of the king'.
65 British Library, London, India Office Records (hereafter IOR), R/5/37 Letters to India 1816 and IOR, R/5/38 Letters to India 1816–1817.
66 Michael H. Fisher, *Indirect Rule in India: Residents and the Residency System 1764–1857* (Delhi: Oxford University Press, 1991), p. 172.
67 IOR, F/4/550/13379, 17 July. Fort William was the headquarters of the Bengal Presidency.
68 *Ibid.*, Gardner to Adam, 17 July. Gardner's use of the terms 'vaccination' and 'inoculation' was often interchangeable.
69 *Ibid.*
70 IOR, R/5/112, Misc letters sent June 1816–Mar 1817, Gardner to Robert Leny, Secretary, Medical Board, 14 September. The Medical Board was in Patna.
71 No mention is made in the letters of using children to carry live lymph. On the role of children as 'agents of eradication' and empire see Lydia Murdoch, 'Carrying the pox: The use of children and ideals of childhood in early British and imperial campaigns against smallpox', *Journal of Social History*, 48:3 (2015), 511–35.
72 Wright, *History of Nepal*, p. 3.
73 R/5/112, Gardner to Leny, 14 September.
74 IOR, R/5/37, Gardner to Adam, 25 September.
75 IOR, R/5/38, Gardner to Adam, 2 November.
76 *Ibid.*, Gardner to Adam, 18 November. Dixon reviewed the older literature and suggested that despite recent exposure to the virus, a vaccinated person would have had an up to 50 per cent chance of a modified attack and the severity lessened. Dixon, *Smallpox*, p. 337.
77 R/5/38., Gardner to Adam, 20 November.
78 *Ibid.*, Gardner to Adam, 17 December.
79 Oldfield, *Sketches from Nipal*, vol. 1, pp. 253–4.
80 G. H. D. Gimlette, *Nepal and the Nepalese* (London: H. F. & G. Witherby, 1928), p. 155. Although slightly later, Alex McKay discusses how vaccination was assimilated into medical practice, despite Tibetan people's resistance to other aspects of biomedicine. Alex McKay, '"An excellent measure": the battle against smallpox in Tibet, 1904–47', *Tibet Journal*, 30/31:4/1 (2005–06), 119–30.
81 Gimlette, *Nepal and the Nepalese*, p. 252.
82 Yogesh Raj, Deepak Aryal and Shamik Mishra, 'Documents related to the early hospitals in Nepal', *Studies in Nepali History and Society*, 21:2 (2016), 347–400.

83 IOR, L/PS/11/59, P2901/1913, Nepal: Report 1912–13, p. 5. The Residency medical reports are brief.
84 IOR, V/24/4346, Reports on vaccination in the Punjab 1910–26.
85 *Ibid.*, Appendix C, Annual report of the Punjab Vaccine Institute for the year 1924–5.
86 IOR, L/PS/11/138, P3494/1918, Appendix 1, Nepal: Residency report 1917–18, p. 7.
87 IOR, L/PS/11/181, P8149/1920, Nepal: Report on events 1919–20, p. 4.
88 Landon, *Nepal*, vol. 2, p. 184.
89 Dr Rita Thapa, interview with author, Kathmandu, 25 May 2017.
90 SEA/CD/14, Ignjatovic, Report on a visit to Nepal 1967, p. 2. No mention was made of how or from where in India the 'vaids' bought their vaccine.
91 For smallpox and immunisation in Britain, see Gareth Millward, *Vaccinating Britain: Mass Vaccination and the Public since the Second World War* (Manchester: Manchester University Press, 2019).
92 Conversation with author, Kathmandu, 18 May 2017.
93 SEA/CD/8, Radovanovic, Report on field visit to Nepal 1961, p. 7.
94 Interview with author, Thame, 9 January 2012.
95 Zangbu, Ngawang Tenzin (as told by), Frances Klatzel (ed.), *Stories and Customs of the Sherpas* (Kathmandu: Mera Publications, 2000), p. 58.
96 Frederick L. Dunn, 'Medical-geographical observations in Central Nepal', *Milbank Memorial Fund Quarterly*, 40:2 (1962), 143–4. See also Carl E. Taylor, 'A medical survey of the Kali Gandak and Pokhara valleys of Central Nepal', *Geographical Review*, 41:3 (1951), 421–37. A Japanese expedition encountered two cases of smallpox but neither the disease nor vaccination is mentioned in the article text. Atsushi Tokunaga, 'Experiences of medical survey in Central Nepal', *Journal of the Indian Medical Association*, 29:6 (1957), 223.
97 USOM became USAID in 1961.
98 George Moore and Berwyn Moore, 'Experience of a US Public Health Officer: 1950s Nepal', *Public Health Reports*, 120:5 (2005), 463–6.

3

Nepal – a nation state

In the 1960s most Nepalis were unaware of the concept of Nepal the nation state as understood in other parts of the world.[1] Three years after the smallpox epidemic in the Mt Everest region, Sir Edmund Hillary, a group mostly of New Zealanders and people from the local Sherpa villages built a small hospital on the edge of the village of Khunde. When the government Assistant Minister for Education, Gyarendra Bahadur Karki, spoke at the hospital opening on 18 December 1966 his speech had to be translated from Nepali, the official language of the nation state of Nepal, into Sherpa.[2] To the majority of the hundreds of Sherpas gathered in the field outside the hospital, the language they spoke was Sherpa and the name Nepal still meant the Kathmandu Valley more than a week's walk away in the central hill region. Through the eyes of the New Zealanders and their guests – the New Zealand, British and US ambassadors who had flown in from Kathmandu by helicopter and landed in a potato field – Nepal was a single nation state.

Like Chapter 2, this chapter similarly takes a wide approach to look at the nation state of Nepal and how this would influence and shape its responses to the global smallpox programme. The ending of the hereditary rule of the Rana family and the return of the monarchy in 1951 brought with it the promise and hopes of modernisation, but the country was ill-equipped for the task. Both a longer and shorter-term lens on the situation in Nepal are relevant as the new order was built on the roots of an older social and political fabric – the smallpox programme in Nepal was successful ultimately because it could work with both. The chapter is in three parts. The first considers the period after 1816 to the late 1940s and asks how and why such a disconnect in perceptions about the nation state of Nepal had arisen. It introduces the nation state of Nepal and outlines the early and limited development of health services. The second section discusses the changing internal and external environment for Nepal after the Second World War to provide the immediate background to the WHO programme. A shorter third section examines the early years of WHO involvement in Nepal.

Towards a nation state

It was not surprising that Sherpas did not understand the English language used by their visitors at the opening of Khunde Hospital, but most also did not understand Nepali. In his seminal article on the formation of the concept of the nation state in Nepal, anthropologist Richard Burghart discussed how 'the Nepalese government legitimates itself on native terms but through foreign eyes'.[3] He focused on government discourse. In the early twentieth century, Prime Minister Chandra Shamsher decreed that the Gorkhali language of the hills was to be the kingdom's official language, but in the 1930s the government began to refer to it as Nepali as the British called it and that it was the language of the 'realm of Nepal' rather than the 'entire possessions of the Gorkha king'.[4] At Khunde, as well as one of the headmen of the adjacent Khumjung village, Ong Chu Lama, having to translate the Associate Minister's speech for the Sherpa onlookers, the disconnect continued because the foreign visitors thought that the cheers at the end of the speech were for Hillary and his efforts to build the hospital. From the press release J. E. (Jim) Farrell, the New Zealand High Commissioner to India who also was accredited as Ambassador to Nepal, learned that they were for the King who was now the centre of political power.[5] The timing was significant because in Kathmandu, as Chapter 7 discusses, the Government and WHO in November 1966 signed an agreement to implement an expanded and nationwide smallpox eradication programme.

How had this situation arisen? The idea of a nation state, considered Burghart, was 'alien' to Nepal.[6] Nepal had emerged as a state in its present form only in the late eighteenth century. King Prithvi Narayan Shah was not alone in such endeavours but was part of a pattern of state building and expansion across a wide region of Asia. New regional powers were emerging. Sandwiched between the British East India Company to the south and China to the north, Nepal's traditional policy was to balance the influence of each. King Rana Bahadur's abdication in 1799 was pivotal to the deep entwining of Nepalese–British relations with factional court politics which divided and weakened the unity of the new state.[7] It was on a 'collision course' with the British over access to trade routes through the Himalaya to Tibet.[8] War broke out in 1814. Despite Nepal's eventual military defeat, the end of its territorial expansion and the highly unpopular imposition of a permanent British resident, the East India Company did not proceed to establish indirect rule. Michael Fisher uses Nepal as a case study of one 'extreme' within the residency system, in which Nepal not only initially rejected the influence of the East India Company but also continued to do so.[9] The residency in the capital Kathmandu did not become the means for British control of Nepal. Nepal, however, became a stable neighbour for the British in India until India gained its independence in 1947.

Nepal was landlocked but had many official and unofficial entry and exit points that facilitated the movement of people and goods. The Treaty of Sagauli brought the war with Britain to an end in 1816 and the demarcation of a defined border in the south, although the line of stone pillars established under the Treaty was a less effective barrier than malaria which thrived in the Tarai region's warmer temperatures.[10] Not until the mid-twentieth century was Nepal's northern border similarly formalised. For centuries people from Tibet had travelled to Nepal and in 1792 the Chinese army attacked Nepal from the north. Geographer Wim van Spengen has analysed trade and trading among the Tibetan and 'Tibetanized' communities of Nepal's northern border, mapping the numerous north–south major trade routes through Nepal prior to 1959 and the intensification of Chinese presence in Tibet.[11]

Social anthropologist David Gellner, however, sees the Nepali relationship with its northern and southern borders as 'not equal and symmetrical', arguing that 'for reasons of history and geography the links to the south are overwhelmingly important'.[12] Nepal's southern border had remained largely open, and people moved freely in both directions. During the nineteenth century, natural population growth led to increasing land pressure in the hills; in many communities, people combined long-distance trade or work in the plains with the subsistence agriculture of their home villages. Recruitment into the Gurkha regiments of the British Army in India was another option. Temporary or permanent migration inside Nepal or beyond its borders was not confined to the hill regions. Many Sherpa villagers participated in long-distance trade, but Dr Kami Temba Sherpa from Thame village recalled how as a boy he would walk to lower altitude villages looking for temporary work.[13] As mountaineering developed, villagers looked for employment with the expeditions. The fluidity is well illustrated by Tenzing Norgay who reached the summit of Mt Everest with Hillary in 1953. Born in Tibet, his mother brought him over the mountains into Nepal. In late 1932, he and a group of eleven others set off for Darjeeling where they hoped to earn money and 'see the world'.[14]

Nepal is ethnically and culturally complex. Sherpa, for example, are Buddhist and their physical cultural landscape resembled communities in Tibet. They were relative newcomers, migrating from Tibet into the largely uninhabited Mt Everest area in the early sixteenth century. While Nepal may not have been colonised by an external power, internally its many peoples since the eighteenth century had been subjugated first by the Shah kings from Gorkha and then after 1846 by the Rana prime ministers.[15] Nepal's Gorkha rulers were Hindu and Nepal a Hindu kingdom which gradually became, as Chief Minister Jang Bahadur proclaimed in 1866, 'the only country in which Hindus rule'.[16] In 1772–73, the Mt Everest region was incorporated into the new kingdom and Sherpa became subjects of the new Hindu rulers paying taxes and observing new laws. In 1854 the Gorkha government brought the different ethnic groups throughout the country under a single hierarchical caste-based civil code, the Mulaki Ain, which reinforced the superiority of the central hill castes.[17]

The remoteness of an area is often used to explain why a service, for example vaccination, does not exist or operates poorly. In Nepal, the functions of the government as Ludwig Stiller and Ram Prakash Yadav pointedly noted in their study of Nepal's planning development were limited. 'Stated briefly: the objectives of the Rana administration were the collection of revenue and maintenance of law and order.'[18] Neither the administration nor the people expected the government to develop state services such as education or health. That the inhabitants of Khumbu, for example, paid a house and land tax illustrated that when the government wanted to it could devise an effective system that could reach even the remotest areas. In the mid-nineteenth century, land revenue provided three-quarters of government income.[19] The rugged terrain and poor communications throughout Nepal meant that while the central administration gave 'strong guidelines' as to how the country was to be run, in practice local administrators needed 'both the freedom and the authority to rule the districts with a minimum of contact with the central administration'.[20] To the people of a district, the district administrator was the government. Despite considerable powers, his basic task was 'to keep things running smoothly. He was not expected to be either an innovator or an organizer.'[21] As the new Gorkha rulers sought to unify the many groups that formed the new nation state they reduced resistance by limiting the conformity they expected. Local customs and traditions were retained. As a result, district administration was 'patchy and arbitrary'.[22]

An extensive ethnography exists about different Nepali health beliefs and practices, but the historiography about health, illness and health services in Nepal is small. Current research reveals that much information from documents about the early hospitals established from the late nineteenth century has a political and economic rather than social focus as the ruling Rana autocracy, while wanting to establish a 'modern' health system, had 'no intention of diverting the monetary flows away from the state coffers'.[23] Most Nepalis lived in rural areas or the few small towns and when sick resorted to their own knowledge and resources or turned to a wide range of healers. Other options were available to those in power. Mark Liechty has shown how Nepal's ruling elite employed 'selective exclusion' to be able to enjoy foreign goods and expertise but to restrict the presence of different groups of foreigners.[24] Part of that desirable foreign expertise was medicine. The first newspaper, the state-owned *Gorkhapatra* established in 1901, had space to include new medical developments.[25]

Although Dixit provides the main account of the development of health services, Marasini's review article emphasised the development of hospitals and dispensaries during the Rana period.[26]

Prime ministers established health facilities 'as a form of charity for the poor'.[27] Established in 1857 on the southern edge of the Kathmandu Valley, the Khokana Leprosy Asylum was the first state health institution, but leprosy had no cure and so people were detained there by the Home Department rather than treated.[28] The first hospital for 'modern' medicine was the Prithvi Bir Hospital in Kathmandu which was built in 1889. Under prime ministers Bir Shamsher (1885–1901) and Chandra Shamsher (1902–29), other hospitals were established in the administrative headquarters of the districts and smaller dispensaries were added in other centres. Some specialised facilities were established in the Kathmandu area. While most emphasis was on institutions and treatment, concern about the threat of epidemics of smallpox and other diseases after the devastating earthquake of 1934 led to vaccine for cholera, typhoid and smallpox being imported from outside Nepal.[29] Staffing presented challenges. Although some Nepalis were sent to India to study medicine, the government engaged qualified Indian doctors to work in Nepal. Acknowledging its developing role in health, in 1933 the government established a Department of Health Services responsible for the promotion, regulation and management of government facilities. These included both modern and Ayurvedic medicine. In 1918 the Nardevi Ayurvedic Hospital was opened in Kathmandu and Ayurvedic dispensaries operated 'parallel' to 'modern' medicine facilities.[30] Some limited training was established for both systems. The 238 compounders (who distributed medicines and gave injections) and 213 dressers (who attended to wounds) who were trained in Nepal over the next thirty years 'effectively ran the hospitals and smaller units under the supervision of the doctors'.[31]

By the 1940s, most Nepalis might have heard of modern medicine, but unless they lived close to a health facility or health worker few were able to access it. Landon enthusiastically described Chandra's personal benevolence, but Stiller suggests viewing development such as in health services also in terms of expediency.[32] Chandra's main concern was administering Nepal, but Stiller believed that the younger generations of the Rana families were returning from their travels in India wanting to see their country develop. High Nepali participation in both world wars further fuelled a desire for change across society in the later years of Rana rule. Some people could also still look outside the country for healthcare. Just over the border in India were several mission-run health services, such as the Duncan Hospital at Raxaul.[33] A railway line existed, although the 24 km railway line built by the British in 1927 connecting Raxaul with Amlekhganj (Bara district) was Nepal's first and only passenger railway line.

Post Second World War

Locating the 1950s in the idea of 'the long 1950s', the events of the decade that saw the end of Rana rule, experiments with democracy and the rise of royal autocratic rule began before and continued after. It was a period of

> social and political flux as patterns of power—both nationally and globally—shifted from long-entrenched colonial dependencies to new, 'modern' inter-state relations. The emerging new global order simultaneously placed Nepal within Cold War constraints and created the conditions for new forms of international patronage, new configurations of national political power, new civic freedoms, new foreign development initiatives in Nepal, new class-based patterns of social organization in Kathmandu, and new commercial opportunities (including tourism) drawing on liberalized trade regimes linking Nepal with the outside world.[34]

Much has been written about the politics, much less about other aspects (including health) and still less on where outside and local sources engage.[35] Yet it was in this melting pot environment of change – but also continuity – that Nepal would come to engage with the world over smallpox. Vaccinating against smallpox aligned with both internal and external needs and expectations of the state.

The outbreak of the Second World War in Europe in 1939 brought about a massive upheaval for people in much of South and South-East Asia. As in the First World War, no fighting occurred on Nepali soil but recruiting for the Gurkha regiments intensified and placed increasing demands on the local population. Heavy recruiting depleted the manpower of the country and later in the war recruiters were urged to go to more remote areas.[36] Across the border in India, Nepali porters became involved in construction projects, including the massive and deadly 'man-a-mile' Ledo Road to supply goods to China.[37] With the retreat of the British from South Asia and the changing global political environment, the small nation state of Nepal was unlikely to remain isolated or unaffected whether from its citizens wanting political change, an estimated 200,000 returning soldiers 'most without pensions, but well trained and many newly literate', or foreign powers 'vying for Nepal's political loyalties in a veritable Cold War auction' with the offer of aid.[38]

Since the First World War, anti-Rana agitation had been developing outside the country among Nepalis living in India, while internally tension among rival groups of the Rana family continued to occupy Nepali politics.[39] In November 1945, Juddha Shamsher (1932–45) resigned as Maharaja, to be succeeded by his more conciliatory nephew Padma Shamsher (1945–48). In 1948 Padma resigned and his cousin Commander-in-Chief Mohan Shamsher (1948–51) took over. The relative calm in the capital, however, was broken when in the early morning of 7 November 1950 India's public broadcaster All India Radio announced unexpectedly from New Delhi that 'Yesterday in Kathmandu His Majesty King Tribhuvan Bir Bikram Shah Dev took political asylum in the India Embassy.'[40] After just over a century of Rana rule, the King's 'startling action' laid down a challenge to the status quo, but Mohan Shamsher had lost control when on 10 November the King left in an Indian Air Force aeroplane heading for Delhi and to deal directly with Prime Minister Nehru. Mohan Shamsher accepted the Delhi Agreement on 1 January 1951 and on 15 February 1951 King Tribhuvan returned to Kathmandu to rule with a coalition cabinet. The King intended to hold a Constituent Assembly, which would draw up Nepal's first real constitution, but this did not take place. An Interim Constitution operated until 1959, during which time ten changes of government occurred and at times King Mahendra, who took over in 1955 after his father's death, ruled directly.[41]

King Tribhuvan promised to modernise, but the administration's structures and resources were ill equipped for the challenges of national development set out in his Social Manifesto in 1951. The new government had to carve out ministries from the old Rana administrative organisation and extend ministerial authority down to the district and village level.[42] Some former departments converted more easily into the new ministries such as Finance or Foreign Affairs. Nevertheless, in 1952 when Minister of Finance Suvarna

Shamsher presented the country's first budget and an estimate of government income and expenditure for 1951, the accounting procedures then in use made it impossible to produce any accurate financial information.[43] Other former departments and offices were grouped loosely into new portfolios. In the first cabinet in February 1951 Yagya Bahadur Basnyat had charge of the Health and Local Self Development Ministry.[44] This combination reflected changes introduced under Prime Minister Padma Shamsher which brought measures aimed at disease prevention under local government through Nepal's then thirty-two districts. These activities included 'inoculation and vaccinations'.[45] As governments changed, so did the groupings and responsibility for health.

The government's aim was the economic transformation of the country which was formalised with the setting up of a National Planning Commission in 1955. Although the original idea came from the Soviet Union where there was full state control, Nepal followed the Indian model.[46] Indian personnel were prominent in Nepal after 1951.[47] From 1956 a series of Five-Year Plans were introduced that included details of the government's proposed expenditure on development projects, guidelines for the private sector and targets for the economy to achieve. Foreign assistance was to be the way for the new government to achieve the desired national development, including health, and an increasing number of countries, agencies, organisations and individuals were to become involved. Eugene Mihaly in his study of foreign aid in the 1960s found that most of the newcomers failed to meet their expected goals.[48] Plans had conceptual flaws and people seriously underestimated the problems of working in Nepal. Different donors had conflicting advice.[49] Another key issue was the sheer inability of the government to cope either with its own plans or with the increasing demands being made by the donors of foreign aid who wanted to contribute to Nepal's development but, in what was considered good development practice, wanted Nepalis to participate.

By appreciating the enormity of the task in Nepal, it becomes possible to comprehend some of the difficulties and frustrations felt by both the donors and the receivers over many aspects of the aid and development processes. International ideas about aid focused on technical assistance to a country, but Nepal had very few appropriately educated people (Appendix 2). It would take time to increase educational levels. The Ranas restricted education, but the state now accepted responsibility and expanded education provision. At the start of the decade there were 310 primary and middle schools, eleven high schools, one college, one teacher training centre, one technical school, a few centres for adult education and a bureau of publications. By 1961 the numbers were 1,237 primary and middle schools, 83 high schools and 4 colleges.[50] Overall population literacy levels had doubled but were still low; 16.4 per cent males and 1.8 per cent females over the age of ten years were recorded as literate – for the census this meant being able to read and write in Nepali.[51] Wide differences also occurred between the large rural and small urban population with the difference between male and female literacy rates also more pronounced. Nevertheless, increases in educational facilities contributed to wider changes taking place in rural Nepal.[52]

The country's communication infrastructure still was extremely limited. At a time when the USA and the USSR were looking to travel in space, most people in Nepal travelled on foot whether for short or long distances. Many routes were north to south in orientation following the contours of the land. No motorable roads existed apart from a few short stretches in the Kathmandu Valley.[53] Although foreign aid was given to develop the road network to improve the country's communication infrastructure, Nepal's topography made this a slow and difficult task and had ongoing implications for the introduction and maintenance of services. Air travel was a way to overcome the difficult terrain and expanded during the 1950s but was expensive; in the mountains in the monsoon, however, flying was often impossible. Telephones were limited, but recent archival research about the development of telephones in Nepal suggests a narrative based not on imperial needs but instead those of the Rana rulers wanting to foster their own interests.[54] A transcript of a conversation between Prime Minister Chandra Shamsher and the British Resident John Manners-Smith reveals that, like vaccination, their introduction in 1915 was initiated by Nepalis rather than the British. The first telephone connection was between the Shah King's palace and that of the Rana Prime Minister, but in 1916 a trunk line was completed to Birganj in the central Tarai. Further expansion to some parts of the country occurred under subsequent Rana rulers and in the 1950s. Radio AM transmission provided an alternative technology to link with the mountainous areas. Such development provided, therefore, some of the earliest national infrastructure. While the number of people who could be trained for the new roles was insufficient, people in the villages became disillusioned with the government when, for example, there was no one to staff the health clinics and provide the services that they wanted and needed.[55] Life expectancy could only be estimated, since births and deaths were not recorded, and was thought to be just twenty-eight years with an infant mortality rate of 255/1,000 live births.[56] The government only provided some healthcare services in parts of the country; most areas had none. Prior to the government's first Five Year Plan in 1956, Nepal had 34 hospitals with just 625 beds, 24 dispensaries and 63 Ayurvedic pharmacies (*aushadhalaya*).[57] Health personnel consisted of basic-level health workers – compounders and dressers – and about fifty doctors who had trained in India. When sick, therefore, most people continued to self-treat or resort to a wide range of other practitioners; most people still lived and died away from any formal healthcare.

In the 1950s global public health interest focused on malaria, which was a much more serious public health and economic concern for Nepal than smallpox.[58] In 1955 the WHO launched a Global Malaria Eradication Programme. Malaria was prevalent in Nepal up to an altitude of about 1,200 m and had long been considered the chief cause of mortality.[59] With international assistance, malaria control efforts in Nepal made some progress; the 1950s was a period of transition establishing the preconditions for the later rapid population growth.[60] Malaria suppression in Pokhara, Nepal's second most important city, enabled the population to grow; to the south, the Tarai's proportion of the national population began to increase as people moved from the hills and new industries were established. Combined with the youthful population this changing demography was significant for the pattern of smallpox occurrence and transmission since smallpox spread more easily among high density populations and the young.

During the 1950s three types of foreign medical encounters became a feature of the medical landscape in Nepal: Christian missions, visitors and international aid.[61] As Pieter Streefland has stressed, in Nepal 'Modern Western medicine has ... many faces'.[62] Each contributed to the introduction and spread of modern medicine alongside that of the government and helped set the stage for the later smallpox programme, but how and what Nepali people thought about modern medicine would be influenced by the version a person experienced. Many newcomers came with little understanding of where they were coming to; while visitor medical encounters were mostly short term, providing long-term healthcare usually was frustratingly slow to develop. Over time the foreigners learned to live and work in Nepal, but the presence of multiple versions of 'the modern system of medicine' that became established in the 1950s continues to shape healthcare.[63]

Missions were the first to arrive.[64] In much of South and South-East Asia, Christianity, missionary work and colonialism for a long time had been intertwined. In Nepal, Christian missionaries had not been allowed to operate inside Nepal since their expulsion in the eighteenth century by King Prithvi Narayan. In the new political and social environment of the early 1950s, Christian missions operating in India near the border wanted to help Nepal's government achieve its aim of providing health services. The proudly Hindu kingdom of Nepal retained its antipathy towards the Christian religion, but in 1952 accepted the Nepal Evangelistic Band's offer to build a hospital at Pokhara. In 1953 it gave permission to what would later be called the United Mission to Nepal (UMN) to build a hospital at Tansen, an administrative centre in Palpa district in the hills of western Nepal, and to start a series of maternity welfare centres in Kathmandu.

Over the next few years mission health services slowly developed and expanded activities. The UMN became the largest mission organisation undertaking medical work in Nepal in the 1950s; its largest facility was the general hospital at Shanta Bhawan in Kathmandu providing outpatient and inpatient services (132 beds). The missionaries, however, also found they had to operate within an increasing range of conditions imposed by the government, partly because their missions were foreign Christian organisations but partly because the government had its own plans for health services. The medical missionaries came from many countries and with backgrounds of working in very different health systems. They had different ideas and philosophies about the level and type of health services missions should be providing in Nepal. Nepal's needs were considerable. Should their focus be on providing basic services or be a model for what is best medical practice? Visitors to Nepal and the medicines they carried became another important vehicle for the introduction and spread of modern medicine.[65] During the late Rana period, a steady if small stream of foreigners received permission from the government to visit Nepal, but a new group of visitors entering Nepal in increasing numbers during the 1950s were the climbing expeditions which were now able to access the high Himalayan peaks from inside Nepal. The Mt Everest area attracted many expeditions and served as a magnet. Some expeditions employed large numbers of local people. Needing to be self-sufficient, they carried with them a range of treatments and medical equipment. Some, such as the successful 1953 Mt Everest expedition, had doctors to look after their own health problems and to treat varying numbers of local people. Other visitors arrived in the country and travelled as individuals or in small groups, also treating or trying to help sick local people when approached. Visitors came, as Ian Harper has written, and 'were exposed to the secrets of the closed land for the first time'.[66] They explored the country, engaged with wider society and some also wrote about their travels and encounters with the geography and peoples of Nepal. Visitors made health in Nepal visible to a wide outside audience. For local populations, treatment opportunities were still limited and fragmentary reflecting the still small number of visitors and their variable health knowledge, the limited time spent in an area and the few places visited.

The third group of encounters came under the umbrella of international aid, whether bilateral agreements between nation states or involving international agencies that came into prominence after the Second World War. While much of the foreign medical aid came from western countries, India's connection with Nepal was well-established and Indian aid established in 1959 Nepal's first Maternity Hospital, at Thapathali, in Kathmandu.

The big newcomer in the wider region was the USA, which was concerned increasingly about the threat of the spread of communism presented by China. Nepal was of strategic importance.[67] Even before Britain had withdrawn from India the USA sent officials to

Kathmandu, but only after the USA officially recognised Nepal's independence was Rana Nepal ready to sign an agreement. India was concerned that American interest in Nepal was a threat to Indian authority in the region. In 1949, against India's wishes, the US officially supported Nepal's unsuccessful bid to become a member of the UN.[68] Nepal, however, was not a new postcolonial nation state. It had kept the British at arm's length and now brought in foreign aid from a range of countries with different political ideologies. The USA was the first country to provide bilateral aid to Nepal, signing an agreement in New Delhi on 23 January 1951 to provide technical assistance under the Point Four Program for 'developing countries' announced by President Harry S. Truman in his inaugural address on 20 January 1949. In January 1952 Paul Rose, the first Director of the United States Operation Mission (USOM), arrived in Nepal with a small team of experts. In the first few years USOM supported a wide array of projects in community development (the Village Development Program), education, malaria eradication and the opening-up of the Rapti Valley as a model development project. Nepal appeared to many as 'an ideal laboratory' and 'a place where nothing had happened before 1950'.[69] Other projects focused on specific activities in health, transportation, communication, agriculture, and industrial and capital development. Both Americans and Nepalis thought that it would only take a few years to set the country 'on the road to economic modernization'.[70] Mihaly was particularly critical of the failure of American aid during the early years. He thought that this was due partly to the technical assistance development model of the Point Four Program whereby a country-wide programme could be run with a small number of technicians and achieve quick results. 'Almost as damaging ... was the astonishing underestimate of how primitive Nepal was.'[71]

Initially few, the number of foreigners involved in aid grew during the 1950s. Like the missionaries, initially such personnel had to learn how to work and live in Nepal. Nepalis also had to find a way to deal with these new outsiders. As the decade progressed, more countries and organisations became involved and the number of foreign aid personnel increased. Nevertheless, their influence in the 1950s was less dominant than it would soon become; whether foreigner or Nepali, the 1950s was a learning time for all and a disappointment for many.

Nepal and the WHO

On 2 September 1953 Nepal became the eightieth member state of the WHO.[72] As Randall Packard has written, the 'postwar vision of health and development was much more pervasive and encompassing'; national and international health policies 'reflected a new realization of the need to extend the provision of health care to entire populations'.[73] For India and South-East Asia, Sunil Amrith has traced a shifting philosophical paradigm of healthcare as a human right to health as a tool for economic development that was evident by the 1950s.[74] The situation was complex when such ideas were translated into practice in different locations and, as Cueto, Brown and Fee discuss in their 'narrative history' of the WHO, in the context of 'fraying European imperialism' and the 'American Cold War vision of the world'.[75]

As a member state, Nepal could attend and participate in meetings of the WHA, which decided on policy. The WHO, however, was alone among the specialised agencies of the UN to have adopted a policy of full regionalisation. Located in New Delhi, the South-East Asia Regional Office (SEARO) was the first of the six WHO regional offices to come into operation, opening in 1948 with Dr Chandra Mani as its Regional Director.[76] Although the names of its attendees were not mentioned, the Government of Nepal was listed as an observer at the meeting of the Regional Committee in 1949.[77] Regional committees were composed of member states and associates. Nepal did not attend the meeting in Bangkok in September 1953, but the following year in New Delhi was represented by J. N. Singha, the First Secretary at Nepal's Embassy.[78]

The WHO regional offices had wide powers and considerable autonomy; they were responsible for drawing up a plan of international assistance for health projects in collaboration with governments and within an allotted budget.[79] They differed from HQ Geneva in their mode of operation largely because they assisted governments directly upon request. After approval and allotment of funds by the WHA, the regional office was again responsible for their implementation. This enabled WHO to begin assisting each country to take the next appropriate step 'towards developing its health services within the limits of its economic, social, and cultural circumstances'.[80] With the large quantity of widely accessible

WHO reports from SEARO, the lens we have on Nepal is often that of the outsider, but the 1969 report from the Directorate of Health Services made the same point about the role of the WHO.[81]

While it was generally agreed that the main role of a regional office was to provide 'more effective contact' between WHO and national governments, at the start it was less clear how this would occur. In its history of the first twenty years, WHO's South-East Asia Regional Office saw itself as 'very largely a field laboratory in which experiment guided the future organisational pattern'.[82] The Region's resources were limited; in the first few years SEARO had to focus initially on 'immediate short-term projects, especially for the control of communicable diseases', and were 'demonstration and training projects in specific areas'.[83] The WHO embraced the technological focus of the new international public health. By 1952 field experience in different countries suggested that achieving effective control required 'mass attacks on a nation-wide scale, employing many auxiliary personnel working under qualified physicians'.[84] Demonstration programmes gave way to mass programmes, such as BCG vaccination for tuberculosis, and for malaria and yaws control. Along with other countries in the South-East Asia Region, Nepal in the 1950s also received aid for health projects from bilateral programmes (the largest being the USA) and the Colombo Plan.[85]

The UN began assistance in Nepal in 1952, although without a resident country representative in the early years its personnel had limited access to those in power and specifically the King.[86] On 13 May 1954, Nepal's government and WHO SEARO concluded a Basic Agreement, which provided the foundation for relations between the two and focused on technical advisory support. It also set the stage for the later smallpox programme.

The first and largest WHO project (Nepal 1) was intended to demonstrate modern methods of malaria control and to build up a 'malaria organisation'.[87] An estimated 5.1 million (57 per cent) Nepalis lived in malarial areas. In 1952 Nepal reported an estimated 3,445,000 cases of malaria with a likewise estimated 38,450 deaths directly due to the disease and the same number indirectly.[88] As others had experienced when beginning work in Nepal, 'considerable' delays 'due to non-completion of essential preliminary arrangements' prevented the project's planned start at the end of

1953. A WHO malariologist arrived in 1954 and began recruiting his team. In contrast to the ambitious nationwide aims of USOM which had 'prompted' the Government to establish an Insect-Borne Disease Control Bureau in August 1954, the WHO project operated in a small area of the Rapti valley in the Inner Tarai (Chitwan district).[89] In 1957, Dr Raymond Stannard from USOM acknowledged the success of the WHO project. The USOM project had focused on large numbers but had inadequately trained people for such a programme and all areas in the US project had to be resprayed. Even the WHO project had not yet trained sufficient people who could then expand and run an operation in another area.[90] In December 1958 Nepal's government (HMG) concluded a plan of operation with both WHO and USOM for country-wide malaria eradication setting up an autonomous Malaria Eradication Board, with HMG having 'full authority' to implement the programme 'in consultation with WHO and USOM representatives' through the Nepal Malaria Eradication Organization (NMEO).[91]

Nepal lacked trained health workers and asked WHO to assist. Project Nepal 2 was a nurses' training project and was 'one of the country's most urgent needs'.[92] Progress was expected to be slow but was 'even slower than anticipated', and not until June 1956 were the first twenty nursing candidates selected and finally enrolled. The third project (Nepal 3) was a school for training health assistants – a new type of health worker – which opened with twenty students on 20 February 1956. Despite the demands of the course, only three students 'abandoned' it; the rest of the students all passed the exams for entry into the second year, which 'gives reason for satisfaction'.[93] As the decade progressed both projects developed. In May 1958 thirteen nursing students who had completed the preliminary course began practical experience in Bir Hospital.[94] New WHO-assisted projects were also introduced for assistance to the Central Health Directorate (Nepal 4), fellowships (Nepal 5) and cholera control (Nepal 7). The WHO was also able to help Nepal's medical profession more widely with access to information. In 1958 the Nepal Medical Association (NMA) – established in 1951 – hosted a lunch party for WHO Director-General Dr Marcolino Candau. 'Following the visit', recorded Hemang Dixit in the Association's history, 'the NMA started getting the WHO publications on a regular basis'.[95] The oscillating fortunes of NMA members and the government in the 1950s, however, is illustrative of the challenges not just for outsiders in Nepal.

During the 1950s, therefore, the government of Nepal and WHO through SEARO had a developing role and relationship, but smallpox was not yet part of this. It was not mentioned by name in the regional summary in the WHO history of its first decade.[96] Smallpox had a long history in the region as an international quarantinable disease and the notification of cases had improved, although Nepal provided no data.[97] It was not that smallpox was unimportant, but tuberculosis and malaria were of more concern. The Regional Committee passed Resolutions regarding smallpox from 1949 onwards. While the Committee in 1953 considered that 'in the South-East Asia Region effective control of the disease is not at present feasible through a world-wide campaign', it still hoped that its member countries would receive WHO assistance for national efforts to control smallpox 'in the same ways as for other WHO assisted programmes'.[98] Vaccine supply was one area where the Regional Office thought it could assist countries through helping to arrange for the supply of vaccine from outside and assisting with local vaccine production. Nepal was dependent on the supply of vaccine from external sources, relying on WHO in terms of both quantity and quality.

In his annual report in 1958, Mani reported that there had been 'no improvement' in the control of smallpox in the region.[99] A regional survey had found that even in areas where total vaccination coverage was claimed by the number of vaccinations carried out, for a variety of reasons the vaccination of infants under one year of age was only about 30 per cent of estimated live births.[100] Nevertheless, at its meeting in New Delhi in September the Regional Committee passed a resolution to support the worldwide initiative for global eradication of the disease and the following year the Regional Director wrote of 'renewed interest' in smallpox.[101] In 1959 the proposed regional budget for 1961 included funding to start a WHO-assisted smallpox control pilot project in Nepal in the Kathmandu Valley.

As with the earlier WHO malaria project, the aim of the pilot was to develop smallpox capability which could then be expanded. It would be, however, brought in at a time of significant ongoing political and administrative changes within Nepal that left the foreigners powerless.[102] In 1960 King Mahendra dismissed the government elected in the 1959 general election and appointed a council of five to assist his administration. He outlawed political parties and prominent political leaders were imprisoned. Reflecting the ascendancy of the monarchy, a new constitution in 1962 introduced a four-tiered structure of government from village to national level of limited elected assemblies (*panchayat*) and divided the country administratively into fourteen zones and seventy-five districts.[103] Known as the panchayat system, this form of government would last until 1990 and would have a major influence on how the smallpox programme developed and operated.

Conclusion

The WHO worked through nation states, but Nepal in the 1950s was ill equipped for the enormous challenges that lay ahead. Governments changed frequently. To outsiders, Nepal had been a single nation state since the latter part of the eighteenth century, but in 1960 most Nepalis were still getting used to the idea. Poor communications and challenging geography made district officials the government for most Nepalis. They raised taxes and kept law and order. In the later nineteenth century, central government began to establish hospitals in Kathmandu and some other centres, but 'modern' health services remained beyond the reach of most people. With the involvement of Nepali troops in various overseas theatres of two World Wars and the new post-colonial environment of much of South and South-East Asia from the late 1940s, more people began to want change. The restoration of the monarchy in 1951 and the ending of Rana rule brought with it hopes for modernisation of a country that was one of the least developed in the world.

By the end of the 1950s health services overall had expanded, although not equally throughout the country and especially not in most rural areas. The Nepali state had extremely limited resources; above all the country lacked qualified personnel to implement the policies and plans that it wanted. The government turned to new groups of outsiders to help, even Christian missionaries. Technical experts were brought in to tackle public health issues such as malaria. All contributed to making Nepal's health environment more visible to the outside world. The big new 'player' in the region was the USA. At a time when foreign presence in healthcare was small and scattered, the Nepali government could try to control or at least direct what was happening. During the 1950s external groups increased their presence which would further consolidate and develop in subsequent years, shifting the balance towards an international development agenda. The 1950s were particularly important because although we see the beginning of this process, we also see a government with a more independent voice as to the healthcare provision it wanted.

The WHO made a slow beginning in Nepal from 1954, working with the government and gradually increasing its presence during the decade. Its biggest involvements were in malaria control and eradication, and health worker training. Although widespread and serious, smallpox in the 1950s was neither Nepal's main health priority nor that of WHO's South-East Asia Regional Office. Nevertheless, as part of the global commitment to worldwide smallpox eradication, SEARO in 1959 allocated funding for a pilot control project in the Kathmandu Valley to begin to develop capability within Nepal. After a delayed start, a mass vaccination programme began in three districts in early 1962, but the following year endemic smallpox became epidemic. Different responses to outbreaks of smallpox in different parts of Nepal would reveal that the nation state existed more on paper than on the ground.

Notes

1 Richard Burghart, 'The formation of the concept of nation-state in Nepal', *Journal of Asian Studies*, 44:1 (1984), 101–25.
2 Louise Hillary, *A Yak for Christmas* (Garden City, NY: Doubleday, 1969), pp. 95–6.
3 Burghart, 'The formation of the concept of nation-state in Nepal', 122.
4 *Ibid.*, 119.
5 Archives New Zealand/Te Rua Mahara o te Kāwanatanga, Head Office, Wellington (hereafter ANZ), ABHS 6949 W4628 NDI 64/14/2 Part 3, Himalayan climbing expeditions & schoolhouse projects, J. E. Farrell, High Commissioner, to Secretary External Affairs, Hillary Hospital Expedition, 23 December 1966.
6 Burghart, 'The formation of the concept of nation-state in Nepal', 101.

Nepal – a nation state 87

7 Bernardo A. Michael, *Statemaking and Territory in South Asia: Lessons from the Anglo-Gorkha War (1814–1816)* (London and New York: Anthem Press, 2012), p. 319.
8 Ludwig F. Stiller, S. J., *The Silent Cry: The People of Nepal: 1816–1839* (Kathmandu: Sahayogi Prakashan, 1976), pp. 330–2.
9 Fisher, *Indirect Rule in India*, pp. 414–22. The origins of the residency system in India lay in the rapid expansion of the Company's activities in India with the first resident appointed in 1764. Residencies were established at different times, and each reflected the different ideas operating at the time.
10 Burghart, 'The formation of the concept of nation-state in Nepal', 114–15.
11 Wim van Spengen, *Tibetan Border Worlds: A Geohistorical Analysis of Trade and Traders* (London: Kegan Paul International, 2000), p. 105.
12 David N. Gellner, *The Idea of Nepal*, Mahesh Chandra Regmi Lecture 2016 (Kathmandu: Himal Books, 2016), pp. 10–12.
13 Conversations with author. With the development of tourism, today the pattern is reversed.
14 Tenzing Norgay (as told to) James Ramsey Ullman, *Man of Everest: The Autobiography of Tenzing* (London: The Reprint Society, 1956), p. 44.
15 Hem Narayan Agrawal, *The Administrative System of Nepal: From Tradition to Modernity* (New Delhi: Vikas, 1976), p. x.
16 Burghart, 'The formation of the concept of nation-state in Nepal', 116.
17 Whelpton, *A History of Nepal*, p. 56.
18 Ludwig F. Stiller and Ram Prakash Yadav, *Planning for People* (Kathmandu: Human Resources Development Research Center, 1993), p. 12.
19 Whelpton, *A History of Nepal*, p. 51.
20 Stiller and Yadav, *Planning for People*, p. 13; Agrawal, *The Administrative System of Nepal*.
21 Stiller and Yadav, *Planning for People*, p. 15.
22 *Ibid.*, p. 14.
23 Raj, Aryal and Mishra, 'Documents related to the early hospitals in Nepal', 348.
24 Mark Liechty, 'Selective exclusion: Foreigners, foreign goods, and foreignness in modern Nepali history', *Studies in Nepali History and Society*, 2:1 (1997), 5–68.
25 Until 1961, *Gorkhāpatra* was weekly.
26 Dixit, *The Quest for Health* (1995); Marasini, 'Health and hospital development in Nepal'.
27 Dixit, *The Quest for Health* (1995), p. 21.

28 Marasini, 'Health and hospital development in Nepal', 308.
29 Brahma Shumsher Jung Bahadur Rana, *The Great Earthquake in Nepal (1934 AD)*, trans. Kesar Lall (Kathmandu: Ratna Pustak Bandar, 2013). It was first published in Nepali in 1934. The author was Director of Hospital Management, but as he was also a member of the elite ruling Rana family Raj urges caution. Yogesh Raj, 'Management of the relief and reconstruction after the great earthquake of 1934', *Studies in Nepali History and Society*, 20:2 (2015), 375–422.
30 Marasini, 'Health and hospital development in Nepal', 309.
31 Dixit, *The Quest for Health* (1995), pp. 138–9.
32 Landon, *Nepal*, 2, p. 183; Ludwig F. Stiller, *Nepal: Growth of a Nation* ([Kathmandu]: Human Resources Development Research Center, 1999), p. 156.
33 School of Oriental and African Studies (SOAS) Library, London, MS 380389/Regions Beyond Missionary Union publications, 1903–52, Dr and Mrs Trevor Strong, *The Duncan Hospital, Raxaul, Bihar, India: An illustrated account of the work of the hospital from October 1948 to April 1952* (London: Regions Beyond Missionary Union, 1952), p. 24.
34 Mark Liechty, Pratyoush Onta and Lokranjan Parajuli, 'Introduction: Cultural politics in the long 1950s', *Studies in Nepali History and Society*, 24:1 (2019), 6.
35 *Ibid.*, 11.
36 Yasmin Khan, *The Raj at War: A People's History of India's Second World War* (London: Vintage, 2016), pp. 228–9.
37 *Ibid.*, pp. 259–64. The actual number of deaths is unknown.
38 *Ibid.*, p. 315; Rose, *Nepal: Strategy for Survival*, p. 177.
39 Whelpton, *A History of Nepal*, pp. 66–7.
40 Stiller and Yadav, *Planning for People*, p. 1. Popular opinion in Kathmandu influenced British and US views of the events of 1950.
41 *Ibid.*, pp. 2–5.
42 *Ibid.*, p. 12. See also Agrawal, *The Administrative System of Nepal*.
43 Stiller and Yadav, *Planning for People*, p. 114.
44 Dixit, *The Quest for Health* (1995), p. 226.
45 *Ibid.*, p. 27.
46 Whelpton, *A History of Nepal*, pp. 125–6.
47 Agrawal, *The Administrative System of Nepal*, p. 311.
48 Mihaly, *Foreign Aid and Politics in Nepal*, pp. 204–7.
49 Agrawal, *The Administrative System of Nepal*, p. 310.
50 Hugh B. Wood, UNESCO Specialist in Educational Planning, Professor of Education, University of Oregon, Eugene, Oregon, USA, and Bruno Knall, UNESCO Specialist in Economic Development,

Institute of World Economics, University of Kiel, Kiel, Germany, 'Educational planning in Nepal and its economic implications: Draft report of the UNESCO mission to Nepal, Kathmandu, January–May 1962', p. 25. www.martinchautari.org.np/storage/files/educationalplanninginnepalanditseconomicimplication1962woodknall-draftreport.pdf.
51 ESCAP, *Population of Nepal*, p. 140.
52 John T. Hitchcock, 'Some effects of recent change in rural Nepal', *Human Organization*, 22:1 (1963), 75–82. www.jstor.org/stable/44124171.
53 Mihaly, *Foreign Aid and Politics in Nepal*, pp. 13–14; Stiller and Yadav, *Planning for People*, pp. 207–24.
54 Martin Chautari, *Early Developments in Telephones and Electricity in Nepal*, Research Brief No. 26 (Kathmandu: Martin Chautari, 2019).
55 Stacy Leigh Pigg, 'Unintended consequences: The ideological impact of development in Nepal', *Comparative Studies of South Asia, Africa and the Middle East*, 13:1/2 (1993), 45–58.
56 Christa A. Skerry, Kerry Moran, Kay M. Calavan, *Four Decades of Development: The History of U.S. Assistance to Nepal 1951–1991* (United States Agency for International Development, 1991), p. 47. These figures are used widely to illustrate a grim picture of health status in Nepal.
57 Hemang Dixit, *Nepal's Quest for Health: The Health Services of Nepal*, 3rd edn (Kathmandu: Educational Publishing House, 2005), p. 28. Some would have been added after 1951. The small number of beds indicates that many of the hospitals were small.
58 In his history to 1950, Bikrama Hasrat mentioned malaria but not smallpox. Bikrama Jit Hasrat, *History of Nepal as Told by Its Own and Contemporary Chroniclers* (Hoshiarpur, Punjab: V. V. Research Institute, 1970).
59 Directorate of Health Services, *A Report on Health and Health Administration in Nepal 1969* (Kathmandu: Ministry of Health, 1970), p. 37.
60 Durga P. Ohja, 'History of land settlement in Nepal Tarai', *Contributions to Nepalese Studies*, 11:1 (1983), 27 https://himalaya.socanth.cam.ac.uk/collections/journals/contributions/pdf/CNAS_11_01_02.pdf.
61 Susan Heydon, 'Missions, visitors and international aid', *Studies in Nepali History and Society*, 24:1 (2019), 73–104.
62 Pieter Streefland, 'The frontier of modern western medicine in Nepal', *Social Science & Medicine*, 20:11 (1985), 1156.

63 This terminology was still used by the Ministry of Health & Population on its website in 2008 when listing Essential Care Services www.moh.gov.np/Reforms/DELIVERY.ASP (accessed 28 February 2008).
64 This paragraph draws on published accounts from those involved at the time and, although fewer than for later periods, archives from the Nepal Evangelistic Band (later called the International Nepal Fellowship) and the United Mission to Nepal (UMN).
65 Susan Heydon, 'Medicines, travellers and the introduction and spread of "modern" medicine in the Mt Everest region of Nepal', *Medical History*, 55:4 (2011), 503–21.
66 Ian Harper, 'Mediating therapeutic uncertainty: A mission hospital in Nepal', in Mark Harrison, Margaret Jones and Helen Sweet (eds), *From Western Medicine to Global Medicine: The Hospital Beyond the West* (New Delhi: Orient BlackSwan, 2009), p. 306.
67 For the wider domestic and international context of US aid in Nepal see Robertson, 'Front line of the Cold War'.
68 Nepal became a member of the UN on 14 December 1955.
69 Tatsuro Fujikura, 'Technologies of improvement, locations of culture: American discourses of democracy and "community development" in Nepal', *Studies in Nepali History and Society*, 1:2 (1996), 301–2.
70 Skerry et al., *Four Decades of Development*, p. 2.
71 Mihaly, *Foreign Aid and Politics in Nepal*, pp. 45–7.
72 WHO, *The First Ten Years*, p. 474. Nepal was present at the first WHA in 1948 as an observer.
73 Randall Packard, 'Visions of postwar health and development and their impact on public health interventions in the developing world', in Frederick Cooper and Randall Packard (eds), *International Development and the Social Sciences: Essays on the History and Politics of Knowledge* (Berkeley, CA: University of California Press, 1997), p. 96.
74 Sunil S. Amrith, *Decolonizing International Health: India and Southeast Asia, 1930–65* (Basingstoke: Palgrave Macmillan, 2006).
75 Cueto, Brown and Fee, *The World Health Organization*, pp. 1, 73. The South-East Asia Region is not a focus.
76 Mani had been a member of the Technical Preparatory Committee.
77 World Health Organization, Regional Office for South-East Asia (hereafter WHO SEARO), SEA/RC2/7 Rev.1 – List of Delegates & Observers, WHO Regional Office for South-East Asia, 1949 https://apps.who.int/iris/handle/10665/131336.
78 WHO SEARO, SEA/RC7/2, Sixth annual report of the Regional Director to the Regional Committee for South-East Asia, July 1953–July 1954, p. 1. www.who.int/iris/handle/10665/126767.

79 Fraser Brockington, *World Health* (Harmondsworth and Baltimore, MD: Penguin, 1958), p. 215.
80 World Health Organization and Brock Chisholm, Work of WHO, 1950: annual report of the Director-General to the WHA and to the UN, p. 2. https://apps.who.int/iris/handle/10665/85609.
81 A report on health and health administration in Nepal, p. 90.
82 WHO SEARO, *Twenty Years in South-East Asia 1948–1967*, p. 56.
83 WHO, *The First Ten Years*, p. 162.
84 *Ibid.*
85 The Colombo Plan for Co-operative Economic Development in South and South-East Asia was launched in 1950 in Colombo, Ceylon. It aimed to help combat the spread of communism by encouraging economic and social development within poorer Asian countries. The original seven members were all Commonwealth countries.
86 Mihaly, *Foreign Aid and Politics in Nepal*, p. 200.
87 WHO SEARO, Sixth annual report of the Regional Director, p. 161.
88 WHO Malaria Conference for Western Pacific and South-East Asia Regions, Taipei, Taiwan, 1954, Information on the malaria-control programme in Nepal, p. 1. https://apps.who.int/iris/handle/10665/64259.
89 Mihaly, *Foreign Aid and Politics in Nepal*, p. 42. See also Thomas B. Robertson, 'DDT and the Cold War jungle: American environmental and social engineering in the Rapti valley of Nepal', *Journal of American History*, 104:4 (2018), 904–30.
90 Mihaly, *Foreign Aid and Politics in Nepal*, p. 43.
91 Report on health and health administration in Nepal 1969, p. 38.
92 WHO SEARO, Sixth annual report of the Regional Director, p. 61.
93 WHO SEARO, Ninth annual report of the Regional Director to the Regional Committee for South-East Asia, July 1956–July 1957, p. 112 https://apps.who.int/iris/handle/10665/126741.
94 WHO SEARO, Tenth annual report of the Regional Director to the Regional Committee for South-East Asia, August 1957–1 July 1958, p. 121 https://apps.who.int/iris/handle/10665/126769.
95 Hemang Dixit, *Fifty Years of NMA* (Kathmandu: Nepal Medical Association, 2001), p. 16.
96 WHO, *The First Ten Years*, pp. 161–3.
97 Frank Fenner, 'Smallpox in Southeast Asia', *Crossroads: An Interdisciplinary Journal of Southeast Asian Studies*, 3:2/3 (1987), 34–48. For the development of global information networks, see Heidi J. S. Tworek, 'Communicable disease: Information, health, and globalization in the interwar period', *American Historical Review*, 124:3 (2019), 813–42.

98 WHO SEARO, SEA/RC6/R5, Smallpox, 1953 https://apps.who.int/iris/handle/10665/131032.
99 WHO SEARO, Tenth annual report of the Regional Director, p. 26.
100 WHO SEARO, *Twenty years in South-East Asia 1948–1967*, p. 174.
101 SEA/RC11/R6, in WHO SEARO, *Twenty years in South-East Asia 1948–1967*, p. 174; WHO SEARO, Eleventh annual report of the Regional Director, p. 7. https://apps.who.int/iris/handle/10665/126742.
102 Sudhindra Sharma, 'Trickle to torrent to irrelevance? Six decades of foreign aid in Nepal', in Dipak Gyawali, Michael Thompson and Marco Verweij (eds), *Aid, Technology and Development: The Lessons from Nepal* (London and New York: Routledge, 2017), p. 59.
103 Whelpton, *A History of Nepal*, p. 101.

4

1963–64 – epidemic smallpox

This chapter, written mostly from the perspectives of local people and foreigners caught up in helping, provides 'snapshots' from different areas in Nepal to illustrate the many and fragmented responses to smallpox in the early 1960s prior to the intensification of the global programme. The epidemic, which broke out in North-East India and East Pakistan in the first half of the year, was the main cause for the increase in cases reported worldwide.[1] Responses in Nepal reflected the enormous challenges presented by the country's geography and very limited infrastructure, broad change occurring within the country, and the wider context of new international and global relations after the end of the Second World War. The chapter identifies the many facets, difficulties and layers in smallpox control – or the lack throughout most of the country – but highlights local adaptation and how people's beliefs influenced their practices.

Each snapshot is different, but all also reveal an already global environment for smallpox in Nepal. In each location, the almost 'accidental' but distinctly different presence of foreigners was important. Nepal did not produce its own vaccine and relied on foreign sources; acquiring vaccine to respond to the epidemic was key. These foreigners were not experts, but foreigners could sometimes get things done or open doors that were difficult or impossible for local people.[2] Experiences discussed in this chapter attest to the commitment of the foreigners who became involved in a particular area either independently, with local officials or with central government, but their wider influence was limited. These accounts also demonstrate community participation and initiative and the expanding if patchy development of Nepali services and programmes amid a changing and uncertain political environment.

The chapter is framed around three localities. Although absent from the official record, a wide range of official and unofficial, written and oral sources exist that not only provide evidence that Nepal experienced widespread smallpox in 1963–64 but also enable us to explore events, experiences and activities from different viewpoints and from the individual to the global. The many older Nepali people today who remember smallpox as a common disease of their childhood are an invaluable source of information. Their accounts together with those of new types of foreigners in Nepal who found themselves involved with an epidemic of a disease that had disappeared from their home countries, richly supplement information from official and more orthodox sources to render the epidemic and events of 1963–64 visible for both Nepal's history and the global smallpox story. Each section has a brief introduction. Collectively, the three snapshots represent a large part of Nepal's very different geography and demography: remote high mountains with a scattered population, the many villages of the middle hills and the densely populated urban capital. They are presented chronologically as the epidemic unfolded in these areas: the Mt Everest region (March–May 1963); the Kathmandu Valley (November 1963–January 1964); and the Lamjung district in central Nepal (late 1963–April 1964).

Mt Everest region

Although Mt Everest was first climbed in 1953, the mountain, the remote surrounding area and its inhabitants retained their fascination for foreign visitors whose numbers were increasing. The small administrative centre of Namche Bazar was beginning to develop, but the area could only be reached on foot or by air. This snapshot details how smallpox could spread in such an environment and that both local people and the foreign visitors understood that it could. Local people were keen to be vaccinated, but as the area had no vaccine, they approached the foreigners for help. This section illustrates the interplay between local people and the outsiders as the epidemic unfolded. The foreigners in this area operated independently, communicating directly with another foreign presence in Nepal – the WHO country representative in Kathmandu. An important aspect of expedition preparation was seeking sponsorship and donations of supplies. The list of companies supporting the large American Mount Everest Expedition (AMEE) was extensive and included the pharmaceutical company Wyeth Laboratories, which in the next section supports Dr Edward Crippen's request for its vaccine.

After Nepal opened to climbing expeditions in the 1950s, Khumbu Sherpas looking for work no longer had to travel to Darjeeling in north-east India. In 1963, hoping for employment with the American expedition, a young Sherpa man walked to Kathmandu where he would have stayed in a crowded poorer part of the city. Most Sherpas were not wealthy. Smallpox was common in Kathmandu, which was also within reach of northern India; it was therefore a transmission point for the disease being spread to other areas. Having found work as a porter, he set off on his return journey. Although he now carried the smallpox virus, he was not yet symptomatic and so not contagious to others; the disease only became evident several days later by which time he was in the hills. Dr Lhakpa Norbu talked of how news of smallpox spread and gripped the villagers with fear. The narrow trails were Nepal's highways. Khumbu people travelled up and down the narrow Dudhkosi valley frequently for trade and to fetch grain, bringing people together and visiting or staying at the same houses:

> I heard that one such trading family from Thamo village contracted the disease from a trailside home-stay in Chhuthok village. After the death of a child, the family disposed [of] the contaminated clothing on a nearby thorn bush. Kids from an adjacent home touched the contaminated clothing and got infected.[3]

Himalayan expeditions in the twentieth century built up a tradition of providing medical care as they travelled throughout the country, especially those with doctors such as the Americans and Hillary's group in 1963. When the AMEE doctors discovered the porter with smallpox, they isolated him and provided what little treatment they could, but he died.[4] Both local people and the two groups of foreigners knew that vaccination was needed, but in this remote area there was neither vaccine nor the health workers to administer it.

Some vaccination had occurred previously from visiting vaccinators, but most people were unprotected.[5] Vaccination was not a usual expedition activity, but separately both AMEE and later Hillary managed to obtain vaccine through the WHO country representative, Dr N. Ahuja, in Kathmandu. Before leaving Namche Bazar, AMEE used the radio at the nearby military checkpost when their own would not work.[6] They vaccinated 'about 500 people' in the area above Namche Bazar, although by the time the vaccine arrived unvaccinated lowland porters had already left the expedition, so facilitating further spread of the disease.[7] The American climbers saw no more cases, and so continued their journey towards Mt Everest, where later the expedition was successful in achieving its climbing goal of putting the first Americans on the summit.

New Zealander Sir Edmund Hillary's group set off from Kathmandu two weeks after the Americans, was much smaller and as the name Schoolhouse implied had a different aim. It had two newly qualified doctors, Philip Houghton and Michael Gill. One of the houses that the sick porter visited was in Surkye village where the group met its first case of smallpox on 26 March. Hillary was a practical person and responded to the situation in his typical fashion. 'We all agreed that a big vaccination programme must be one of our jobs during the course of the expedition' and set about organising it. Some of Hillary's earlier activities in Nepal had earned the displeasure of Nepal's authorities, but this time his expedition's vaccination activities were to create a favourable impression with the government in Kathmandu.[8] The expedition had reached the higher village of Khumjung and over the next two days Houghton vaccinated – 'scratched' – between five and six hundred villagers on his own.[9] Later he enlisted the help of some of the other expedition members.

One of the worst hit villages was Thamo, situated in another valley. Lhakpa was related to one infected family; when his uncle and aunt discovered their children had smallpox, they immediately left Thamo and moved to an isolated area. Although relatives helped deliver food supplies to a nearby location, they avoided direct contact for fear of contamination. Three of the four children died. Fear also led to villagers reacting badly towards a lama who visited a bereaved family. In Sherpa society a lama is treated with considerable respect, but villagers barred him from entering their village.

Smallpox affected both rich and poor alike and another infected household was that of the headman from Thame village further along the valley. Their two daughters died, but the youngest son survived.[10]

One day, wrote Lhakpa, 'a bearded westerner in shorts, apparently a doctor' visited Upper Thame village to immunise the children.[11] Lhakpa described how his parents' home became 'a default vaccination center' and how his father 'got very uptight when a crowd began to arrive for vaccination at our home. He was fearful of already infected people arriving and tried to close the door unsuccessfully.'[12] They did not know how the vaccination had been organised. Today Lhakpa is a respected Sherpa cultural authority; he comments that Sherpas, at that time, practised a variety of traditional healing systems such as religious rituals, blessings, supplication of spirits, driving out of evil spirits and taking herbal remedies to heal illnesses, but smallpox did not have a local cure. 'Therefore, people willingly took part in the immunization program which prevented it from spreading further.'[13] The head lama of the area's main monastery at Tengboche had been vaccinated as a child.[14] The only opposition, Hillary noted, came from a group of monks at Thamo who had recently come over the high glacial pass from Tibet and believed that their extra religious practices should protect them. None developed smallpox 'and their status in the village increased enormously' wrote Hillary, adding that 'We were impressed.'[15]

For most people, vaccination was their first encounter with 'modern' medicine, and they believed that having the vaccination was an effective course of action.[16] A woman, now a Buddhist nun, recalled almost fifty years after the epidemic that as everyone feared the disease they were not scared. People were apprehensive, but they subjected themselves to the painful procedure, she said, because they expected it to work.[17] Reflecting that a few people were already vaccinated, a villager in Thame commented that 'He had the smallpox injection before the epidemic – that was why he didn't get it.'[18]

Writing a contribution for the book to celebrate fifty years since Hillary's first school was established in Khumjung in 1961, Ang Jangbu Sherpa, who subsequently became a pilot, described his memories of being a young boy during the smallpox epidemic and so provides a rare written and published account of local people's experiences. 'We were not even permitted to talk about it, for fear of bringing bad luck.'[19] His mother sent him to get a vaccination from the foreigners who had arrived in Lukla, several hours' walk away.

> She prepared a potato pancake as a packed lunch and gave me lengthy instructions to make sure that I wouldn't get contaminated along the way. First she wanted to make sure that I got there in time to get the life-saving inoculation. She then told me to avoid meeting people along the trail. In order to do this, I had to step off the trail and into the bush every time I saw someone coming from the opposite direction. While inside the bush, I would get busy collecting plants ... This delayed my trip and I nearly missed the vaccination.

At Lukla, 'adults were displaying scars about the size of a coin on their upper arms to encourage the younger kids. I thought it was quite attractive. After braving the jab myself, I was quite disappointed because of the pain and fever that followed.'

Hillary also recorded how the epidemic spread more widely in the district to the lower and more populous Solu area and how he began to get requests from many villages for help. One of his senior Sherpas, Nawang, whose home was near the village of Junbesi, five days' walk away, heard his children were ill. Nawang was worried, but – providing another example of ongoing variolation – his concern was 'aggravated by the fact that local quacks use the system of vaccinating with the actual pox from sick and dying people ... The quacks get ½ a rupee for each vaccination'.[20] Hillary, in an illustration of his developing relationship with Sherpas that would occupy the rest of his life, sent Nawang with enough vaccine to vaccinate his whole village.

Hillary, however, was also the victim of a trick.[21] He wrote how a well-dressed young man came to Khumjung with a petition from the panchayat of Jubing, a mixed Nepali and Sherpa village three days' walk away, saying that there was a lot of sickness and could Hillary give them some vaccine. The man said he had previous vaccinating experience and when Houghton tested him appeared competent. As Hillary's group was very busy with the epidemic, Hillary asked the military checkpost captain at Namche if the army's medical orderly could go with him. The orderly was said to be ill, and the man departed alone with the vaccine. Two days later Hillary learned that the man had written the petition himself and that he had accepted money from his neighbours on the promise that he would get vaccine. A month later Hillary was visited by the district police commissioner – was Hillary vaccinating and charging people? The next morning a policeman was sent to arrest the young man. A few weeks later the policeman returned to see Hillary; he had gone to Jubing village, but the young man had vanished, and the policeman had not been able to find him. Hillary also learned that the young man had only taken 'forty-seven rupees (six dollars)' for his vaccination services and had vaccinated many other people free of charge. For Hillary, that was the end of the matter.

In late April, after they had finished vaccinating, Hillary's expedition proceeded with its original objectives to bring piped water to the villages of Khumjung and Khunde and build schools at Thame and Pangboche. Some of the group managed some climbing. By the time the successful American expedition returned to Namche on 26 May the epidemic was under control. Finally, when the rest of Hillary's expedition left in June, his two doctors stayed for a further three months running a medical clinic from a room in Khumjung *gompa* (temple). The following year Hillary returned to build more schools but also provided further vaccination to those who sought it.[22] Expedition medical care was short term, but Hillary's involvement in the area was fast becoming long term. In 1966 he built the small hospital in Khunde, which offered vaccination as a permanent service.[23] The head lama at Thamo, who had declined a vaccination during the epidemic, came and blessed the hospital on its opening.

Kathmandu Valley

In the early 1960s, the 450,000 people who lived in the Kathmandu Valley included the residents of three ancient cities and multiple townships and villages. The largest city was the capital Kathmandu. The Valley was also the most densely populated part of Nepal. In 1963, a smallpox epidemic in Kathmandu was reported to international health authorities. As in other parts of the country most people with smallpox were looked after at home. In this section the influence of foreigners and the world of foreign aid is seen through the experiences and activities of Dr Edward Crippen of the United States Agency for International Development (USAID) who was able to access high level government and other influential personnel to secure a large supply of vaccine.[24] Ironically, Crippen appears to have become a victim of the Cold War. The epidemic was before US support for smallpox and a thawing in relations between the USA and the Soviet Union.

Although the first cases of smallpox from Nepal appeared in international statistics in the *Weekly Epidemiological Record* (WER) in 1961, no further cases were reported until 1963, when fourteen cases and three deaths were notified during the period 28 April to 4 May.[25] All are listed from Kathmandu which – under WHO's disease prevention International Sanitary Regulations – was declared an infected area on 22 May.[26] Case numbers and deaths in Nepal appeared in the *WER*, albeit irregularly, over the following weeks and months (Table 4.1). In early December, the number of smallpox cases and deaths surged. A 'special note' identified that a 'severe epidemic of smallpox is raging in Katmandu' where 3,112 cases were notified during the week ending 14 December.[27] No more cases were recorded after 25 January 1964, although Kathmandu remained classified as an infected area.[28] The high number of notifications for December was later revised downwards to a much lower

Table 4.1 Notified smallpox cases and deaths, Kathmandu, April 1963–January 1964

	Cases	Deaths
1963		
28 Apr–1 Jun	43	6
2 Jun–29 Jun	41	12
30 Jun–3 Aug	32	18
4 Aug–31 Aug	43	26
1 Sep–28 Sep	31	12
29 Sep–26 Oct	83	51
3 Nov–7 Dec	102	16
1964		
8 Dec–4 Jan	445	124
5 Jan–25 Jan	58	4

Source: *Weekly Epidemiological Record*.

total of 319 cases with 112 deaths, although these were still significantly higher than for other periods.[29]

Nepal was not alone in its limited reporting; international officials regularly noted the low level of notifications. The poor situation in Nepal, however, merited a note in the *WER* in its review of global smallpox in 1964 that the figures for Nepal were 'very incomplete'.[30] This would continue to be an issue. While the large number of notifications from Kathmandu in December 1963 was substantially lowered, the earlier high figure was perhaps more realistic. Newspapers in the capital, *The Rising Nepal* and *The Motherland*, reported 'as high as 100,000 cases in Nepal and over 25,000 deaths' and asked what the government was going to do.[31] Although these figures appear high, they do reflect that with variola major the proportion of deaths to cases was high. It could not be known with any accuracy as to what was happening in Kathmandu or elsewhere except that smallpox outbreaks were occurring in different regions. Shortly after his arrival, Crippen saw children on the streets with smallpox; most instances were in the middle of the day when less seriously ill children came out of their cold houses into the winter sunshine.

In the steep hillside Newar town of Kirtipur, to the south-west of the Valley, smallpox was widespread. Streets were narrow; houses surrounded a courtyard and people often had to pass through one house to reach another. 'Everyone along the street had someone who died of smallpox', recalled one mother, as she spoke of the 'terrible suffering'.[32] Other mothers separated the child who had smallpox from the rest of the family or sent uninfected children elsewhere, but she could not as four of her children had the disease at the same time. Whatever she knew about smallpox and how to care for her sick children, she had learned through personal and family experience and knowledge. She had not been to school and was not aware of information from posters or radio. On the fourth day of the sickness, she walked down from her house to Ajimatha (place of Ajima) situated among rice fields at the confluence of three roads. Here she made an offering to the goddess Ajima. Ajimatha was in line of sight of the hilltop temple of Swayambu several kilometres away where she went on the tenth day with further offerings. The journey took all day. Only if a child was very sick, recalled another mother, might a healer be called to come to the house to perform the necessary rituals and say mantras to 'calm' the disease.[33] One Ayurvedic healer who specialised in smallpox rituals went to people's homes but another healer who said he had inherited spiritual powers from his father expected people to come to him.[34] Both 'massaged' the site of the disease but said that they did not expect to get smallpox.[35]

Only the government-run Bir Hospital in Kathmandu – Nepal's main hospital – had an Infectious Diseases Unit. An article in the *Journal of Nepal Medical Association* analysed 100 cases of smallpox admitted to Bir Hospital during the epidemic.[36] Of these, twenty-eight died in hospital and five people left hospital against medical advice in a critical condition. The authors, who were doctors at the hospital, noted that most cases came from Kathmandu. Only a few came from Patan (Lalitpur) and Bhaktapur just a few kilometres away, attributing this to transportation problems. Yet, when the epidemic broke out in the Kathmandu Valley towards the end of November 1963 the worst affected area was in the town of Thimi in Bhaktapur district where it was estimated that by late December there had been 'between 200 and 600 deaths'.[37]

Thimi had a population of 14,000 and bordered the district's main town. Vaccination activities had been focusing on the municipal areas and had not yet reached Thimi. To help with the epidemic, the Director of Health Services sent students from the Auxiliary Health Workers School and student nurses to Thimi. Dr Ram Bhadra Adiga, the dermatologist at Bir Hospital, wrote that he was 'ordered to take over the entire command'.[38] His account of the epidemic provides a rare and valuable Nepali government health perspective and insight from someone, albeit at a senior level, who was actively involved. 'On the first day of my assignment, while touring Thimi, I could hardly find a house which did not have a case of smallpox. It was the first time in my life that I saw so many cases in one place.' The following day was a religious holiday. Pilgrims travelled around the Valley but had to pass through Thimi. 'This was a good opportunity to contact these people, hence all the roads in Thimi were blocked and everybody using the road was vaccinated. We had to vaccinate 1,500 people on that day alone.' Compulsory vaccination was introduced at Bhaktapur Bus Station. 'All those using public transport were vaccinated. Over 7,000 people were vaccinated by this tactic.' Reference to motorised transport illustrates Nepal's changing environment. Further compulsory vaccination was introduced around Thimi and 'all those who did not have smallpox were vaccinated'. They also distributed leaflets and showed films.

> If the doors were left open by mistake, orders were issued to search the house for any inmates. Only those who were absent, who could run faster than us, or who kept their doors closed escaped vaccination. Local Magistrates, Police and Panchayats were approached for help, and they all did their best.

The epidemic in the Thimi area was controlled in 'about three weeks', with 'over 29,000' people being vaccinated. Vaccination activities then continued through the staff of the Smallpox Control Pilot Project.[39]

Further government initiatives also took place in early 1964. Each February, holy men from India travelled on pilgrimage to Kathmandu for the Shivaratri festival, but Nepali health officials had 'long felt' that these holy men were the source of the recurrent smallpox epidemics in Kathmandu and ordered their compulsory vaccination, which was carried out.[40] The Government also passed legislation to make smallpox vaccination compulsory for children under the age of twelve years.[41] How this was to be achieved was not specified. Nevertheless, despite the epidemic, for the Government smallpox was still but one of a range of communicable diseases; on the same day it passed another law 'to control epidemics of infectious diseases'.[42]

From the early 1950s, the USA was active in Nepal with specific projects, but in 1963 it also responded to a call to assist with the epidemic. A brief mention in Skerry, Moran and Calavan's authoritative history of US assistance to Nepal is one of the few published references to the epidemic.[43] The authors interviewed Crippen but his own account provides more detail and emphasises the important context within USAID and Nepal that shaped this 'non-project' activity. Just before his departure for Nepal, the Agency's Washington staff informed him that USAID's basic policy was now economic development. 'In effect, they told me my mission in Nepal was to reduce USAID's commitment in health.'[44]

During the months since his arrival in Kathmandu, Crippen had continued to notice people with smallpox. Confidentially, the medically qualified Prime Minister Dr Tulsi Giri had approached the US

Embassy physician who asked Crippen about obtaining some of the American 'Dry-Vac' (Dryvax) smallpox vaccine for his family. Such an approach was very much in line with past requests to the British. 'We did, and others began asking for it.'[45] The wives of American Mission personnel became alarmed 'because so many of their servants and their children were sick with smallpox and had died'.[46] To Crippen, it was clear that despite a vaccination programme in the Valley, it was not stopping the epidemic and the government was 'receptive to help, especially in the form of Dry-Vac vaccine'. This vaccine was more heat stable and in a country with little refrigeration was better suited to Nepali conditions.[47]

Complicating the situation was the Government, which was downplaying the epidemic. Tourism in Nepal was in its infancy but was developing; declaring an epidemic could be detrimental. News of the epidemic had already reached the international press through some coverage of both the earlier American and Hillary expeditions' activities. A friend sent an article to Crippen from the *Washington Post*, which had picked up Hillary's story. The epidemic was also mentioned – albeit very briefly – in the English national press, where it was reported that Hillary's sponsors had told him to halt his expedition's building and climbing activities 'while he fights a smallpox outbreak'.[48] At the end of September the *New York Times* reported on the spreading smallpox epidemic in the Kathmandu Valley.[49] Crippen showed the *Washington Post* article to the Director of Health Services, Dr Dinesha Nanda (D. N.) Baidya, who replied that 'It's above me'. The wording is significant – it was not the Director's decision to make. His inability – and unwillingness – to make this decision reflected Nepali process, the political uncertainty of the time and the very hierarchical structure of government, the bureaucracy and society. Above the director was the minister, the prime minister and the king. A royal coup in 1960 brought a halt to many of the political and administrative changes of the 1950s. Although the four-tier administrative structure of 'a partyless panchayat democracy' set up under the new 1962 Constitution suggested representation, the king wielded absolute power.[50]

Crippen approached the Mission's Director, John Roach, about offering to help Nepal with Dryvax.[51] The Director 'refused to provide anything not already approved in the health budget'.[52] Crippen, however, thought that the American pharmaceutical firm Wyeth, which manufactured Dryvax, might donate the vaccine. Roach then agreed to support the proposal on the conditions that the vaccine was donated and that the Government in requesting the vaccine confirmed that there was an epidemic. The next day Roach received confirmation of the epidemic and an urgent request for Dryvax vaccine.[53] In less than a week, 200,000 doses of the vaccine and 200,000 scarifying needles donated by Wyeth Laboratories arrived from Washington in Kathmandu. His description of 'double-pointed' needles suggests they may have been the new bifurcated needles that were being developed.[54] Pan American Airlines transported the supplies by air to Calcutta in India and then Royal Nepal Airlines to Kathmandu.[55]

The next stage was to develop a plan 'within HMG's Health Department' for the vaccine's distribution; from USAID's standpoint it was primarily to be used outside the Kathmandu Valley in US-supported clinics as WHO was responsible for vaccination in the Valley, using vaccine provided by the Soviet Union.[56] Word spread quickly about the new vaccine's arrival. 'Due to the excitement generated by the program, the Mission allowed me to distribute vaccine to the more remote areas of Nepal by helicopter,' wrote Crippen.[57] The Director of Health Services accompanied him on these trips. Crippen gave as an example how they delivered 2,000 doses 'at a mountain top clinic a day's walk from Kathmandu'. Whether this needed to be delivered by helicopter was questionable, as in the context of wider Nepal a one-day walk was hardly remote and three days later the doctor in charge was in the Director's office requesting another 3,000 doses as he had used up the first supply. Skerry et al. mention that by May 1964 700,000 doses had been distributed through the Department of Health infrastructure, and the epidemic had been quelled.[58] The further 500,000 doses, however, came from different sources. Crippen's account related that

> the Director of Health informed me that Nepal had received 200,000 doses of freeze-dried vaccine from Pakistan. A week later he announced another donation of 200,000 from the United Arab Republic. WHO ... brought in 100,000 more doses.[59]

Such significant international and national involvement makes the omission of the epidemic from the official narrative even more surprising.

Crippen left Nepal in early June 1964 and returned to the USA to Alabama where he became the city of Mobile's County Health Officer. The context surrounding his 'End of Tour Report', however, was not the usual process. The memorandum from Robert L. Cherry, Public Health Advisor, Near East/South Asia Region, does not indicate to whom it was sent but details that 'This report was prepared after his return to the States at our request. For some reason he had been advised by the Mission that it was not necessary for him to prepare such a report.'[60] Cherry praised Crippen's work highly. This omission could relate to the change in priorities for the US aid programme. In another paper Crippen wrote about a conversation with the Minister of Health, Dr Nageshwar Prasad Singh, who said that he 'was under the impression that your government under President Kennedy didn't want to support any health project under [its] new economic development strategy for Nepal'.[61] While the USAID history refers to the Mission being able to secure large donations of freeze-dried vaccine from Pakistan and the United Arab Republic, Crippen's family understand that their father incurred Washington's displeasure because, although Crippen did not know this at the time, the source of the vaccine from Pakistan was in fact the Soviet Union.[62] In the political environment of the Cold War, this was unfortunate.

Lamjung, central Nepal

Crippen's involvement also provides a link to responses to the epidemic in the Lamjung district (Map 1). Lamjung is in the mid-hills and has a mixture of castes and ethnic groups with a high concentration of Gurung, many of whom were former Gurkha soldiers with the British and Indian Armies. The section highlights social and cultural differences in responses to the epidemic as well as a patchwork of developing health services and providers. Another kind of foreigner was also present in the area. In contrast to the temporary nature of a foreign expedition passing through an area, young US Peace Corps volunteers arrived to spend two years working in rural development. As news spread of cases of smallpox, local panchayat officials approached Donald Messerschmidt and Bruce Morrison to help. They were taken to see Crippen about vaccine. In contrast

1963–64 – epidemic smallpox

to Hillary in the Mt Everest region, Messerschmidt and Morrison described how the vaccination programme was organised and delivered through local organisations and how they worked with local officials and community leaders. Their efforts were not mentioned, however, in the Peace Corps' later account of its involvement with the global smallpox story.

As the Indian states of Bihar and Uttar Pradesh were also experiencing smallpox epidemics in 1963, it was highly likely to be present in Nepal's Tarai region as people moved freely across the border.[63] The hospital in the town of Birgunj, which was situated near the border and linked by rail with Raxaul in Bihar, carried out smallpox vaccinations among outpatients through a health unit with a staff of three – a 'health specialist', a health assistant and an auxiliary health worker.[64] Unit staff also undertook house-to-house visits. Nevertheless, when WHO medical officer, Dr Valentin E. Vichniakov, visited in late 1964, he reported that during the past year staff had 'only' given about 3,000 smallpox vaccinations.[65] Such a number does not suggest the presence of a widespread epidemic, but the number of vaccinations would also have depended on having the vaccine to undertake a campaign and the vaccine supply in the country was limited at this time.

Nevertheless, smallpox was spreading north beyond the Tarai. Pokhara, which was situated in the central hill district of Kaski on a north–south trade route, was growing rapidly in the early 1960s. American Dorothy Mierow, who arrived in Nepal with the first group of Peace Corps volunteers in 1962, went to Pokhara in 1963. She described how some Tibetan refugees had walked back into Nepal from India and were in 'the last stages of smallpox'.[66] They stopped at a well in the bazaar for water. A local woman was at the tap at the same time, was infected but recovered. The Tibetans died in their tents. Having left their homeland, most Tibetans in Nepal were living in very poor conditions.[67]

Nepal was one of the first countries to receive the Peace Corps volunteers. Within two months of his inaugural address in January 1961, President John F. Kennedy had issued the executive order that led to the establishment of what became known as the Peace Corps.[68] It was not a new idea and Republicans dismissed the initiative as the 'Kiddie-Corps', but the ensuing Peace Corps Act passed through Congress and was signed by Kennedy on 22 September.

Volunteers were 'to provide trained manpower to developing countries and increase understanding of America in these countries and vice versa'.[69] For the individual volunteer, their time overseas was an intense personal experience with often lifelong effects and associations. Mierow 'lost my heart to Pokhara and its people' and spent more than thirty years in the country.[70] Collectively, the volunteers were part of a global programme.[71] The Peace Corps was an integral part of the ideas that framed Kennedy's foreign policy; they were 'to exemplify the virtues of American society through their humanitarian deeds and democratic values'.[72] Peace Corps volunteers, although they may not have thought of themselves that way, would help in America's struggle to contain communism in the developing world.

Nepal's very limited health infrastructure, its geography and people's health needs presented opportunities and challenges for other groups on a long-term or short-term basis. In some areas, the new foreign Christian missions had an agreement with the government to provide health services and during 1963–64 gave additional support. On 21 June 1963, Jonathan Lindell, Executive Secretary of the United Mission to Nepal (UMN), wrote to the Department of Health Services in Kathmandu that medical workers at Amp Pipal village in Gorkha district had requested smallpox vaccine.[73] At this time the mission operated out of a one-roomed dispensary. A child, wrote Lindell, was brought into the dispensary who was very ill with smallpox and staff feared that an epidemic would spread in the district. Little vaccine was available in Gorkha, and the staff had requested as large a quantity of vaccine as possible.[74] Small outbreaks were occurring in the district, but 'prompt action' and vaccinations being carried out, brought the spread 'quickly' under control.[75] How quickly is not mentioned, but another account indicated that the epidemic was still active during the first few months of 1964.[76] The amount of vaccine received was also not detailed. At Tansen in Palpa district UMN staff made 'several visits to villages with smallpox cases for vaccination and advice'.[77] In January, two nurses from Shining Hospital, which was run by the Nepal Evangelistic Band mission in Pokhara, helped the local authorities by carrying out a vaccination campaign for 2,000 people in Argum on the edge of Pokhara.[78] The epidemic was also continuing in other mission areas. At the dispensary at Okhaldunga in eastern Nepal (Sagarmatha zone), staff gave health talks and vaccination where there were recent cases of smallpox.[79] As with other examples, none of these cases was reported internationally in the *WER*.

Messerschmidt and Morrison were part of the second group of Peace Corps volunteers to arrive in Nepal. Peace Corps policy was that the volunteers were expected to live as the local people – usually a great contrast to what they were used to at home. Messerschmidt's published account written much later revealed the youthful aspirations and attitudes typical of many foreigners in Nepal at this time – and especially those in rural areas where they were often on their own.[80] His account reflected the ethnic diversity that made up Nepal's population; the two different reactions from Gurung villagers also emphasises the need to beware generalising about cultural responses.

Messerschmidt and Morrison began hearing stories in early December 1963 of smallpox in the villages. People told them that smallpox regularly came to Nepal via the trade route from north India and so this was just the latest outbreak.[81] A common theme of the accounts from both the Mt Everest and the Lamjung areas was that local people asked the foreigners for help. 'When village leaders approached district officials to do something about it', wrote Messerschmidt, 'they, in turn, asked us for help.'[82] Many of the requests came from the area's northern villages where there were ex-soldiers of the Indian Army. After India's independence from Britain in 1947, some of the Gurkha brigades went into the British Army while others became part of the Indian Army. During their Christmas break in Kathmandu, Messerschmidt and Morrison went to see the Peace Corps Country Director who took them to Crippen at USAID for assistance with obtaining vaccine. Crippen, in turn, took them to the Health Department. In January, Director Baidya 'entrusted' the two volunteers with vaccine to take to 'their village health assistant'.[83]

Messerschmidt and Morrison submitted their reports to the District Panchayat Officer who then forwarded them to government authorities in Kathmandu and on to the Department of Health Services. They indicated the large scale of activities and importantly the cooperation that was taking place at a local level:

4–5 days of nearly every week were spent planning and impl[e]menting the program, including conference with village leaders and Jilla [district] Panchayat Development Officer and staff over the numerous requests that flooded the office; trekking and vaccinating in a majority of Gaun [village] Panchayat areas; arranging vaccination supplies to be sent to local Soldier's Board and HMG [His Majesty's Government] Dispensary persons; several week long trips to Kathmandu and Pokhara for vaccination supplies; training PDWs [panchayat development workers] in vaccination and program organization procedure to work with village Panchayat leaders, etc.[84]

In total, 23,773 people, mostly children under the age of ten years old, were vaccinated between January and April 1964.[85]

In his later magazine article, Messerschmidt wrote about the human side of the campaign – both about themselves and the communities. After their break, he and Morrison returned to Kunchha, headquarters of Lamjung district, to begin vaccinating. They went to Amp Pipal mission – a day's walk away – to learn how to vaccinate.[86] The two Peace Corps volunteers faced a challenge. Their supply of vaccine was limited, but parents 'insisted' that all children should be vaccinated 'believing that any unvaccinated ones would catch the disease from their vaccinated siblings and friends'.[87] Messerschmidt and Morrison were puzzled. With variolation, however, people were given the actual smallpox virus and so unvaccinated people were at considerable risk of getting smallpox, also suggesting that variolation might still be being practised in the area or had been in the recent past.[88] More vaccine was needed urgently, but after three days and no reply to their message Morrison set off to walk – since there were no roads – for two days to Pokhara from where he could get a plane to Kathmandu on one of the two flights per week provided by Royal Nepal Airlines.

While the only health worker in the Mt Everest region in 1963 was the military orderly at the check post in Namche Bazar, Messerschmidt recounted that a porter arrived 'unexpectedly' at the small village health post run by the Indian Soldiers Board carrying vaccine but sufficient for only fifty doses. Since 1947, the Defence Wing of the Indian Embassy in Kathmandu provided welfare support for the veteran Gurkha soldiers of the Indian Army who had returned to Nepal. An ex-soldier, who was a compounder, staffed the post. Although district officials and Messerschmidt advised him to wait until more vaccine arrived, he responded to local people's pressure and gave it. The vaccine did not 'take'. Villagers were unhappy and then angry at the situation. More than a week passed without any news about extra vaccine, but when Morrison finally returned, he brought enough for 12,000 people 'and a promise of more if we needed it'.[89]

Messerschmidt's account suggested some local tension. Although he and Morrison began vaccinating the next morning at the school, it was locked and there were no tables or hot water. They set up under a tree. Villagers were keen to be vaccinated and local police helped keep order. First, each child's forearm was scrubbed with soap and water with some children who had a very dirty or infected arm receiving a further wash with the local alcohol, *raksi*, as an antiseptic. This initially upset some of the Brahmin parents until they understood it was used for cleaning and not consumption.[90] Most vaccinations were given on the lower left forearm because the great majority of the children wore tight-fitting, long-sleeved shirts, which would have had to have been cut off to vaccinate the upper arm. As Hillary had also found, families had little or no money and children wore clothes until they outgrew them, or they fell apart.[91] Over two days they vaccinated 4,500 children. They then trained other Peace Corps volunteers and local people to run vaccination camps around the district. On one occasion further vaccine supplies arrived by helicopter. As with the Mt Everest area epidemic, news again reached overseas. Messerschmidt's family wrote to him that they had heard on the radio about a 'load of vaccine shipped in. Hope nothing serious.'[92]

Messerschmidt also noted an additional and valuable benefit from their involvement in that 'we gained a strong working knowledge of the Gaun (village) Panchayats, their leaders and villagers who in return came to know us and our role in the Lamjung Panchayat'. This led to further requests for help with projects. Nevertheless, the two Peace Corps volunteers in March 1964 were rebuked in a letter by Dr Mark Rhine, the Peace Corps physician for Nepal, for not following correct procedure. Measures for disease prevention were the responsibility of local government and vaccination outside the Kathmandu Valley was the responsibility of the local health officer – although this was not made clear to Messerschmidt and Morrison earlier.[93] They had operated 'with the full concurrence' of the district (jilla) panchayat and had worked with local staff developing and implementing the campaign. That the letter was copied to the WHO Representative in Nepal, Crippen, the Director of the Panchayat Development Office, and Peace Corps Representatives – although not to anyone in the Directorate of Health Services – suggested that the vaccination campaign was caught up in national politics and bilateral aid relations, and around the development and role of panchayats and central and local power. By this time, Messerschmidt and Morrison had nearly finished their vaccination campaign – which they duly did.

Conclusion

These snapshots from three very different areas of Nepal illustrate the many and fragmented responses to smallpox in the early 1960s. Drawing extensively on people's experiences and unpublished sources, they clearly tell us that the disease was much more widespread than was reported and enable us to look at other areas as well as the capital Kathmandu. These sources provide much new and valuable, in-depth information.

While each scenario is very different, common themes emerge. Unsurprisingly, responses reflected the enormous and varying challenges of the Nepali human and physical environment in different parts of the country at the time of the epidemic and are set in the wider context of changed international and global relations after the end of the Second World War. The ability of authorities to respond was extremely limited, even in the capital. Also evident is how Nepal was changing and the early importance of developing tourism. Placing people's perspectives at the forefront, both local Nepalis' and the foreign visitors', highlights the multiplicity of perspectives of those involved, process and layers of bureaucracy. In each location despite some differences in attitudes and practices vaccination was supported by local populations. In each location vaccination services were limited, irrespective of whether other health services were available, but communities take the initiative and approach foreigners for help in obtaining vaccine. In this chapter the distinctly different presence of foreigners was important in each of the localities but as smallpox becomes a government programme supported by the king and the supply of vaccine is ensured by the WHO the number of foreigners involved decreased.

Notes

1. *Weekly Epidemiological Record* (WER), 39:31 (31 July 1964), p. 375.
2. Although a decade later, see Schnur, 'Innovation as an integral part of smallpox eradication'.
3. Dr Lhakpa Norbu Sherpa, written communication to author, July 2017.
4. Gilbert Roberts, 'Health and medicine', in James Ramsey Ullman, *Americans on Everest* (Philadelphia, PA: J. B. Lippincott, 1964), p. 347.
5. M. B. Gill, 'The Sherpas: A survey of an isolated mountain community' (Department of Preventive and Social Medicine dissertation, University of Otago, 1961), p. 16; Dr Kami Temba Sherpa, personal communication.
6. This Indian check post was one of a number deployed along the Nepal–China border.
7. Ullman, *Americans on Everest*, p. 82 and Roberts, 'Health and Medicine', p. 348.
8. ANZ, ABHS 6949 W4628 NDI 64/14/2 Part 2, Himalayan climbing expeditions & schoolhouse project, Ian McIntosh, Department of External Affairs, Wellington to Hillary, 21 September 1963.
9. Linear scarification of one or two superficial scratches was the simplest method.
10. Hillary, *Schoolhouse in the Clouds*, p. 44. In Sherpa society, the youngest son inherits and has the responsibility of looking after his parents in their old age.
11. L. N. Sherpa, written communication to author, July 2017. The doctor most likely was Houghton who wrote in his diary about visiting the village. Philip Houghton, email communication, 20 July 2014.
12. L. N. Sherpa, written communication to author, July 2017.
13. *Ibid.*
14. Ngawang Tenzin Zangbu, *Stories and Customs of the Sherpas*, p. 58.
15. Hillary, *Schoolhouse in the Clouds*, p. 47.
16. Susan Heydon, 'Medicines, travellers and the introduction and spread of "modern" medicine in the Mt Everest region of Nepal', *Medical History*, 55:4 (2011), 503–21.
17. Interview (26) with author, January 2012.

18 Interview (1) with author, January 2012.
19 Lhakpa Norbu Sherpa (ed.), *Khumjung Secondary School: Celebrating 50 Years of Education (1961–2011)* (Lalitpur: Golden Jubilee Celebration Committee, 2011), p. 33.
20 Auckland War Memorial Museum/Tāmaki Paenga Hira, MS-2010–1 Sir Edmund Hillary personal papers, Ed Hillary – letter book, March – April 1963, 16 April 1963. This is not mentioned in the book.
21 Hillary, *Schoolhouse in the Clouds*, pp. 47–9.
22 ANZ, EA W2824 118/13/13/13 Part1, Sir Edmund Hillary, Himalayan Schoolhouse Expedition report on 1964 activities, p. 1.
23 Heydon, *Modern Medicine and International Aid*, p. 121.
24 Formed in 1961, it replaced USOM.
25 WER, 38:21 (24 May 1963), p. 262. The system relied on state self-notification.
26 *Ibid.*, p. 260.
27 WER, 38:51 (20 December 1963), p. 631.
28 WER, 39:8 (21 February 1964), p. 87.
29 WER, 39:7 (14 February 1964), p. 76. The WHO's *Epidemiological and Vital Statistics Report* 17 (1964) lists 404 cases and 120 deaths for December 1963, p. 157.
30 WER, 40:11 (19 March 1965), p. 126.
31 Edward F. Crippen, 'Smallpox, Nepal 1963 ... Prelude to eradication?', paper presented to the International Health Society, program: Immunization strategies past and present, Las Vegas, Nevada, 30 September 1986, pp. 2–3. I am very grateful to Don Messerschmidt and Dr Crippen's family for copies of different drafts of this paper.
32 Interview (3) with author, May 2017. This was the first time her son had heard her talk about these times.
33 Interview (4) with author, May 2017.
34 Interviews (4) and (5) with author, May 2017.
35 The second healer was vaccinated as a child in a hospital.
36 M. R. Pandey, I. L. Acharya and A. Moyeed. 'Clinical survey of small pox', *JNMA*, 2:1 (1964), 8–11. Dr Pandey was the Journal's first editor.
37 World Health Organization, Expert Committee on Smallpox, Meeting 1964, Geneva, Switzerland, Smallpox/WP/12, Review of smallpox situation in the world, 1963, prepared by the Secretariat, p. 3 https://apps.who.int/iris/handle/10665/67663.
38 [B.] B. Adiga, 'Smallpox epidemic in Nepal (1963–1964)'. I am very grateful to Dr Crippen's family for a copy.
39 See Chapter 5.
40 Crippen, 'Smallpox, Nepal 1963 ... Prelude to eradication?', p. 9.

41 Law Enacted to Provide for Vaccination for the Prevention of Smallpox among Children (Smallpox Control Act); Law No. 27 of 2020 B.S. (28 February 1964), published in *Nepal Gazette*, vol. 13:29 (Extraordinary) of Falgun 16, 2020 B.S.
42 Law Enacted to Control Epidemics of Infectious Diseases (Infectious Diseases Act); Law No. 28 of 2020 B.S. (28 February 1964), published in *Nepal Gazette*, vol. 13:29 (Extraordinary) of Falgun 16, 2020 B.S.
43 Skerry et al., *Four Decades of Development*, p. 137. The American Mount Everest Expedition (AMEE) and the smallpox epidemic in the region were, however, nearly nine months before the Kathmandu epidemic peak.
44 Crippen, 'Smallpox, Nepal 1963 ... Prelude to eradication?', p. 1. For this refocusing, see Skerry et al., *Four Decades of Development*, pp. 8, 135.
45 Crippen, 'Smallpox, Nepal 1963 ... Prelude to eradication?', p. 3.
46 *Ibid.*, p. 4.
47 *Ibid.*; Crippen, 'When there was smallpox', 2 July 1998. I am very grateful to Dr Crippen's family for a copy. Unfortunately, many family papers were lost in a house fire.
48 *Daily Telegraph and Morning Post*, 4 April 1963, p. 15.
49 ProQuest Historical Newspapers: The New York Times, 'Smallpox spreading in Nepal', Special to the New York Times, *New York Times (1923–Current File)*, 29 September 1963.
50 Agrawal, *The Administrative System of Nepal*, p. 355.
51 Crippen, 'Smallpox, Nepal 1963 ... Prelude to eradication?', p. 3.
52 *Ibid.*, p. 4.
53 *Ibid.*
54 As Crippen was writing later, he may have inadvertently referred to the new needle.
55 Crippen, 'When there was smallpox'.
56 HMG was commonly used to denote His Majesty's Government.
57 Crippen, 'Smallpox, Nepal 1963 ... Prelude to eradication?', p. 7.
58 Skerry et al., *Four Decades of Development*, p. 137.
59 Crippen, 'Smallpox, Nepal 1963 ... Prelude to eradication?', p. 8.
60 Robert L. Cherry, M.D. M.P.H., Public Health Advisor, Near East/South Asia Region, Washington, DC, 30 September 1964 (Crippen family papers).
61 Crippen, 'When there was smallpox'.
62 Don Messerschmidt, email communication, 26 September 2018. Messerschmidt met two members of Crippen's family at a reunion, talked about this book, and later visited where he was given copies

of these documents to pass on. Skerry et al. considered that USAID's overall involvement in Nepal was more humanitarian than about security. Skerry et al., *Four Decades of Development*, p. 365.
63 Basu, Jezek and Ward, *The Eradication of Smallpox from India*, p. 41.
64 SEA/WHO, SEA/Smallpox/8, Dr V. E. Vichniakov, WHO Medical Officer, Field visit report on Smallpox Control Pilot Project, Nepal WHO Project: Nepal 9, 22 October–5 November 1964, 9 March 1965, p. 7.
65 SEA/Smallpox/8, Vichniakov, Field visit report 1964, p. 7.
66 Dorothy Mierow, *Thirty Years in Pokhara* (Kathmandu: Pilgrims Book House, 1997). See also Jagannath Adhikari and David Seddon, *Pokhara: Biography of a Town* (Kathmandu: Mandala Book Point, 2002).
67 Ann Frechette, *Tibetans in Nepal: The Dynamics of International Assistance among a Community in Exile* (New York/Oxford: Berghahn Books, 2002).
68 James F. Fisher, *At Home in the World: Globalization and the Peace Corps in Nepal* (Bangkok: Orchid Press, 2013), pp. 1–2.
69 *Ibid.*, p. 2.
70 Mierow, *Thirty Years in Pokhara*, p. vii.
71 Fisher, *At Home in the World*.
72 Michael E. Latham, *Modernization as Ideology: American Social Science and 'Nation Building' in the Kennedy Era* (Chapel Hill, NC: University of North Carolina Press, 2000), p. 110.
73 Other spellings are Ampipal or Amppipal.
74 Divinity library of Yale University library, New Haven, Connecticut, United Mission to Nepal (UMN) archives, Record Group No. 212 (hereafter UMN RG 212), Box 73 H020101, J. Lindell to Department of Health Services, 21 June 1963.
75 UMN RG 212, Box 78 H020701/0003, Amp Pipal.
76 Donald A. Messerschmidt and Robert Bruce Morrison, Interim report phase one smallpox vaccination program Lamjung District, West Zone #3, Nepal, 3 March 1964 (Messerschmidt personal papers). I am very grateful for a copy of this and a further report and for valuable help with this section.
77 UMN RG 212, Box 78 H020701/0005, Tansen.
78 Divinity library of Yale University library, New Haven, Connecticut, International Nepal Fellowship (INF) archives, Record Group No. 214, AO30101/0005/000, Annual report of the Shining Hospital for 1964.
79 UMN RG 212, Box 78 H020701/0002.
80 Don Messerschmidt, 'The scourge of smallpox: Nepal 1964', *ECS Nepal* 74 (July 2010) http://ecs.com.np/features/the-scourge-of-smallpox-nepal-1964.

1963–64 – epidemic smallpox

81 Bruce Morrison, email communication to Messerschmidt, 15 May 2018.
82 Messerschmidt, 'The scourge of smallpox: Nepal 1964'.
83 Crippen, 'Smallpox, Nepal 1963 ... Prelude to eradication?', pp. 7–8. Although Crippen's and Messerschmidt's accounts differed over the amount of vaccine, this timeline fits with the USAID narrative. Messerschmidt and Morrison's interim report noted that vaccine was limited in the beginning.
84 Donald A. Messerschmidt, Brief outline of activities – US Peace Corps volunteers Lamjung District, Gandaki Zone, West #3 October, 1963 through July 15, 1964.
85 Messerschmidt, email communication, 8 May 2018. This was in Lamjung district and one community in the neighbouring Tanauh (Tanahun) district.
86 Bruce Morrison, 15 May 2018.
87 Messerschmidt, 'The scourge of smallpox: Nepal 1964'.
88 Messerschmidt and Morrison heard stories about this.
89 Messerschmidt, 'The scourge of smallpox: Nepal 1964'.
90 Messerschmidt, email communication 14 April 2018.
91 *Ibid.*
92 Messerschmidt, unpublished narrative, 2006, p. 5 (Messerschmidt personal papers).
93 17 March 1964, Messerschmidt, email communication, 7 May 2018.

5

Engaging global policy – from control to eradication

This chapter investigates another aspect of foreign involvement in Nepal with smallpox in this period – the WHA's goal of smallpox eradication. It highlights that the key external relationship for Nepal's central government was at a regional level with WHO's South-East Asia Regional Office (SEARO). While the official and other histories of smallpox eradication are most concerned with the period after 1967 when the WHO launched its intensified smallpox eradication programme, I argue that the joint Government of Nepal/WHO Smallpox Control Pilot Project, which started in three districts of the Kathmandu Valley in early 1962 and was operating at the time of the epidemic in 1963, provided the foundation for Nepal's implementation of the global programme. Despite dismissive criticism of Nepal's pilot control project in the official history, the later intensified eradication project agreed to and signed by Nepal's government and WHO in November 1966 was built on the experiences – both positive and negative – with the pilot. Also, a local initiative in 1965 in another part of the country demonstrated better than the pilot project that higher immunisation targets were achievable and how.

The chapter is in three parts. The first examines the issue of whose responsibility it was to deal with implementing the global smallpox programme and situates Nepal within global and regional perspectives and debates about smallpox, control and eradication. The WHA passed resolutions in 1958 and 1959, but the next stage was how to achieve this. Views differed. Despite the WHA's global commitment to smallpox eradication, little funding was provided to undertake this work; implementation would be the responsibility of the different member states. Smallpox, however, was just one of many communicable disease issues facing the South-East Asia Region. The second section discusses the pilot project. A key and repeated theme identified in the field visit reports of regional WHO staff to Nepal was that despite the number of vaccinations carried out the need to raise immunisation coverage (estimated percentage of the population who have received a specific vaccine) remained. The final part introduces a 1965 local initiative, coordinated by the Biratnagar branch of the Nepal Medical Association (NMA), to vaccinate all children in Morang and Sunsari districts in the Tarai. Involvement of the panchayats and community participation contributed to the project achieving better coverage than the pilot.

Smallpox control – whose problem?

At the beginning of the 1960s Nepal's government provided some smallpox vaccination services, but coverage was very incomplete. Although the government more than doubled its expenditure for smallpox activities between 1962 and 1965, the annual amount was just US$2,447 rising to US$5,334 (Appendix 3).[1] As in the First Five Year Plan period (1956–61), the Second (1962–65) maintained the emphasis on curative health but also gave more attention to preventive activities.[2] These included not only smallpox but also programmes for tuberculosis and leprosy control.

Smallpox control in Nepal presented many challenges, unimaginable in much of the world. Indeed, whether the target was smallpox, or another disease, was not the point. Although discussing Nepal's wider economic development, Whelpton suggests that 'the intractability of the problems rather than the nature of a particular regime may have been the most important factor retarding progress'.[3] With limited methods of communication, how would the government or any other organisation know what was happening throughout the country when cases of smallpox arose? Even less likely, how would the government be able to direct timely responses, coordinate and monitor the situation? How would it communicate with its mostly rural population? Very low levels of literacy meant that people could not read information, although Radio Nepal periodically issued notices regarding vaccination services.[4] Most people, however, could not afford or did not have access to radios.

The health education section of the Ministry of Health had a fully equipped cinema van funded through foreign aid, but Nepal had few roads outside the Kathmandu Valley.[5] Even within the Valley, travel was difficult. With the country's challenging geography, how would the necessary supplies be transported to where they were needed? How would vaccine be stored? The vaccine then in use needed refrigeration, but Nepal had limited power and few refrigerators. Who would pay? The nation state of Nepal had very limited financial resources. With few trained health workers, who would or could vaccinate? Vaccination activities in the Mt Everest and Lamjung areas had demonstrated that others could be shown how.

In 1962 Dr Marcolino Candau, WHO Director-General, outlined the worldwide smallpox situation in his report to the Fifteenth WHA.[6] Although his previous two reports had mentioned smallpox as a major problem in Nepal, this was the first time that international statistics listed cases. The five cases and two deaths were not from the capital Kathmandu but from Pokhara where an outbreak in 1961 occurred particularly among Tibetan refugees. In his South-East Asia Region summary, Candau also referred to Nepal as one of four countries that had either 'planned or initiated eradication programmes and have requested WHO assistance'.[7] The others were Afghanistan, India and Thailand.

With intensified Chinese presence in the Tibetan region, many people were coming over the mostly mountainous border into northern Nepal, although it is more likely that the cases of smallpox in 1961were in Tibetans travelling back into Nepal from India. Pokhara was on their route. The PRC was not a member of WHO and so did not provide information but had carried out its own major vaccination campaigns.[8] WHO later learned that no new community cases of smallpox in the Tibet (Xizang) Autonomous Region (TAR) were reported after 1960.[9] Many routes existed through the mountains and imported cases of smallpox from Nepal into the TAR in 1962 and 1964 were identified in border areas not far from the Pokhara region.[10]

Candau, drawing on the 1960–61 annual report of the Regional Director to the Regional Committee, noted that 'A vaccination campaign in the area and quarantine restrictions on travellers to and from the affected area soon brought the situation under control'.[11] Disease notifications were listed in WHO's *Weekly Epidemiological*

Record and on 1 April 1961 'West Nepal' was declared a newly infected area.[12] Four cases were notified on 26 March and two deaths on 1 April. A further case was notified for the week 9–15 April.[13] No other cases were recorded, and from 6 September 1961 West Nepal was no longer listed as an infected area.[14]

Government smallpox control activities were organised as part of its communicable disease services, but the government continued to face many challenges as it tried to develop and expand. Other agencies and people also became involved. The WHO in Kathmandu was one of these, but in the Pokhara area in 1961 Christian missions and the Indian Soldiers Board provided a range of health services alongside the limited government activities. Whether the government or another organisation notified the cases of smallpox in 1961 to the WHO, or why only these ones since smallpox existed elsewhere in the country, was not mentioned. Nor was who carried out the vaccination campaign or from where the vaccine came. Dr Graham Scott-Brown joined the Nepal Evangelistic Band in 1960 and 'about' 1961 they ran a 'smallscale' vaccination programme in the villages near Pokhara.[15] The situation with the Tibetans was politically sensitive and in 1961 the International Committee of the Red Cross opened a delegation in Kathmandu to help the refugees. In Pokhara it had a depot for supplies and nearby at Hyangya a transit camp for several hundred refugees.[16]

Candau's gaze was wider than Nepal or the South-East Asia Region. He presented the worldwide situation in the context of slow progress over the previous four years. In 1962 he noted that 'more than ever before concerted action at both national and international levels' was needed.[17] The great majority of cases were from India and Pakistan, but he urged countries that no longer had smallpox to maintain their levels of immunity in the population. 'The international importance of the eradication programme is indicated by the fact that in 1961 and 1962, thirteen importations of smallpox from endemic countries occurred in Europe. A number of these importations led to serious outbreaks.'[18] Candau had raised an important point. Although quarantine had long been an international health focus and people had always travelled, the introduction of air travel made travel times shorter and enabled larger numbers of people to move around the globe. Travel that had taken days or weeks now took hours. The smallpox virus, therefore, could be transported more easily. Not only might it be brought from an endemic country to one that did not have smallpox, but also more people were travelling from non-endemic to endemic countries. By the early 1960s increasing numbers of individual people and groups were beginning to visit Nepal.[19] While people could fly into Kathmandu, much of the rest of their time would be spent travelling on foot along trails and through villages and small towns. These visitors were supported by local Nepalis carrying equipment and supplies.

The Director-General considered that the ability of endemic countries to afford the current smallpox control strategy of a mass vaccination programme varied 'according to the degree of development of the health services concerned'.[20] From this perspective, Nepal would be at the lower end of any scale of ability. Views differ about Candau's level of enthusiasm for smallpox eradication, but 'given a potent vaccine and sufficient funds to implement widespread campaigns it is within the capacity of all those countries to rid themselves of the disease'.[21] Smallpox prevention and control had effective vaccines – especially the newer freeze-dried vaccines that were more stable in warm environments, but the slow progress was due 'in great part to the lack of financial resources'. Candau estimated that

> the sum of $10 million for additional aid for the programme, representing 10 per cent. of the sum of $100 million estimated in 1959 as the total cost is therefore probably reasonably accurate since it is thought that most endemic countries could themselves find 85 to 90 per cent. of the cost.[22]

In other words, by far the greatest financial input had to come from individual countries.[23] The limited WHO funding would be used for transport, equipment and training. No extra funding was voted to support the new initiative; expenditure on smallpox 1959–66 represented just 0.2 per cent of the WHO's regular budget and 0.6 per cent of the total funds at its disposal.[24] In marked contrast, funds for the malaria programme 1959–66 represented 10.8 per cent of WHO's regular budget and 27.2 per cent of all funds at WHO's disposal.[25]

Could smallpox be eradicated? Should resources be directed towards eradication rather than control? Programmes already carried out in both low and high-income countries demonstrated that eradication was technically feasible.[26] The new global programme's objective was 'to maintain the smallpox-free status of all countries already free of the disease, while intensifying existing vaccination efforts in the endemic regions'.[27] Like many places, Ceylon (Sri Lanka) had a resurgence of smallpox during the Second World War but regained control and eliminated endemic smallpox in 1951.[28] Vaccination was carried out as part of general health services. Those in favour argued that if smallpox was eradicated worldwide all the money spent on its control and vaccination would no longer be necessary. Between 1960 and 1965 eradication efforts were intensified worldwide with programmes initiated in Afghanistan, Burma, Nepal, Pakistan, Saudi Arabia, Sudan, Thailand and Yemen, and in several countries in the African Region and the Americas. In India, individual states developed pilot projects before introducing a national smallpox eradication programme in 1962.[29] The USSR provided over five hundred million doses (vaccine required to give one vaccination to one person) of freeze-dried vaccine to India and other countries in Asia and Africa.[30] While the WHO Director-General's report indicated that progress was up and down and slow, the later official history suggested that when 'the situation is viewed in retrospect, it is evident that much was achieved by a number of countries' and that these achievements 'were, however, largely unknown to WHO Headquarters staff, so that the Director-General's reports were perhaps more pessimistic than was warranted'.[31] Approximately 25 per cent of the world's population lived in mainland China where the WHO had later learned about 'the elimination' of smallpox 'in 1961 or thereabouts'.[32]

In New Delhi, Regional Director Mani's focus was on the South-East Asia Region and its member states.[33] While Mani was pleased that communicable disease control was progressing and health services were expanding, he was concerned about weaknesses and deficiencies around many issues such as supervision, staffing, shortages, reporting and records, laboratory services and maintenance.[34] Rapid expansion and low resources led to a proliferation of low-quality services. He wanted the 'special programmes' integrated into basic health services which 'must' be strengthened to absorb them.[35] This could be done programme by programme and might be possible now for malaria, yaws and leprosy which had achieved their objectives. Smallpox would come later. Mani's annual report, therefore, conveyed a message that smallpox was not SEARO's priority. Although smallpox remained widespread, it was part of the general problem of communicable diseases which remained endemic at high levels and demanded 40–50 per cent of the Region's total expenditure for most years.[36]

Cooperation and involvement with WHO through SEARO nevertheless offered a way for Nepal and other member states towards achieving their goals for improvement and better services for their populations. 'In general', Candau commented for smallpox, 'governments in this region have elected to proceed by means of pilot projects to establish methodology and to enable estimates of costs to be determined before embarking on eradication programmes'.[37] In Nepal the government decided to launch a pilot project and approved NRs 60,000. At the end of 1960 it requested WHO assistance. The proposed SEARO programme and budgetary estimates for 1961 included provision in Nepal for two years for a sanitarian (environmental health officer), and $4,000 for supplies and equipment.[38] In August 1961, Dr M. Radovanovic, Regional Adviser on Communicable Disease, made his first visit to Nepal. While part of his short visit was to review the cholera situation since the 1958 outbreak, the other was to assist the government in drafting 'a plan of action' for a Smallpox Control Pilot Project.[39] Radovanovic discovered that there were no statistical data to assist him but learned from the Directorate of Health Services and the Directorate of Statistics that smallpox was endemic throughout the country and periodically epidemic, with the next epidemic expected in spring 1962.

The Smallpox Control Pilot Project – Nepal 9

'There is serious limitation of resources as compared with the enormous need in the field of public health', wrote Radovanovic.[40] 'Public health it would appear', he continued, 'is at present given low priority on account of competing requirements in the fields of agriculture, irrigation, communications, etc.' Following 'detailed' discussions at the Directorate of Health Services, it was agreed that any plan should 'above all, be realistic in terms of achievements'.[41]

Engaging global policy 125

The plan was finalised towards the end of 1961 and began operation in the Kathmandu municipality in February 1962.[42] The Smallpox Control Pilot Project was housed in two rooms of the Singha Durbar Secretariat Building, where importantly there were refrigerators to store vaccine but it was separate from the government's immunisation services. The aim was to create 'a relatively small but solid nucleus of smallpox activities' over the following two years in the Kathmandu Valley.[43] This is key to understanding its significance for implementing the global programme. No project in Nepal yet had the nationwide coverage which would be required if eradication was to succeed. During the first year the pilot would cover the three municipalities of Kathmandu, Lalitpur and Bhaktapur (population 200,877) and four adjacent townships of Thimi, Nakadesh, Deopatan and Kalimati (population about 50,000).[44] In its second year the project would incorporate the remaining 200,000 people in 752 villages together with revaccination in the Valley's urban areas. Revaccination was advised every five years.[45] A final report was to be prepared 'along with draft recommendations for a programme for the years to come'.[46]

Except for the account of Dr Adiga, our view of the pilot is largely through the top-down and outsider lens of the various WHO SEARO documents as we have little else originating from the project, from the government or a wider Nepali perspective.[47] Reports from visiting overseas officials, such as Dr Albert Zahra in May 1962, commonly noted the need to gain 'first-hand experience' of the situation in Nepal.[48] The significance of this bias in the sources is illustrated by the differing conclusions drawn. From a regional perspective the pilot in Nepal was a very small part of SEARO's overall work. When it was mentioned in the official history, the verdict was that the 'programme was poorly funded, poorly supervised and poorly executed and with the additional impediment of resistance to vaccination progress was slow'.[49] In Nepal, the authors of the 1969 Directorate of Health Services report took a different view and commented that the 'operations of the pilot project proved very successful'.[50] It was the Valley's largest communicable disease programme – and therefore Nepal's; it had improved the situation and was being extended in phases to other parts of the country.

The first stage in implementing the pilot was for the government and WHO to meet 'their respective commitments' for the joint project as outlined in the plan of operations.[51] In Radovanovic's draft, August to November 1961 was designated the 'preparation phase'. Family registers were to be completed, equipment, supplies and transport assembled, personnel trained and health education and publicity undertaken.[52] This would be followed by a vaccination programme. The plan was ambitious. The greater 'commitment' came from the Government, which provided one medical officer, Dr Tej Lal (T. L.) Shrestha, one part-time health educator, Chiranjibi B. Thapa, one chief inspector, Chini Kaji Sthapit who was a sanitarian, five sanitarian-aides, as vaccination inspectors, twenty-five vaccinators (nineteen male, six female), three clerks, two peons (the lowest rank in the health bureaucracy) and one driver.[53] In line with support given elsewhere, WHO's smaller commitment was one overseas male public health nurse (L. Ramos), 100,000 doses of freeze-dried vaccine and one vehicle.[54] Lymph vaccine was to be used in urban areas as this could be stored, while the vaccine to be supplied by WHO was to be used in the villages. Following their recruitment, the inspectors and vaccinators received a one-week intensive training course in vaccination techniques, recording and reporting before commencing vaccinating children in schools.

Zahra's report provides considerable information about the project and its operation during the first three months and is useful for setting the scene. Before and after vaccination activities the health educator and other project staff carried out health education and publicity with assistance from the Ministry of Health's health education unit. As the Valley had some roads, a mobile van with loudspeaker, suitable posters and films could be used as well as the press and radio where available. A total of 15,174 vaccinations were given during the period. Each municipality was geographically divided into neighbourhoods (*tol*), each tol into blocks and each block into groups of houses. With assistance from the Directorate of Statistics and 1961 census information, project staff designed and completed 'a useful' family register. The vaccinator then filled in the names and ages of any other household members, past vaccinations, pock marks, type of vaccination carried out at the visit (primary or revaccination) and batch number of the vaccine used. Despite the initial intention to use liquid vaccine, Zahra wrote that only freeze-dried vaccine was used.[55] It was given by the multiple pressure method and Zahra observed the vaccination technique was used correctly 'and the vaccinators seen at work were using it with confidence'. Each inspector allotted the weekly work to his team of five vaccinators, supervised their work and checked, with the help of the completed household register, on all their vaccinations by revisiting the house on the third or fourth day to read the results of the revaccinations and on the eighth or ninth day after the primary vaccinations. He also vaccinated previous absentees, whenever possible. The results were then recorded. The inspectors read 12,802 (84 per cent) of the vaccinations performed and of these 11,949 (93 per cent) were reported as successful 'takes'. 'This indicated a potent vaccine and a satisfactory vaccination technique.'

From WHO's perspective, the daily average of ten vaccinations per vaccinator was low. Project objectives would not be achieved 'unless the vaccination coverage is raised to over 80 per cent, preferably to over 90 per cent, in view of the fact that the teams are working in a densely populated urban area in which smallpox has long been endemic'.[56] Suggestions, such as intensifying health education and publicity and simplifying the way the teams worked, were made, but when Radovanovic visited to review the first year's achievements and discuss the second year he was similarly concerned with the low coverage. Although he had thought the targets to be realistic, only about 20 per cent had been achieved. The average output of seven to ten vaccinations daily was 'definitely disquieting'.[57]

Some of these points had been made in Zahra's earlier report, with little progress seeming to have been made since then. Discussions with project staff revealed several issues. The initial project leader had left for a fellowship abroad and his replacement was about to do likewise, but no replacement had yet been made. Frequent staff transfers were a general and ongoing problem. The project was also waiting for the appointment of five more vaccinators and one inspector, but it was also proving difficult to keep good vaccinators in view of the permitted salary scale and that no daily allowance was possible. Vaccinators had to be taken by car from their residences to place of work, which in the case of Bhaktapur was seven or eight miles. Given the poor state of the roads, this was no easy journey. From local people's perspectives, the vaccinators were not identifiable and vaccination times clashed with when they were at work. In discussion with the Director and Deputy Director of Health Services it was agreed to have smaller vaccination field teams who would wear uniforms, and vaccination times would change to a morning session and an evening one when most people would be at home. Appointments would be expedited, and action was to be initiated about daily allowances as this would be 'particularly important when the project activities were expanded to rural areas'. Director Baidya also asked 'that possibilities of assigning a WHO medical officer to the project be explored'.

The pilot project was running into problems and already behind schedule. It was agreed that for year two activities should continue to be carried out in the three municipalities and that project sub-headquarters should be established at Lalitpur and at Bhaktapur. Both should be in hospitals, and that the medical officers and other staff would assist. Approval was needed for extra staff, but each municipality would have two inspectors and ten vaccinators. Although the focus would continue to be the urban areas, 'preliminary experience' of working in rural areas should be obtained by covering a few nearby villages in the Lalitpur and Bhaktapur areas. Finally, project staff would submit 'a comprehensive review' of the project's first year to the Directorate and WHO at the end of March 1963 and a follow-up report on action taken on the points made in his report would be given to the government and the WHO 'towards the end of June 1963'. The next WHO field visit was in October/November 1964, but Dr Vichniakov's report did not mention the receipt of any reports arising from the previous visit.[58] By this time, however, D. N. Baidya had been replaced as Director and Dr Bharat Raj (B. R.) Baidya was acting Director.

Dr Adiga's paper was written around this time.[59] Once the epidemic in the Thimi area was under control, the pilot project continued activities with its normal staffing complement. Much of the paper was devoted to practical issues such as method of operation, people's beliefs and vaccination acceptability. Adiga was the son of a former High Priest at the holiest of Hindu temples of Pashputinath on the bank of the Bagmati River. He analysed people's responses in different villages and considered that educational level was more important than religion or community. Success against smallpox could be achieved in a few years, he believed, through a multifactorial approach of legislation, health education 'propaganda', panchayats at all levels acknowledging their responsibilities towards controlling infectious disease, air transport for difficult terrain, dedicated workers who must be supported and a seasonal programme avoiding the difficulties of the rainy season.[60]

Vichniakov did not mention Adiga. Interestingly, given the subsequent lack of official recognition of the epidemic, Vichniakov set the scene for his report by writing that the last major outbreak of smallpox in Nepal was in the Kathmandu Valley at the end of 1963 and that there were no statistical records.[61] The evidence for the existence of widespread smallpox was visual. The percentage of people in the valley with pock marks ranged from 2.4 in infants and 14.1 in adults, making an overall average of 10.8 per cent. Of the 798 people Vichniakov examined, he observed that 103 had pock marks (12.9 per cent). Allowing for those who would have died, he estimated that 'at least a seventh or eighth of the total population in the valley suffer from smallpox'. He also reported that a 'good number' of people with pock marks on their faces can be seen in 'many areas' of the country.

Little appeared to have changed. The project office was still situated in two rooms in Singha Durbar and no mention was made of any sub-headquarters. As the initial WHO nurse had finished in October 1963 and T. O. Crisp, a WHO sanitarian, started with the project in January 1964, it appears that there were no WHO staff involved with smallpox in Kathmandu at the peak of the epidemic in November/December. National staff had increased in number from thirty-six to forty-two, indicating that the previously suggested new positions had been sanctioned. Unfortunately, the health educator had been assigned to the Malaria Eradication Organization 'for a few months'. All staff, including the vaccinators, were still working without uniforms. While he observed that only the multiple pressure technique was being used and that it was being done correctly, his description of the method of work suggests that some of the recommendations to simplify procedures also had not been implemented. Although the figures indicated that the daily number of vaccinations done by each vaccinator had increased to thirty-seven, Vichniakov observed an average of six to eight per vaccinator per day. 'This low output of work by the project staff does not require further emphasis.' The vaccination figures and percentage of immunological coverage of the population of the valley were also still of concern. Although the vaccinated and revaccinated rates were better for children than adults, from random samples of family registers even the greatest success of 53.6 per cent in Bhaktapur was still well below the target 'if smallpox is to be controlled'. As with previous field visits, the discussion and recommendations followed the lines of 'further and constant' efforts required to raise vaccination coverage if they were to meet the target. Proper storage of the vaccine was also a concern.

Looking to the future, Vichniakov discussed with the Director of Health Services about extending the programme to other areas but learned that plans were underway already. The Director indicated that the most suitable area for such expansion was the Rapti valley and that this programme would have its own staff and start in mid-1965.[62] While road communications with other parts of the country were 'poorly developed', two 'jeepable roads' ran from the area which was near the main road from Kathmandu south to the Indian border and potential economic markets. Formerly 'a malarial and largely uninhabited expanse of jungle famed for big-game hunting', the Rapti valley had become the focus of much (particularly US-supported) development activity including better health services.[63] Vichniakov had visited Hitaura health centre where the sanitarian informed him that 'there should be no great resistance to a vaccination campaign in the Rapti valley'.[64] Between April 1963 and April 1964 he had visited 38 villages and given a total of 8,878 vaccinations – a rate, as Vichniakov commented, that was higher than the project area. Rather than house-to-house visits, people came to 'collecting points' such as schools, bazaars and meeting places. As discussed in Chapter 4, this timeframe also coincided with the presence in Nepal of epidemic smallpox and extra US-organised supplies of freeze-dried vaccine.

A few months later, in March–April 1965, Vichniakov returned to lead a team of WHO and national staff in an assessment and evaluation of the project.[65] The team comprised Vichniakov, Dr T. L. Shrestha (Directorate of Health Services), Crisp (WHO smallpox control officer) and Sthapit (Smallpox Control Pilot Project).[66] The evaluation was not unexpected. Unlike the later totally negative interpretation of the project in the official history, the report noted some positive aspects. For example, the project had adequate freeze-dried vaccine and vaccinator kits. These, as Vichniakov listed in his earlier report came from various sources.[67] Although a donation of lymph vaccine was received from India, no mention was made of using it. Had adequate supplies not been obtained for a project in the Kathmandu Valley, later expansion of activities nationwide would have been even more challenging as Kathmandu was the central distribution point. Although the project's experience with its vehicle was presented more negatively, in the wider context of transport in Nepal it should not have been a surprise. At the beginning the project had an old Land Rover, but from the end of 1963 it no longer worked. A vehicle was then obtained on loan from the malaria programme and in April 1965 WHO supplied a new Land Rover. The Senior Supervisor used the one lightweight motorcycle while each of the seven supervisors had a bicycle. In practice, as Nepal had so few roads, using vehicles would not be the way to carry out a nationwide vaccination programme.

The team looked at the success rate among revaccinated people in a technical college and a girls' school. In both, students had been vaccinated or revaccinated during the first year of the project and were now being revaccinated. The average success rate of 61.4 per cent was considered high and the team concluded that the vaccination technique was correct and the vaccine potent. The family registers were found to be up to date. Project staff adopted two main approaches to community vaccination – house-to-house visits and vaccination of organised groups at collecting points (schools, colleges, government and private offices, clinics and block posts on the main roads leading into the city). Sufficient family register forms were printed in advance and then filled in by the vaccinators as part of their day-to-day work. When the project was assessed, vaccination staff were visiting households for the third time to complete repeat primary vaccinations and to revaccinate as many members of the families as possible.

Between 6 March 1962 and 27 March 1965, project staff vaccinated 325,489 people (Figure 5.1).[68] During the course of the assessment, it became clear that the figures represented the volume of work rather than people needing to be vaccinated. The assessment team visited households and examined 493 people. They also incorporated information from the family registers and believed that they had a sample that would 'represent the community as a whole'. They found that of the people requiring primary vaccination, 61.2 per cent had been vaccinated since the launching of the

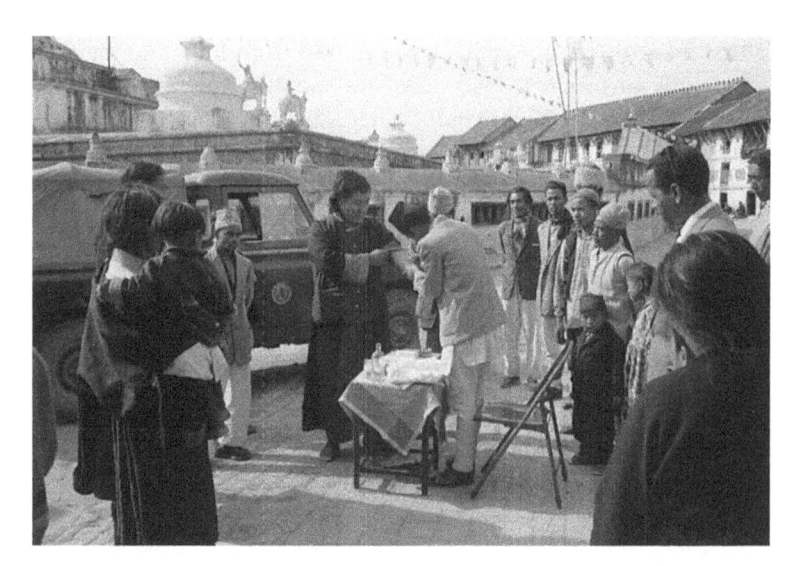

Figure 5.1 A vaccination team near Boudhanath Stupa, a place of pilgrimage in the Kathmandu Valley. The first person to be vaccinated was a lama.
Source: © World Health Organization/Philip Boucas, 1965.

project with the highest rates of the unvaccinated being in the very young or older age groups. Only 58.6 per cent of those requiring revaccination had been done during the same period with the highest rate in the five to fourteen years group. The level of coverage (the percentage of those successfully vaccinated or revaccinated) had been a major concern of SEARO since the earliest field visit report. Immunological coverage by the project vaccinators was found to be only 54.4 per cent, while immunological protection (the percentage of persons protected by successful vaccination, revaccination, or an attack of smallpox) was higher at 65.7 per cent. The examination findings were compared against the family registers and were 'very close to the figure found by the assessment team in the field'.

Overall, the team concluded that the level of immunological coverage and protection was inadequate and that 'further energetic efforts are required to achieve the target of 100% primary successful vaccinations and 85–90 per cent revaccinations'. The higher targets reflected the view of the WHO's Expert Committee on Smallpox which considered that the lower accepted target of 80 per cent was sometimes insufficient.[69] Again illustrating the importance of acknowledging that the Government and WHO operated with different perspectives, the evaluation report – despite government plans to extend the smallpox programme – recommended keeping all project staff in the Valley until targets had been reached and gave suggestions as to how to improve people's acceptance. Most of the world's cases came from the South-East Asia Region, although each country differed considerably; India reported the largest number of cases, while smallpox had almost disappeared from Thailand. Progress was variable in each country. Regional Director Mani was cautious, therefore, about plans in Nepal to extend the existing programme. 'Owing to insufficient resources, and the difficulty of communications, this may take a longer time.'[70]

In 1966, following the visit of a short-term WHO consultant Dr David Yarom from Israel, the previously entitled Smallpox Control Pilot Project was developed into a revised plan of operation for Smallpox Eradication and Control of Other Communicable Disease. It was signed by the Government on 4 November and WHO on 25 November, superseding the 1962 plan and an addendum in 1965.[71]

A local initiative: vaccination in Morang and Sunsari Districts

A key element that was emerging as important in Nepal was the use of panchayat vaccinators. In Yarom's draft plan, overall policy and planning was retained at Directorate level in Kathmandu but also aligned with the wider administrative reorganisation taking place in the country which had been divided into seven areas each with two zones. Yarom considered that the 'Ministry's acceptance of wider use of panchayat workers is an important step towards a wide acceptance of the eradication programme' and wrote of their 'better sense of community participation and a possibility of their use in health education'.[72] The panchayat vaccinators were partially paid by local village councils, but government vaccinators were also to be recruited and trained locally. Supervisory staff would be drawn from existing staff as well as recruited. Although not referred to in any of the WHO or project reports, the Lamjung vaccination campaign in early 1964 had operated closely with the local panchayat.

The non-project smallpox campaign that SEARO was aware of was in Kosi (or Koshi) zone where in 1965 vaccinators in Morang and Sunsari districts in the Tarai were recruited from among primary school teachers who received a short training in two government hospitals. 'It is of importance to note here', wrote Yarom, 'that teachers or persons carrying authority in their own surroundings prove to be much more efficient in vaccinations and could protect around a 100 persons a day.'[73] This was vastly better than the experiences of the pilot operating out of the Kathmandu Valley. Stiller and Yadav did not use health services as an example in their study of planning development, but the contents of early issues of the *JNMA* provide an overview of topics, ideas, and activities.[74] First published in September 1963, the journal wanted to reach all doctors as health services in Nepal continued their nationwide expansion. As noted in Chapter 1, the authors of a 1966 article wrote that success for the smallpox eradication programme required 'active' community participation and of the 'very encouraging' result of utilising locally recruited vaccinators in the programme tried in the Morang and Sunsari districts the previous year.[75]

We know much more about this campaign from the autobiography of Dr Prasai.[76] His account provides a rich description of the plan and the wider context of how 'things' operated in Nepal. In 1965, when an outbreak of smallpox occurred in the districts of Morang and Sunsari, Prasai was a junior medical officer at Biratnagar, the Morang district centre. In his previous posting at Doti (Seti zone) in the Far-Western region of the country, 'I had seen a small outbreak of smallpox that had taken the lives of many children. No action had been taken by the government to bring that under control.' Despite the many challenges, Prasai thought that if other countries could eradicate smallpox, 'then why not in Nepal?' Being 'encouraged by such an experienced senior officer' as Dr B. R. Baidya, who had been Prasai's former chief at Biratnagar Hospital and was now acting Director of Health Services based in Kathmandu, Prasai set out to develop a plan. He went to see Dr Buddhi Man (B. M.) Shrestha, a dental surgeon, whose relative Dil Bahadur (D. B.) Shrestha of Sunsar was Minister of Health. 'On the basis of that relationship' they sought the support of the Minister for the proposal to vaccinate all children in Morang and Sunsari over a period of three to four months. 'Things worked out the way we had hoped.'

Engaging global policy 135

In May, the Biratnagar Branch of the NMA decided to launch a 'compulsory vaccination programme' against smallpox on market days 'in and around' Biratnagar and the Rani Mills Area.[77] This began on 9 June and 'about 2000' people were vaccinated. The programme was to last initially for a month but 'with a view to extend the period if necessary'. In September, the Branch resolved 'unanimously' that Prasai and B. M. Shrestha, should prepare 'a comprehensive plan' to combat the 'annual epidemic' of smallpox in Morang district to submit to the zilla (district) panchayat.[78] As a reminder that smallpox was not the only public health issue, a second resolution similarly was passed unanimously for all members 'to actively extend their co-operation in the inoculation programme' to combat the 'present' epidemic of cholera. At the October meeting, the Health Minister, D. B. Shrestha, expressed his support and offered 'all possible' government assistance. The Branch approved the plan in November and authorised Prasai and B. M. Shrestha to implement it.[79]

The vaccination programme was to take place in all the village panchayats in both districts and would be coordinated by the Biratnagar Branch of the NMA, of which Prasai was secretary.[80] The District Officer agreed to provide the 'necessary support' for the programme and his administration would inform the village panchayats to 'also cooperate accordingly'. District panchayat administration at Dharan and Biratnagar would cooperate with the training centres sited there and issue the 'necessary directives' to the village panchayats. Each was to select someone who had passed class eight or 'if possible, a school teacher' and send them to Biratnagar Hospital for training. On completion, they would be sent to the vaccination centres set up in each village panchayat and would go out to the different villages with vaccine to vaccinate the children. Each village was to pay fifty paise for each child vaccinated and the village panchayat would pay a total of Rs 300 to each vaccinator for their services.[81] The 'minimum' requirements for the programme were 'evenly distributed' among the concerned village panchayats, district panchayats, municipality, Medical Association and the hospital. The plan also gained the support of Dr Damber Bahadur Karki, the Medical Officer at Dharan Hospital. The Department of Health Services gave permission to use Biratnagar and Dharan hospitals as vaccinator training centres with Karki, B. M. Shrestha and Prasai as instructors. Out of the 116 vaccinators trained, eleven were female.[82] 'All the plans were in place, but the main problem was the supply of vaccines.'[83] This was to be provided by the WHO through the Department of Health Services, but a change of leadership occurred in Kathmandu. Baidya was transferred from the post of Acting Director back to Biratnagar and Dr Mahendra Prasad was appointed Director. 'As these two individuals were not on good terms, we thought it most likely that the new Director would not give support to what we were about to start and perhaps even stop it. Such action was a likely possibility in the Nepal of those days.'[84] Before the end of the training programme, 300,000 doses of vaccine were requested, but they only received 20,000 doses 'which were totally inadequate'. It should be noted that the WHO only supplied 200,000 doses for the whole country. Prasai sent further letters to the Director for vaccines, 'which annoyed him'. 'Our plan of action to vaccinate all the children of our area did not tally with the plans of Singha Durbar.'[85] Nevertheless, Prasai and his colleagues were not the only people in Kathmandu concerned that Nepal needed more vaccine. A team, including doctors from the Department of Health Services, the Public Health Officer, Dr Bainetya Nanda (B. N.) Vaidya, and Vichniakov from SEARO went to Biratnagar on 10 December.[86] They visited the areas where the programme had started operating 'and were impressed', recorded the Branch News. 'The training imparted to the vaccinators, the organisation and the efficiency of the vaccinators were appreciated and they have assured us of all possible help required to make this project a success.'[87] They also reported that the plan should not be restricted to Sunsari and Morang 'but should be carried out all over the country'. Those who had opposed the request for 300,000 doses of vaccine, writes Prasai, 'were at a loss for words'.[88] The project became a reality, but unfortunately no further accounts of the project were reported in the Biratnagar Branch News after Prasai left for London on 30 December to undertake higher studies in clinical pathology.[89] A 1967 field report from SEARO's Smallpox Eradication and Epidemiological Advisory Team referred to 'the inspiring leadership of the zonal medical officer and the dentist'.[90] Since December 1965, panchayat vaccinators had carried out 210,000 vaccinations and that government vaccinators were now 'mopping up' and completing vaccinations in the remaining parts of the districts.

Conclusion

Despite the WHA's global commitment to smallpox eradication, little funding was provided for the WHO to undertake this work meaning that implementation became the responsibility of member states. Smallpox remained widespread within the South-East Asia Region, but it was viewed as part of the wider problem of high levels of communicable diseases.

Despite the ongoing concerns around the level of coverage, the Smallpox Control Pilot Project begun in early 1962 in the Kathmandu Valley provided the foundation for the implementation of the WHO's global smallpox programme in Nepal. It began as a limited small control project with the aim of building up a core of activities from which it could later expand. Working through SEARO, both the WHO and the government gained from their joint involvement – the former through experience on the ground of conditions in Nepal and the latter through being able to access resources and expertise and to offer increased health activities. Both drew different conclusions from the project, reiterating the importance of considering the implementation of the worldwide smallpox programme from multiple perspectives.

The pilot only operated in three districts in the Kathmandu Valley and so other vaccination activities continued elsewhere in Nepal. These came under the responsibility of the local medical officer, but with few resources were mostly limited. A small supply of vaccine was one barrier; Nepal did not produce its own vaccine and was dependent on external sources. The Morang and Sunsari district project, however, showed that the initiative and drive did not have to come from an overseas organisation, from central government or from Kathmandu. Wider community involvement and support was important. This initiative drew on different personnel, implemented training and addressed funding issues, but most importantly its vaccinators had a much higher daily rate of activity. It showed what was possible.

Notes

1 These dates coincide with the operation of the pilot project.
2 Dixit, *Nepal's Quest for Health* (2014), pp. 156–7.
3 Whelpton, *A History of Nepal*, p. 79.
4 Prasai, *Afu Lai Farkera Hereko* (Looking Back at Oneself), p. 139.
5 SEA/Smallpox/8, Vichniakov, Field visit report 1964, p. 7.
6 World Health Assembly, 15 (1962), Smallpox eradication: report by the Director-General, World Health Organization https://apps.who.int/iris/handle/10665/135762.
7 WHA 15, Smallpox eradication: report by the Director-General, p. 11.
8 Chen, 'China in the worldwide eradication of smallpox'.
9 WHO/SE/79.151, World Health Organization, 'Smallpox eradication in the Autonomous Region of Tibet in the People's Republic of China' https://iris.who.int/handle/10665/68284.
10 Fenner et al., *Smallpox and Its Eradication*, pp. 1258–9.
11 WHA 15, Smallpox eradication: report by the Director-General, p. 13. See also WHO SEARO, SEA/RC15/2, Fourteenth annual report of the Regional Director to the Regional Committee for South-East Asia, p. 10 https://apps.who.int/iris/handle/10665/130700.
12 WER, 36:15 (14 April 1961), p. 158.
13 WER, 36:16 (21 April 1961), p. 169.
14 WER, 36:36 (8 September 1961), p. 95; WHO, *Epidemiological and Vital Statistics Report*, 16:4 (1963), p. 284.
15 Dr Graham Scott-Brown, email communication with author, 10 August 2017. Their archives are limited for this period.
16 International Committee of the Red Cross, *International Review of the Red Cross* 22 (1963), pp. 17–18.
17 WHA 15, Smallpox eradication: report by the Director-General, p. 1.
18 *Ibid.*, p. 2. In Britain vaccination and revaccination rates were low, although increased in areas when cases of the disease occurred. Millward, *Vaccinating Britain*, chapter 2. Vaccination in the USA was not routine and most of the population was unprotected, including Henderson's family. Scabs in the refrigerator, www.zero-pox.info/more.htm (accessed 4 April 2018). They were vaccinated before they left for Geneva.
19 The Department of Tourism began keeping statistics about the tourist numbers from 1962 when there were 6,179 arrivals. Hari Prasad Shrestha and Prami Shrestha, 'Tourism in Nepal: A historical perspective and present trend of development', *Himalayan Journal of Sociology & Anthropology*, V (2012), 54–75.
20 WHA 15, Smallpox eradication: report by the Director-General, p. 2.

Engaging global policy 139

21 *Ibid.*
22 *Ibid.*, p. 20.
23 Bhattacharya highlights India's financial challenges at the time. Bhattacharya, *Expunging Variola*, pp. 71–2.
24 Fenner et al., *Smallpox and Its Eradication*, p. 384.
25 *Ibid.*, p. 382.
26 See for example in Bolivia: Harald Frederiksen, Nemesio Torres Munoz and Alfredo Jauregui Molina, 'Smallpox eradication', *Public Health Reports*, 75:9 (1959), 771–8.
27 WHO, *The Second Ten Years of the World Health Organization, 1958–1967* (Geneva: World Health Organization, 1968), p. 106.
28 Fenner et al., *Smallpox and Its Eradication*, p. 348.
29 Basu, Jezek and Ward, *The Eradication of Smallpox from India*, p. 21.
30 WHO, *The Second Ten Years*, p. 106.
31 Fenner et al., *Smallpox and Its Eradication*, pp. 403–5.
32 *Ibid.*, p. 404.
33 In 1962 the People's Republic of Mongolia became a member.
34 SEA/RC15/2, Fourteenth annual report of the Regional Director, p. vii.
35 *Ibid.*, p. viii.
36 WHO, *The Second Ten Years*, p. 17.
37 World Health Assembly, 17 (1964), Smallpox eradication: Report by the Director-General, World Health Organization. https://apps.who.int/iris/handle/10665/136501 (accessed 4 February 2019).
 In Indonesia eradication plans were not yet envisaged, while Thailand operated a countrywide vaccination campaign.
38 WHO SEARO, SEA/RC12/3 Proposed programme and budget estimates for 1961, 1959. https://apps.who.int/iris/handle/10665/204573 (accessed 6 February 2019).
39 SEA/CD/8, Radovanovic, Report on field visit to Nepal 1961, p. 1. A vacancy existed for a second position.
40 *Ibid.*
41 *Ibid.*, p. 2.
42 SEA/WHO, SEA/Smallpox/4, Dr A. Zahra, Field visit report on Smallpox Control Pilot Project, Nepal, WHO Project: Nepal 9, 23–26 May 1962, 10 August 1962, p. 3.
43 SEA/CD/8, Radovanovic, Report on field visit to Nepal 1961, p. 1.
44 *Ibid.*, p. 2.
45 World Health Organization. (1959). Smallpox vaccination technique. Geneva, Switzerland; World Health Organization https://apps.who.int/iris/handle/10665/67140 (accessed 3 March 2019).
46 SEA/CD/8, Radovanovic, Report on field visit to Nepal 1961, p. 2.

47 Adiga, 'Smallpox epidemic in Nepal (1963–1964)'.
48 SEA/Smallpox/4, Zahra, Field visit report on Smallpox Control Pilot Project, 1962, p. 1.
49 Fenner et al., *Smallpox and Its Eradication*, p. 795.
50 Report on health and health administration in Nepal 1969, p. 62.
51 SEA/Smallpox/4, Zahra, Field visit report on Smallpox Control Pilot Project 1962, p. 1.
52 SEA/CD/8, Radovanovic, Report on field visit to Nepal 1961, p. 3.
53 For the important role of the peon see Judithanne Justice, 'The invisible worker: The role of the peon in Nepal's health service', *Social Science & Medicine*, 17:14 (1983), 967–70.
54 SEA/CD/8, Radovanovic, Report on field visit to Nepal 1961, pp. 4, 5.
55 WHO/Smallpox/9, Smallpox vaccination technique, 3 July 1959.
56 SEA/Smallpox/4, Zahra, Field visit report on Smallpox Control Pilot Project 1962, p. 3.
57 SEA/WHO, SEA/Smallpox/5, Dr M. R. Radovanovic, Regional Adviser on Communicable Diseases, Field visit report on Smallpox Control Pilot Project, Nepal WHO Project: Nepal 9, 25–7 February 1963, 22 March 1963, p. 2.
58 SEA/WHO, SEA/Smallpox/8, Dr V. E. Vichniakov, WHO Medical Officer, Field visit report on Smallpox Control Pilot Project, Nepal WHO Project: Nepal 9, 22 October–5 November 1964, 9 March 1965.
59 Adiga, 'Smallpox epidemic in Nepal (1963–1964)'.
60 *Ibid.*, p. 9.
61 SEA/Smallpox/8, Vichniakov, Field visit report on Smallpox Control Pilot Project 1964.
62 *Ibid.*, Vichniakov, Field visit report on Smallpox Control Pilot Project 1964, p. 9. In 1960 this area was considered for part of the pilot project. SEA/PHA/15, Nath, Assignment report on assistance to Central Health Directorate 1960, p. 11.
63 Mihaly, *Foreign Aid and Politics in Nepal*, p. 89.
64 SEA/Smallpox/8, Vichniakov, Field visit report on Smallpox Control Pilot Project 1964, p. 7.
65 SEA/WHO, SEA/Smallpox/9, Dr V. E. Vichniakov, WHO Medical Officer, Assessment and evaluation of the Smallpox Control Pilot Project in Kathmandu Valley by a team of WHO and national staff (WHO Project: Nepal 9), March–April 1965, 18 March 1966. Vichniakov, along with Zahra and Radovanovic, was involved with some of the evaluation of the Indian pilot projects. I am grateful to Namrata Ganneri for this information.
66 Shrestha was the initial pilot project medical officer.

Engaging global policy 141

67 SEA/Smallpox/8, Vichniakov, Field visit report on Smallpox Control Pilot Project 1964, p. 4.
68 SEA/Smallpox/9, Vichniakov, Assessment and evaluation of the Smallpox Control Pilot Project 1965, p. 3. Some vaccinations were carried out outside the Valley, but numbers are unclear as no other information is given. The figures in a table in Shrestha, Robinson and Friedman's analysis and the official history are different again.
69 World Health Organization, *WHO Expert Committee on Smallpox: First Report* (Geneva: WHO Technical Report Series no. 283, 1964), p. 26. Dixon was rapporteur.
70 WHO SEARO, Seventeenth annual report of the Regional Director, p. 14.
71 SEA/WHO, File 447, Box 185, Revised plan of operation for Smallpox Eradication and Control of Other Communicable Diseases, Nepal (Previous title: Smallpox Control Pilot Project), p. 1. For Nepal, the plan of operation also included the control of other communicable diseases.
72 SEA/WHO, File SPX–1, Box 544, Dr David Yarom, WHO short-term consultant on smallpox eradication, Draft report on a visit to Nepal, 7–28 August 1966, p. 11.
73 Yarom, Draft report on a visit to Nepal 1966, p. 9. No mention is made about vaccine, but a note in pencil in the margin asks what vaccine is used.
74 Stiller and Yadav, *Planning for People*.
75 Vaidya and Gurubacharya, 'On smallpox'. Gurubacharya was project chief in 1966–67.
76 Prasai, *Afu Lai Farkera Hereko* (Looking Back at Oneself), pp. 139–43. I am again very grateful to Professor Hemang Dixit for bringing this to my attention and for his translation. Professor Dixit also followed up with Dr D. B. Karki, 6 June 2023.
77 Biratnagar Branch News, *JNMA*, Suppl 3:3 (1965), 13.
78 *Ibid.*, Suppl 3:4 (1965), 17.
79 *Ibid.*, Suppl 4:1 (1966), iv.
80 See also Dixit, *Fifty Years of NMA*.
81 100 paise to 1 Nepali rupee.
82 Biratnagar Branch News, *JNMA*, Suppl 4:1 (1966), v.
83 Prasai, *Afu Lai Farkera Hereko* (Looking Back at Oneself), pp. 139–43.
84 *Ibid.*
85 *Ibid.*
86 Biratnagar Branch News, *JNMA*, Suppl 4:1 (1966), iv. Vaidya was subsequently the first author of an article in the *JNMA*. Vaidya and Gurubacharya, 'On smallpox'.

87 Biratnagar Branch News, *JNMA*, Suppl 4:1 (1966), v.
88 Prasai, *Afu Lai Farkera Hereko* (Looking Back at Oneself), pp. 139–43.
89 Biratnagar Branch News, *JNMA*, Suppl 4:1 (1966), v.
90 SEA/WHO, File SEARO 30, Box 211, Dr J. Keja and Dr F. G. L. Gremliza, Smallpox Eradication & Epidemiological Advisory Team, Quarterly field report second quarter 1967, 1 July 1967.

6

Vaccination and global strategies

Vaccination lay at the centre of the global smallpox programme. Although the goal changed from disease control to disease eradication and the strategy later shifted away from mass vaccination to surveillance and containment, vaccination remained important throughout. Rather than aiming to vaccinate everyone, surveillance and containment – or 'ring' vaccination – involved the active searching for cases, rigorous isolation of cases and vaccination and surveillance of close contacts to contain outbreaks.[1] Scientific knowledge about smallpox was increasing and therapies investigated, but the situation remained that the disease could be prevented but not cured. In Nepal, some groups were perceived as 'resistant' or 'against' vaccination, but in practice most Nepalis accepted it – and irrespective of whether it was global policy or whether the aim was control or eradication. People's ideas might differ, but in general most thought that smallpox vaccination worked; when the disease was present in a community vaccination was even more acceptable. Health services were expanding by the early 1960s, but, as discussed in earlier chapters, vaccination was still not available for most people. Eradication as a strategy had general features in its favour because smallpox was a disease with no intermediate host and effective vaccines existed, but any scaling up of a programme in Nepal would face enormous implementation challenges.

Why did the change from control to global eradication matter? While control is the reduction of a disease to an acceptable level, eradication is the permanent removal worldwide. A control programme requires continued intervention measures, but after a successful eradication programme they are no longer necessary.[2] In 1962 WHO Director-General Candau appealed to member states that no longer had a problem with smallpox to keep up their level of immunity, saying that this expense would no longer be necessary if smallpox was eradicated.[3] Inevitably, seeking to find every last case worldwide would require a higher level of focus and effort from those involved in implementing the programme. In 1965, as the Eighteenth WHA discussed a 'comprehensive plan for a global eradication programme', existing smallpox programmes were national programmes.[4] They varied enormously. Smallpox was widespread in Nepal, but it probably made little difference whether the goal was control or eradication and whether it was with or without outside assistance or direction as Nepal was not yet in a position to implement any nationwide programme.

During most of the 1960s the worldwide smallpox strategy was to vaccinate as many people as possible to achieve a level of herd immunity within a population that interrupted the transmission of the virus and inhibited spread of the disease. That could be achieved as an integral and routine part of a country's health services (horizontal approach) or as a separate mass vaccination programme (vertical approach) initiated often at the time of an outbreak.[5] Smallpox vaccines existed in different forms; lymph vaccines, however, were cheaper to produce than the newer dried vaccines, but the latter were more stable in warmer climates. Vaccine quality, distribution and techniques of administration were also improving. Nevertheless, until 1967–68, neither the potency nor the methods of vaccination were standardised making it difficult to estimate efficacy or how long protection lasted.[6] Since its introduction, vaccination acceptance, as numerous studies have noted, varied between and within countries. As Greenough, Blume and Holmberg write in their comparative study, mass immunisation 'should not be considered a neutral practice'. A country's capacity to produce its own vaccine has 'frequently played a role in building and sustaining national sovereignty'.[7] Nepal had to rely on outside sources for vaccine.

This chapter argues that issues concerning smallpox vaccination and vaccination behaviour could be both separate and linked and need to be considered as such. Faulty vaccine, for example, was related to technical aspects of the vaccine and problems of storage and distribution in Nepal, but these issues also influenced people's attitudes to vaccination and how they responded. The chapter is in two parts. The first considers the vaccine and takes a logistics approach. Broadly, thinking logistically means considering not only vaccine and vaccine supply, but also that the vaccine needed to be in the right place at the right time.[8] To achieve eradication in Nepal an adequate supply of an appropriate vaccine was required, and this then had to be distributed throughout the country so that people could be vaccinated. Smallpox logistics would be considered critical to the successful implementation of the intensified global programme after 1967.[9] This section shows that logistics was important before 1967 and the many challenges affected plans for developing the programme in Nepal after 1967. Later success was built on the earlier struggles which had to be overcome or worked around. The second part of the chapter discusses vaccination acceptance in the 1960s and explores people's attitudes and practices. Success would only be achieved if people who needed vaccination were vaccinated. Vaccination behaviour was – and remains – complex and multi-faceted and requires a more 'sensitive' approach beyond acceptance and non-acceptance. Social scientist Pieter Streefland and colleagues suggested a framework of acceptance, social demand and non-acceptance.[10] Particularly helpful is the concept of 'vaccine hesitancy', which recognises a continuum of attitudes and practices and acknowledges that 'hesitant' people may 'refuse some vaccines, but agree to others, delay vaccines, or accept vaccines but are unsure of doing so'.[11] Being hesitant was – and is – not the same as refusal.

Smallpox logistics

A mass vaccination campaign required a suitable vaccine and method of delivery, an appropriate supply, a storage and distribution system, people to administer the campaign from those at the centre to those in the field vaccinating and people to be vaccinated. Endemic smallpox in general was more firmly entrenched in areas of high population density and to interrupt transmission a higher proportion of the population needed to be vaccinated. When a campaign was integrated into the health service it could be incorporated into existing infrastructure but when it was separate it had to develop its own. At a WHO inter-regional smallpox conference in New Delhi in November 1960, Dr Harald Frederiksen, a programme officer of the Division of International Health, Public Health Service, in Washington, discussed the merits of eradication versus control and provided a case study of the achievements of the programme in Bolivia. In 1957–58 he was Director of the Servicio Cooperativo Interamericano de Salud Pública, which was a joint agency of the Republic of Bolivia and the USA.[12] Bolivia had had a very high attack rate (percentage of an at-risk population who contract a disease) for smallpox and was one of the main endemic foci in the Americas. A mass vaccination campaign was undertaken supplementing existing routine programme activities. Despite the country's many challenges around climate, its low-density population, illiteracy among the indigenous Indian population, limited communication and underdevelopment, eradication through mass vaccination was shown to be feasible.

The New Delhi conference participants came from many countries of the wider Asian region. Country reports confirmed that the problem of smallpox varied, and that attitudes and approaches differed. While globally most smallpox cases occurred in the WHO South-East Asia Region, in Ceylon (Sri Lanka) the disease was no longer endemic. A former British colony, it adopted vaccination early and had a long-established vaccination programme, but after an outbreak in 1957 of nineteen cases in Kalpitya it carried out mass vaccination of about 2.25 million people.[13] In the Federated States of Malaya (Malaysia), which was a member of the WHO Western Pacific Region, mass vaccination was used to maintain a high level of herd immunity and there were no endemic foci.[14]

A key reason that enabled the establishing of either a smallpox control or eradication vaccination programme was that a suitable vaccine existed. In practice, there were different smallpox vaccines. In Bolivia, lyophilised (freeze-dried) vaccine supplied from Paris and Lima was used and routinely tested for potency. 'At no time was the vaccine refrigerated. Some of the vaccine had been stored for as long as 1 year before use.'[15] Although the country's climate ranged from tropical to alpine, most of the population lived on the cooler highland plateau. Ceylon had a warm climate but used the slightly cheaper and easier to produce glycerinated vaccine lymph from the Medical Research Institute in Colombo. The vaccine was found to maintain its potency at seven days and was issued weekly, being able to be distributed to the most remote areas in two to three days.[16] Thailand, however, had set up a facility with the help of the United Nations Children's Fund (UNICEF) to produce freeze-dried vaccine for use in remote rural areas.[17] Malaysia produced glycerinated lymph but had no personnel trained to produce dried vaccine. In a mass campaign during a localised epidemic in Kelantan State in 1959, it had used dried vaccine obtained from other countries.[18]

At the start of the 1960s Nepal was using a liquid vaccine that was supposed to be kept frozen to retain potency. This was difficult. Nepal's mostly warm climate, rural population, difficult communications, and lack of refrigeration suggested that a vaccine more suited to Nepal's conditions was needed. While the initial discussions for the pilot project referred to lymph vaccine, in May 1962 Zahra wrote in his field visit report that 'Freeze-dried smallpox vaccine exclusively is being used'.[19] Vaccination undertaken outside the pilot continued to use the lymph. At its meeting in September 1963, the Regional Committee 'RECORDS that one of the chief difficulties facing the countries of the Region and delaying maximum coverage of populations within the shortest possible time is in providing a potent and stable vaccine in adequate quantity'.[20] As was evident in 1963, many Nepalis preferred freeze-dried vaccine which they knew was better suited to Nepali conditions. With a lack of refrigeration throughout the country and poor communication it was not possible to supply remote areas within the seven days' timeframe needed with liquid vaccine to retain high potency at room temperature. In the Mt Everest region, the American climbers sent their unused vaccine to Hillary, but in the cold of the high mountains in March and April temperature was probably not an issue. Hillary did not mention storage in his report or book and later sent some vaccine down to the lower altitude and therefore warmer Solu district. Hillary also considered the Russian vaccine much more potent than the Swiss because of the very visible reactions.[21] The Russian vaccine being supplied for the pilot project was freeze-dried, but neither Prasai nor Yarom tell us what type of vaccine was secured for use in the Tarai in 1965.

The next logistical consideration was for the government to secure an adequate supply. The procurement stage made Nepal dependent on its relations with external 'others' as the country did not produce its own vaccine. Many of the member states of SEARO manufactured their own vaccine or were being assisted to by WHO. In 1961 Nepal was continuing to obtain vaccine from the Vaccine Institute at Patwadangar in Uttar Pradesh.[22] With its large population India had vaccine institutes throughout the country. In the initial plan for a smallpox control pilot project, Nepal's Directorate of Health Services was to approach institutions in Calcutta (Kolkata) and Madras (Chennai) as well as Patwadangar 'to ensure sufficient quantities of lymph vaccine required to be sent at regular intervals'.[23] The first part of the pilot project was to be carried out in the municipal areas of the Kathmandu Valley where it was considered that 'Adequate facilities for the safe storage of vaccine lymph already exist in Kathmandu'.

In his report in late October/early November 1964, Vichniakov outlined the various outside sources that had supplied vaccine to Nepal. Out of 609,000 doses, only a gift of 10,000 doses from the Government of India was wet lymph vaccine and was also of unknown date.[24] All the rest was freeze-dried. The first 100,000 doses, received in September 1961, were a gift of the Netherlands and came in 100-dose phials which were later reconstituted when ready for use in the field. The remainder was Russian vaccine, supplied in twenty-dose phials by WHO in December 1962, September 1963, February 1964 and March 1964.[25] From the perspective of the global programme, the focus was on the pilot project in the Kathmandu Valley, but some vaccination was occurring in other parts of the country. During 1964, USAID and the governments of Pakistan and the United Arab Republic contributed 400,000 doses for use elsewhere in Nepal outside the pilot project area.[26] Where this sizeable amount of vaccine was used was not recorded.

In addition to the vaccine, other supplies also had to be procured. Radovanovic's initial report outlined the pilot project's needs:

> A total of 30 vaccinators' kits (for 25 vaccinators and 5 inspectors) will be provided (including a bag, needles in a container, small vaccine carrier, a one-pint thermos with wide mouth, metal spirit lamp, hand towels, small aluminium wash-basin, nail clippers, nail brush, bottle for spirit and bottle for zinc boric powder). In addition ... other material such as cotton wool, stationery, five bicycles (for inspectors) etc., will be supplied by 1 October.[27]

Supplies were part of WHO support; in the later evaluation of the pilot project the team commented that such supplies 'have been available in adequate quantities'.[28] Such supplies were essential; when people went out they had to carry everything they would need with them. If something was missing it was usually not possible to replace or substitute, particularly in rural areas.

The 1960 conference revealed the variety of approaches used to tackle the problem of smallpox in each country and their use of different vaccines and reasons why. Some also mentioned the technique adopted. A 1959 WHO document indicated that 'There are various acceptable methods, the scratch and the multiple pressure techniques being those more commonly used.'[29] During the 1963–64 epidemic, Hillary's group and Messerschmidt and Morrison used the scratch technique, as did the ex-Gurkha compounder at the Indian Soldiers Board health post. The pilot project used the multiple pressure technique. Other methods were being developed; the jet injector, which was used in Brazil and west and central Africa and was popular because of the large numbers of people that could be vaccinated in a day, was not used in Nepal.

Foreign aid was becoming in the 1960s 'a way of life' in the capital.[30] Although in the 1950s foreign organisations and their personnel were learning to work and live in Nepal, the pendulum in the 1960s was shifting to their greater influence.[31] American education adviser Hugh Wood surveyed bilateral donors about their priorities in giving assistance. Only the Chinese replied that they would let Nepalis decide according to Nepal's plan and priorities. The other donors replied that 'We think we know best what kind of aid we can give' and thought that their governments would consider that if the Nepalis were allowed to decide 'This would reduce the need for our technicians and management.'[32] The number of agencies and personnel was increasing, but the US continued to have the largest presence. The British Council began operating in Nepal in mid-1959 and in its first progress report in 1960 commented that 'The U.S.A. got in on the groundfloor on Nepali education and is pushing its own textbooks and methods.'[33] It looked to find ways to support activities. In 1963, 'On behalf of the World Health Office in Kathmandu the Council gave 14 public showings of films on Smallpox during a "drive" against the disease.'[34] Stiller and Yadav have suggested that 'If there is any weakness' in Mihaly's influential study 'it lies in his tendency to overplay the political aspect of foreign aid. Foreign politics never assumed the importance in Nepal his book suggests.'[35] This may have been the motive for donor nations, but they were unsuccessful in 'using foreign aid to inject their own political beliefs into Nepalese politics'.[36]

Having identified a suitable vaccine and procured a supply, the next steps in the logistics chain were to bring it into Nepal, store if needed and then distribute it to where it would be used in the field. All vaccine was brought first to Kathmandu. One of the reasons for the pilot project office's location in Singha Durbar was that there were refrigerators that could store vaccine. With the introduction of freeze-dried vaccine, storage requirements changed but were still necessary. In 1964 Vichniakov found that 200,000 doses of freeze-dried vaccine were being kept in one of the rooms of the project office and he had 'strongly' recommended that they should be kept in a more suitable place.[37] Arrangements 'were needed to keep the bulk of the freeze-dried vaccine under proper conditions, at the temperature of 4 to 6 degrees (not more than 10 degrees) in a cool, dark place'.[38]

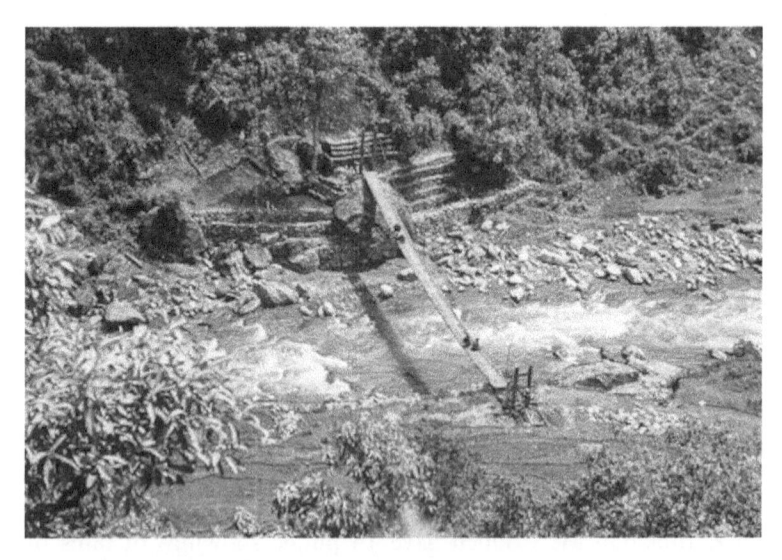

Figure 6.1 Bridge under construction over the Parajuli river, Dailekh district in Bheri zone in western–central Nepal. Inaugurated on 30 June 1971, the bridge was completely destroyed by a monsoon flood on 10 September 1971.
Source: Alan Fairbank, Nepal Peace Corps Photo Project.

Transportation into the field posed major challenges. In the same annual report that informed the Director-General of WHO about the cases in Nepal in 1961, SEARO Regional Director Mani considered Nepal's situation and wrote that 'In view of the difficulties of terrain, poor communications and shortage of medical and auxiliary health personnel, the Government does not expect to be in a position to embark on a country-wide eradication campaign before 1965'.[39] When Messerschmidt and Morrison required sufficient vaccine Morrison walked for two days before catching an infrequent flight to Kathmandu. Although there was a telephone, a message had to be transmitted 'over and over again, one after the other, through 14 operators'.[40] Even if a message reached its intended recipient the potential for error was considerable. Morrison then walked back with the vaccine in his pack. If conditions were challenging in the cool and dry months, working in the monsoon became 'nearly impossible' wrote Adiga.[41] He gave the example of a trip to the village of Duku in the Kathmandu Valley.

> We had to cross the Bagmati River thrice and dried up rivulet in order to reach that village in winter. In the rainy season, it is impossible to cross Bagmati River and the rivulet becomes a rapid. The boulders come down as bullets and bigger than cannonballs. ... Landslides are very common in rainy season.[42]

Adiga also supported the use of aircraft because of the terrain. In early 1963 Hillary was supplied by air, although even if the pilot had wanted to land the plane he could not because there was no suitable flat land near Khumjung village. Air transport was much quicker. Had this not been used it could have been two weeks of walking, or perhaps one week if using a runner, before the vaccine could have reached the intended recipients. In the spring the temperature was warming up. Adiga acknowledged the high cost of air transport but believed that if the country was serious about eradicating smallpox helicopters and small planes became necessary.[43] Crippen had also used flights to distribute the donated vaccine he had secured.[44] The revised plan of operation signed in November 1966 did not mention the provision of such services, although they had been the cause of correspondence from SEARO. Both the Regional Director and HQ in Geneva agreed that helicopters were not necessary for the 1967 stage of the programme.[45] Indeed, the Regional Director's comment was much stronger – 'thoroughly unrealistic'.[46]

The lengthy time for written communications to travel between Nepal, New Delhi and Geneva also illustrates the potential for misunderstanding. The letter from Dr Yagya Raj (Y. R.) Joshi, Nepal's Director of Health Services, to Yarom in 1966 mentioned that helicopters for transporting people and materials 'in the difficult regions of our country would greatly speed up the work'.[47] The Regional Director's correspondence with WHO HQ recorded 'I am sorry Dr Yarom got involved in this; he apparently was in favour which surprises me.'[48] This was then sent by Dr Isao Arita at HQ to Yarom who had returned to Jerusalem. Yarom replied to Arita that the topic was discussed with Joshi. 'No commitments were made and the need for a thorough study of helicopter practicability was stressed.'[49] Yarom continued that in his draft report 'no supply of a helicopter was recommended as it appeared unrealistic at this stage'. A week later Arita replied in a more personal letter to Yarom about how there had been 'some misunderstanding' and that they had known there was no commitment.[50] Yarom's letter had now been sent to SEARO. While the tone of some of the correspondence creates the impression of the Nepali request being unreasonable, in the wider context of Nepal air transportation was a valid option that was being used increasingly. Helicopters could land in a much smaller area than a small plane. Even if using lymph, helicopters could have transported the vaccine nationwide had there been an infrastructure in place to support a vaccination campaign. Air transportation was expensive – but so was lengthy travel over difficult terrain. Hillary built the airstrip at Lukla in the Mt Everest area in 1964 for such reasons, which facilitated the building of Khunde Hospital in 1966.

The third area that was a challenge concerned the shortage of health personnel at all grades. The number of Nepalis in 1951 with sufficient schooling that enabled them to take up training in different areas of health was small, but significant progress had been made by 1961 in terms of students attending school and the special training programmes being started (Appendix 2).[51] Unsurprisingly, the greatest gains were being made in primary education and this would take time to follow through into secondary schooling and then further education. The inadequate supply of high school graduates was compounded by the popularity of college arts and science courses.[52] Wood noted a 'somewhat universal disdain for vocational education'.[53] 'A relatively small but significant part' of both secondary and higher education was being undertaken overseas. By 1961, out of 2,163 scholarships awarded 418 – the second highest category – were in health.[54] Of these, 258 had returned but only 65 were known to be employed. In Nepal, twenty-four nurses had been trained by 1961 at the Nurses Training School, three at the United Mission Hospital and sixty-five health assistants at the Health Assistants School.[55] With no medical school in Nepal, doctors trained overseas. Some also obtained fellowships to gain new skills or to specialise. Adiga and Prasai both went to the UK. While the low number of health personnel was an issue, the situation was also more complex. Adiga mentioned, for example, that terrain difficulties meant that travel was slow to reach villages and so 'Camping facilities for the workers must be provided.'[56] References throughout the pilot project reports were made to the need to pay allowances which until resolved would continue to be an issue. Prasai and those organising the scheme in Morang and Sunsari districts recognised and importantly addressed or worked around such concerns. Its vaccinators were not trained health workers and were paid by the village panchayats rather than the government.

Vaccination acceptability

Mass vaccination was the main strategy for much of the 1960s. 'The importance of public vaccination should be stressed' urged the manual that accompanied the global intensified programme.[57] Although the number of vaccinations given through Nepal's pilot project increased, field visit reports from WHO officials repeatedly expressed concern at the low level of immunological coverage – well below the lowest desired level. They raised several issues surrounding vaccination activities and made suggestions for improvements, including those to facilitate vaccination uptake. Reports from the eradication programme in the 1970s focused on opposition to vaccination that they saw essentially in terms of it being associated with strong religious beliefs.[58] The emphasis on 'strong' explained how a person could be Hindu but not opposed to vaccination. Nevertheless, the earlier reports clearly emphasised that religious beliefs were not the only problem and that there were other 'real difficulties', as Zahra wrote in 1962.[59] A Kathmandu study used as reading material for a regional WHO workshop on health education in 1967 reinforced that view, as do people's stories and recollections.[60]

In their description and analysis of Nepal's programme, Shrestha, Robinson and Friedman divided the country into the three geographic belts which, they said, 'broadly speaking' had their own ethnic and cultural composition.[61] Attitude to vaccination was mostly written about in terms of religious beliefs and practices. In the north, the majority of people in the mountainous Himalayan areas were Buddhist and their language and culture Tibeto-Burman. 'In general they have no particular cultural response to smallpox and they readily accept vaccination.'[62] To the south, many Nepalis in the Tarai were ethnically similar to their Indian neighbours and had family connections across the border. 'The cultural response to smallpox found in the Terai is similar to that seen among Indians living in the border areas and frequently includes religious objections to vaccination.'[63] Seasonal migrants from India in the wealthier eastern Tarai made up a significant part of the area's agricultural and industrial workforce and were responsible for the importation of cases of smallpox into Nepal. Many of these migrants were classed as 'tribals' who worshipped 'Shitala Mai, the Goddess of Smallpox'.[64] In the eastern part of the central hill region, a tradition of military service existed 'for which vaccination is a prerequisite', while to the west vaccination was not available until 1972.[65] Although Hinduism was the state religion, it was only mentioned in the description of the people of the 'Middle Hills'.[66] Their religion, it was noted, also included elements of Buddhism and some people were Buddhist. The region, which contained the Kathmandu Valley, had more economic development than other parts of Nepal and except for 'certain sections' of the Newar people did not have 'strong religious beliefs concerning smallpox which might prohibit them from accepting vaccination'.[67]

As noted in Chapter 1, Shrestha made a point of emphasising that only some Newar resisted vaccination.[68] Dr Rita Thapa was one of very few women in senior health positions. She was appointed Chief of Nepal's Maternal–Child Health and Family Planning Project and recalled that on one occasion Adiga went out but was met with sticks. 'The people said the goddess was angry and if they worshipped the goddess they would be OK.'[69] She contrasted the smallpox and malaria projects and the way they operated. 'With the malaria project you just went and sprayed or whatever – no cultural concern.' She suggested to Adiga that he say to people 'Why don't you worship the goddess and then vaccinate?' This again illustrates the need not to conflate religious beliefs with refusal. This led to an incorporation rather than confrontation strategy of identifying in a community people's beliefs and then to 'go and do what was needed'.

Adiga's paper provides a detailed account of his own and his vaccinators' varied experiences during the epidemic in what he regarded as four 'typical' villages. Harisiddhi, in Lalitpur District and named after its famous temple, was a village mostly of farmers. 'One cannot even enter that village with shoes on. No vaccination was allowed as it was supposed to be against the wish of Harisiddhi.' Most of the more than 150 deaths were children. Adiga continued: 'This was indeed too much for us. We forced our way in that village despite [of] the consequences. With lots of arguments and threat, we finally succeeded in vaccinating for the first time in history. Even then the 29 priests of the temple refused vaccination point blank.'[70] He finished by commenting that no deaths from smallpox were reported after the campaign. The second village that he wrote about was Khokana, which was known for its oil making and the Sikali Devi temple. Over 100 people had died and again most were children. For Adiga, 'the saddest experience of the campaign' was the only daughter of a female farmer who lost both eyes.

> Fortunately the muldhami (chief priest) who had a lot of pox marks was also the teacher in the local school and was of philanthropic nature. He along with the village headman took vaccination in front of everybody and pronounced that there is nothing in religion against vaccination. Believe it or not 1,100 people followed the example. This indeed was the biggest reward for us.[71]

In the southern part of a third village, Tokha Chandeshwari, which was situated near Tokha TB sanatorium, cases of smallpox had occurred, but not in the northern part where people 'used to take vaccination. It is here that we came across a lady of 90, hale and hearty for her age. She along with a farmer age of 70 became volunteers and saw to it that every body took vaccination in her part of the village.'[72] The fourth was Sanu Gaun where all but about thirty people refused vaccination. Those who accepted were all relatives of the *pradhan panch* (leader of the local panchayat).

For Adiga, education was the solution to counter people's 'superstitions'. Local beliefs rather than religion were the problem. The inhabitants of the village of Thaiha, which was next to Harisiddhi, were 'Shresthas (Educated Newars) who have always been taking vaccination, they did so even during our visit'.[73] Only one death occurred in that village. Many Newar in Sankhu were Buddhist, but unlike many other Buddhists rejected vaccination.

> They were so clever that they closed all the doors and remained inside, a few of them even jeering during our visit. One young chap had used lipstick to mimic vaccination. He fortunately was exposed and vaccinated. They fooled us all right but not the smallpox for according to reports people are still dying of smallpox in Sankhu.[74]

In contrast, once the *talukdar* (landtax collector) of the Buddhist Tamang village of Bihebar was convinced about vaccination 'then it was an easy task' to carry out vaccination. 'It was here that they were on the point of keeping us for three weeks as that was the custom related to the [Bardyas].'[75] When using actual smallpox matter as in variolation, this isolation was to prevent the further spread of the disease.

While people were more likely to accept and want vaccination when there was an epidemic, as had been found in the Mt Everest and Lamjung areas, other factors could also be important. While Zahra in 1962 had reported that the overall average vaccination coverage in the Kathmandu Valley project area was 19 per cent, it varied according to locality, ranging from a low of 1 per cent 'indicating non-acceptance of vaccination by the population' but to nowhere higher than 33 per cent.[76] Zahra thought that a number of factors contributed to why the numbers were so low, but the wording of his report is also significant. The reasons he suggested were:

> the long-established unpopularity of (or even resistance to) vaccination, particularly the non-acceptance of the need for re-vaccination; inherent belief that smallpox is caused by the visitation of a goddess, and consequently not feared; the fact that the pilot project is being conducted in a congested city among people who are both urban and

rural in their activities, and hence out of home the largest part of the day in shops, offices, or the fields.[77]

Religious or local beliefs, therefore, were part of a wider spectrum of concerns; even here belief in the goddess was viewed not so much as the goddess being opposed to vaccination, but that people consequently did not fear the disease. In Bhaktapur, a WHO official persuaded some children to be vaccinated by giving them a brightly coloured pin with an image of the goddess Sitala. When other children saw it they also wanted their own and soon long lines of children were eager to be vaccinated.[78] Other factors were lack of knowledge such as not appreciating the importance of revaccination, while some were very practical such as the unsuitable timing of vaccination activities in the context of people's daily lives.

A deeply felt point for people was when to vaccinate. While the previous section in this chapter discussed practical aspects related to timing such as the monsoon rains and difficulty travelling, other aspects related to people's beliefs such as which months of the year to vaccinate and the phase of the moon. The initial pilot project staff training course in 1962 was limited to one week rather than six 'to expedite the start of vaccination activities' because 'according to popular belief, February and March are propitious months for vaccination; after March, vaccination is, apparently, not so readily accepted by the people'.[79] The goddess Sitala usually paid her regular visit in the spring.

Messerschmidt wrote about his contrasting reception in two remote Gurung villages in early 1964.[80] Although requested to visit he was surprised by the cool welcome at one. While staying with the headman and being told that they could begin vaccinating at the school in the morning only a few children from 'poor Blacksmith families' appeared. This was a rare reference to people who today would be referred to as Dalits. Blacksmiths were members of an occupational caste – *kami*. 'Inexplicably, no Gurung children came.' No reason was given. The next day, at another village, Messerschmidt found out why. They were given a warm welcome and treated as honoured guests, but the village elders who were all retired Gurkha soldiers were having a serious discussion. While it might be thought that as ex-Gurkhas and exposed to the outside world their belief in vaccination should have overridden local cultural beliefs, they were also respected village elders whose decisions were important. Finally, the headman told them that it was not a 'propitious' time to vaccinate, and they should wait a few days until the moon reappeared. To risk 'anything as supernaturally powerful as vaccination' was 'inauspicious' and could anger the goddess Sitala. On their fourth day in the village, they were told they could begin vaccinating. 'As befits a village of Gurkha soldiers, everything was in order. Tables and chairs were set out, there was ample hot water for washing arms, and the elders kept a registry, ticking off the name of each person in queue to be immunized.'[81] Everyone showed up, including both blacksmiths and Gurung, and they vaccinated 'all 600 of them'. Earlier in the campaign vaccine was limited and they wanted to vaccinate those most susceptible and especially children, but now they had a better supply of vaccine and this was the last village on their list.

People's responses to vaccination, therefore, were many and varied; different strategies were needed to address different issues. Zahra thought that initially there would be opposition until people and local leaders realised the importance that the government attached to smallpox control; he also noted that at the beginning the community was not involved. An article in the *WHO Chronicle*, based on the Director-General's report to the Seventeenth WHA on the progress of WHO's smallpox eradication programme in 1963, noted at 56.8 per cent the low coverage of the pilot project in Nepal. Nepal was the only country where 'community resistance to vaccination' was mentioned; it was followed by the statement that 'health education efforts have accordingly been intensified'.[82] Pilot project staff promoted vaccination before commencing activities. The Health Education Unit had a van – a symbol of the new foreign aid coming into the country, although with such few roads and narrow congested streets in the towns its use was more limited.[83] Most of Nepal's population could not be reached by such a method of communication. The vaccination teams, however, did not give advance information or warning of their visits 'for fear that the household members might then either purposely keep away or close their doors to them'.[84] Lack of community involvement in the pilot project area contrasted with operation of the programme in Morang and Sunsari. As the authors of an article in the *JNMA* noted, 'As with every other public health programme, smallpox eradication cannot be achieved without community participation.'[85]

They envisaged an active participation not only as recipients but also being involved in the organisation and implementation of the programme.

Not mentioned in Zahra's earlier list of reasons was that people could fear vaccination because of earlier bad experiences. While my interviewees in Kirtipur talked about infected arms, Messerschmidt and Morrison often heard the story that vaccinators travelled around and charged people to be vaccinated but parents then found that children who were vaccinated came down with virulent smallpox. We 'had to promise over and over that our vaccine would *prevent* and not *cause* smallpox'.[86] In the Mt Everest region a woman, who had been vaccinated a few days earlier, died. She had probably already contracted the disease when she was vaccinated – and so the vaccine would not have been as effective – but that was not an appropriate explanation to the local Sherpa inhabitants. They believed the vaccine had killed her.[87] Vichniakov mentioned two further reasons: that people were 'afraid of being "sick" after vaccination' and that many people 'remember that they were vaccinated in their early days by means of the dangerous method of variolation, performed by non-medical persons (so called "smallpox specialists") and do not wish to repeat the experience'.[88] Radovanovic had noted that, although the multiple pressure vaccination technique was being used, in some cases too large a vesicular reaction after primary vaccination was observed 'presumably due to a very potent freeze-dried smallpox vaccine' and these could more easily be prone to secondary infections.[89] Such side effects, their discomfort and lack of treatment options for people did not promote support for vaccination.

People's concerns about vaccine and vaccination methods were not unreasonable worries, although vaccine quality was being improved and new techniques were being tried to address such problems. From 14 to 20 January 1964, the first Expert Committee on Smallpox convened by the WHO met in Geneva to review particularly the control and prevention of the disease and recent developments. It made several recommendations including those relating to vaccine and the method of delivery. In the November 1964 edition of the *WHO Chronicle* these appeared as the last point of an article about the committee's report: 'development of smallpox vaccines as potent as those at present available, but causing slighter reactions and fewer complications'.[90] The wording is significant. While the article indicated that there were issues surrounding vaccination, the actual 1964 report of the Expert Committee was more explicit about their relevance. 'The multiple pressure or the single-scratch method of vaccination should be used universally and the more traumatic methods should be given up.'[91] In other words, the Committee took seriously the impact of people's concerns about vaccine and the method of vaccination. People I talked with vividly described the infections and pain from earlier methods and how the newer methods were less traumatic.[92]

In November 1967, the reading material for the first item of a WHO workshop in New Delhi on the 'Methodology of Planning, Implementation and Evaluation of Health Education' was 'A study of the knowledge, beliefs and attitude of the people relating to specific problems encountered in the smallpox eradication programme in Nepal'.[93] The date the survey was undertaken was not given but relates to the situation in the mid-1960s. While the role and value of health education was not in question, project staff in Nepal had decided that it was important to investigate the different beliefs and attitudes that they had encountered and had developed a structured questionnaire for interviewing people in two city panchayats and two rural areas. Health education staff went from house to house and individually interviewed 120 people (67 urban, 53 rural), male and female, aged between 17 and 75 years. Participants were both Newars and *Parbatiya* (hill people) and most had limited literacy. Most also worked in the fields.

People were asked about their knowledge of smallpox and vaccination. The survey found that people generally knew that children under the age of six months could get smallpox; the older the participant the stronger the correlation. Most also believed that one vaccination was sufficient to give lifelong protection, although people under the age of thirty years were more aware of the need for revaccination and so their children tended to be vaccinated more than once. The great majority preferred to have vaccination during the period mid-January to mid-May and gave a variety of reasons: the moderate temperature; when very cold the rash 'will not appear satisfactorily'; tradition; the rainy season was 'not good' for vaccination; and if done later would disturb their farming. Most also thought they did not need to report a suspected case to either the health department or the panchayat office. Although not a question, some also mentioned that even if vaccinated, a person could still get smallpox. Overall responses from people in urban and rural areas were similar.

The authors of the study report concluded that while the survey was simple it 'contributed a good deal to know the general outlook of the people regarding the smallpox problem'.[94] The interviewers considered that people were receptive to the idea of vaccination and that although 'they had preserved the impression of their traditional ways regarding practices' ideas were changing, especially among the younger population. More information, education and training were suggested. In this transitional period community education should be given through a variety of means of 'good practices' and should be started before vaccination began in an area. Also, if people preferred vaccination during a specific season, staff efforts should focus on this time, even making use of temporary staff. Panchayat workers and the community should be helped to begin reporting suspected cases to the health authority. Future occasional surveys should also be undertaken. As the intensified programme got underway, improving vaccination coverage, therefore, was more complex than just a straightforward introduction of the technology.

As a final thought, this discussion has equated thinking about vaccination with smallpox, but other vaccines existed and were being considered in Nepal. In the Mt Everest region no further cases of smallpox had occurred since the epidemic, but tuberculosis was a major health problem and in 'a region of poverty people cannot afford to spend long periods of time away from their homes and work'.[95] Organising a treatment programme 'sufficiently long term' to effect a cure and prevent the development of resistant organisms was a challenge in 1967 for John McKinnon, Khunde Hospital's first volunteer doctor from New Zealand. He had begun a scheme to give simultaneous BCG and smallpox vaccinations to the approximately 1,200 people of the villages of Khunde, Khumjung and Namche Bazar. Sherpas were 'enthusiastic recipients' of smallpox vaccination and did know about BCG against tuberculosis, and he hoped that by giving them together they would also accept BCG. His successor, Dr Richard Evans, thought that measles vaccination would be worthwhile but was expensive and not readily available while the triple vaccination required for DPT (Diptheria–pertussis–tetanus) would be a major problem 'as Sherpas invariably do not attend for follow-up purposes'.[96] Attitudes and practices were context and vaccine specific.

Conclusion

Whether looking from a global, national or individual perspective, the 1960s was a pivotal period in managing smallpox. Although the global goal shifted from control to eradication and programme implementation required increased effort, the strategy for much of the decade in countries where smallpox was present remained mass vaccination; this was carried out through national programmes with the aim to increase herd immunity and so interrupt the transmission of the virus. Smallpox was a disease that could be prevented rather than cured. As the inter-regional smallpox conference in 1960 in New Delhi illustrated, the problem and responses to the disease varied considerably. The smallpox situation in Nepal was not presented at the conference, but Nepal was one of the countries where the disease was still endemic.

If the global goal of eradication was to be achieved, programmes required tools, and people needed to be vaccinated. From a logistics perspective, any vaccination programme required a suitable vaccine, an adequate supply, a storage and distribution system, personnel to administer the programme at all levels from the centre to those in the field giving the vaccination and people to be vaccinated. At the beginning of the decade vaccination was not available for most Nepalis. Opportunities expanded but also highlighted challenges that needed to be overcome or worked around. Freeze-dried vaccine was better suited to Nepal's climate and the lack of refrigeration for storage throughout most of the country.

While most Nepalis accepted vaccination, improvements to the vaccine and methods of delivery facilitated acceptance and illustrate how technical aspects, people's experiences and their responses were interlinked. The efficacy of the freeze-dried vaccine increased people's trust while less traumatic methods of delivery were also preferred. Resistance for religious reasons was also more complicated than the idea of equating belief in the goddess and vaccination refusal. Other reasons for low immunisation coverage could include practical reasons such as people being at work at the time the vaccinators came. These were issues that could be worked around. One idea that continued to be important was Nepali people's preference for vaccination at certain times of the year, and programmes adapted to accommodate this belief.

Much had been learned about vaccination in Nepal when the revised plan of operation was signed at the end of 1966 to begin implementation of the global intensified programme in 1967. Even if the smallpox programme in Nepal appeared limited, the experiences and developments of the early part of the decade provided the foundation for the new initiative. The next chapter examines the early transition towards a nationwide programme in practice as well as name.

Notes

1. WHO, 'Surveillance-containment operations'.
2. Dowdle, 'The principles of disease elimination and eradication'.
3. WHA 15, Smallpox eradication: report by the Director-General, p. 2.
4. Fenner et al., *Smallpox and Its Eradication*, p. 408.
5. For a discussion of the ongoing debate, see Anne Mills, 'Vertical vs horizontal health programmes in Africa: Idealism, pragmatism, resources and efficiency', *Social Science & Medicine*, 17:24 (1983), 1971–81.
6. Fenner et al., *Smallpox and Its Eradication*, p. 590.
7. Paul Greenough, Stuart Blume, and Christine Holmberg, 'Introduction', in *The Politics of Vaccination*, p. 2.
8. John Wickett and Peter Carrasco, 'Logistics in smallpox: The legacy', *Vaccine* 29S (2011), D131–4; Baptiste Baylac-Paouly, 'Confronting and emergency: The vaccination campaign against meningitis in Brazil (1974–1975)', *Social History of Medicine*, 34:2 (2021), 632–49.
9. Wickett and Carrasco, 'Logistics in smallpox'.
10. Pieter Streefland, A.M.R. Chowdhury and Pilar Ramoz-Jimenez, 'Patterns of vaccination acceptance', *Social Science & Medicine*, 49:12 (1999), 1705–16.
11. Heidi J. Larson, Caitlin Jarrett, Elisabeth Eckersberger, David M.D. Smith and Pauline Paterson, 'Understanding vaccine hesitancy and vaccines and vaccination from a global perspective: A systematic review of published literature, 2007–2012', *Vaccine* 32 (2014), 2150.

12 SEA/WHO, File 824, Box 50, SEA/SPX/conf.5, Smallpox Conference – November 1960, H. Frederiksen, Eradication versus control of smallpox, 10 November 1960.
13 SEA/SPX/conf.14, Smallpox Conference – November 1960, P. Rajasingham, Smallpox in Ceylon, 15 November 1960.
14 SEA/SPX/conf.11, Smallpox Conference – November 1960, S. Narayanan, Malaya and smallpox, 15 November 1960.
15 Frederiksen, Muñoz and Molina, 'Smallpox eradication', 774.
16 SEA/SPX/conf.14, Rajasingham, Smallpox in Ceylon.
17 SEA/SPX/conf.12, Smallpox Conference – November 1960, Pramem Chandavlmol, Smallpox in Thailand, 15 November 1960.
18 SEA/SPX/conf.11, Narayanan, Malaya and smallpox.
19 SEA/Smallpox/4, Zahra, Field visit report on Smallpox Control Pilot Project 1962, p. 2.
20 13 September 1963. World Health Organization. Regional Office for South-East Asia (1963). SEA/RC16/R4 – Need for freeze-dried smallpox vaccine. WHO Regional Office for South-East Asia. https://apps.who.int/iris/handle/10665/130635.
21 Hillary, *Schoolhouse in the Clouds*, pp. 42–3.
22 SEA/CD/8, Radovanovic, Report on field visit to Nepal 1961, p. 2.
23 *Ibid.*, p. 4.
24 SEA/Smallpox/8, Vichniakov, Field visit report on Smallpox Control Pilot Project 1964, p. 4.
25 The report says February1963, but this was probably a typographical error as the list of dates appears chronological.
26 SEA/Smallpox/8, Vichniakov, Field visit report on Smallpox Control Pilot Project 1964, p. 4.
27 SEA/CD/8, Radovanovic, Report on field visit to Nepal 1961, p. 4.
28 SEA/Smallpox/9, Vichniakov, Assessment and evaluation of the Smallpox Control Pilot Project 1965, p. 3.
29 WHO/Smallpox/9, Smallpox vaccination technique, 3 July 1959.
30 Stiller and Yadav, *Planning for People*, p. 51.
31 Heydon, 'Missions, visitors and international aid'; Heather Hindman, 'The everyday life of American development in Nepal', *Studies in Nepali History and Society*, 7:1 (2002), 99–136.
32 Skerry et al., *Four Decades of Development*, p. 94.
33 The National Archives, Kew (hereafter, TNA), BW129/5, British Council: Registered Files, Nepal, Nepal: Representative's annual reports, W. Lyndon Clough, Progress Report 31 March 1960, p. 3.
34 *Ibid.*, Representative's annual report 1962/63, p. 3. Science, agriculture and medicine, Appendix C – Arts & sciences.
35 Stiller and Yadav, *Planning for People*, p. 54.

36 *Ibid.*
37 SEA/Smallpox/8, Vichniakov, Field visit report on Smallpox Control Pilot Project 1964, p. 4.
38 *Ibid.*, p. 9.
39 WHO SEARO, Fourteenth annual report of the Regional Director, p. 10.
40 Don Messerschmidt, email communication, 24 November 2018.
41 Adiga, 'Smallpox epidemic in Nepal (1963–1964)'.
42 *Ibid.*, p. 9.
43 *Ibid.*
44 Crippen, 'Smallpox, Nepal 1963 … Prelude to eradication?', p. 7.
45 SEA/WHO, File 828, Box 210, C. Mani, Regional Director, to Director, Communicable Disease (CD), HQ, 21 September 1966; Director, CD, to Regional Director, SEARO, 27 September 1966.
46 *Ibid.*, C. Mani, Regional Director, to Director, Communicable Disease, HQ, 21 September 1966.
47 *Ibid.*, 26 August 1966.
48 *Ibid.*, 21 September 1966.
49 *Ibid.*, 5 October 1966.
50 *Ibid.*, 12 October 1966.
51 Wood and Knall, 'Educational planning in Nepal and its economic implications', p. 27.
52 *Ibid.*, p. 35.
53 *Ibid.*, p. 61.
54 *Ibid.*, p. 65.
55 *Ibid.*, p. 59.
56 Adiga, 'Smallpox epidemic in Nepal (1963–1964)', p. 9.
57 World Health Organization. (1967). Handbook for smallpox eradication programmes in endemic areas. Geneva, Switzerland: World Health Organization. 4.9.1.3 Education of the public, pp. iv–22. https://apps.who.int/iris/handle/10665/67940.
58 SME/77.1, Shrestha, Robinson and Friedman, *The Nepal Smallpox Eradication Programme*, p. 10.
59 SEA/Smallpox/4, Zahra, Field visit report on Smallpox Control Pilot Project 1962, p. 3.
60 WHO, SEA/HE/WS/RM 21, Workshop on the Methodology of Planning, Implementation and Evaluation of Health Education, 30 October 1967, A study of the knowledge, beliefs and attitude of the people relating to specific problems encountered in the smallpox eradication programme in Nepal.
61 SME/77.1, Shrestha, Robinson and Friedman, *The Nepal Smallpox Eradication Programme*, p. 10.
62 *Ibid.*, p. 11.

63 *Ibid.*, p. 10.
64 *Ibid.*
65 *Ibid.*, p. 11.
66 In the 1971 census 89.4 per cent of Nepal's population identified as Hindu; 7.5 per cent Buddhist; 3 per cent Muslim; 0.1 per cent other. *Ibid.*, p. 8.
67 *Ibid.*, p. 10.
68 SEA/WHO, File 1239, Box 666, Professor P. N. Shrestha, Institute of Medicine, Tribhuvan University to Dr P. Micovic, WHO Programme Co-ordinator and Representative, Kathmandu, 26 November 1984.
69 Interview with author, Kathmandu, 25 May 2017.
70 Adiga, 'Smallpox epidemic in Nepal (1963–1964)', p. 6.
71 *Ibid.*
72 *Ibid.*
73 *Ibid.*
74 *Ibid.*, p. 7.
75 *Ibid.*
76 SEA/Smallpox/4, Zahra, Field visit report on Smallpox Control Pilot Project 1962, p. 2.
77 *Ibid.*
78 Don Messerschmidt, email communication, 16 May 2018.
79 SEA/Smallpox/4, Zahra, Field visit report on Smallpox Control Pilot Project 1962, p. 1; SEA/CD/8, Radovanovic, Report on field visit to Nepal 1961. In Sichuan, variolation and then vaccination was done in spring. Liu, 'Relocating Pastorian medicine', p. 51.
80 Messerschmidt, 'The scourge of smallpox'.
81 *Ibid.*
82 'World incidence of smallpox', *WHO Chronicle*, 18:10 (1964), 378.
83 See Stacy Leigh Pigg, 'The credible and the credulous: the question of "villagers' beliefs" in Nepal', *Cultural Anthropology*, 11:2 (1996), 160–201.
84 SEA/Smallpox/5, Radovanovic, Field visit report on Smallpox Control Pilot Project, Nepal 1963, p. 3.
85 Vaidya and Gurubacharya, 'On smallpox', 343.
86 Don Messerschmidt, email communication, 16 May 2018.
87 Michael Gill, *Mountain Midsummer: Climbing in Four Continents* (London: Hodder and Stoughton, 1969), p. 177. We found that more than thirty years later such beliefs continued to be held in some areas in Khumbu and it took trust before a parent would let us vaccinate their child.
88 SEA/Smallpox/8, Vichniakov, Field visit report on Smallpox Control Pilot Project 1964, p. 6.

89 SEA/Smallpox/5, Radovanovic, Field visit report on Smallpox Control Pilot Project, Nepal 1963 p. 3.
90 *WHO Chronicle*, 18:11 (1964), 422.
91 WHO Expert Committee on Smallpox (1964) First report, p. 31.
92 Interviews with author, Kathmandu and Kirtipur, May 2017.
93 SEA/HE/WS/RM 21, A study of the knowledge, beliefs and attitude.
94 *Ibid.*, p. 7.
95 Khunde Hospital, Annual reports 1967–83, J. R. McKinnon, Health problems of Khumbu: A review of the first nine months work at Kunde Hospital, report to the Minister of Health, His Majesty's Government of Nepal, 6 October 1967. This report was later published as 'Health problems of Khumbu: A review of the first nine months work at Kunde Hospital', *JNMA*, 5:3–4 (1967), 20–6 and 'Health problems of Khumbu in Nepal: The work at the Kunde Hospital', *New Zealand Medical Journal*, 67:40 (1968), 140–3.
96 Khunde Hospital, Annual reports 1967–83, R. Evans, Hillary Sherpa Hospital Report, 23rd August 1968 to February 27th 1969 to Dr Gauri S. L. Das, Director of Health Services, Ministry of Health, 8 March 1969.

7

A time of transition

During 1966, the global smallpox programme received new impetus by the decision in May of the Nineteenth World Health Assembly to intensify the global effort and to increase WHO's participation. Smallpox was now concentrated in three principal parts of the world: South America – particularly Brazil; Africa – all countries south of the Sahara; and Asia – Afghanistan, India, Indonesia, Nepal and Pakistan.[1] In Nepal, 'the lack of communications and the sparsity of health services has handicapped remedial measures in the past' commented the authors of the Directorate of Health Services 1969 report about smallpox.[2] Although communications in Nepal were still rudimentary and the health system limited at the time of the report's compilation, the fractured and patchy responses to smallpox of the early part of the decade had been replaced – in line with the new global policy – by a national plan in 1967. Implementation was far from being nationwide by 1969 and challenges acknowledged at all levels outside and inside the country, but the programme was intensifying and reaching an increasing number of areas.

This chapter is about the transition years in Nepal when global and national smallpox policies began to come together in intent and practice. A joint revised plan for smallpox eradication and control of other communicable diseases was agreed to and signed by the Nepali government and WHO in November 1966 but was followed by a modified implementation plan in 1967 solely concerned with smallpox. Both were nationwide and built on the foundations of the pilot project, which had already begun to expand beyond the Kathmandu Valley, and the local initiative in Morang and Sunsari districts in the Tarai. The chapter is in two parts. The first reviews smallpox in Nepal around the start of the intensified global programme when the disease was still endemic in many parts of the country and a diagnosis that healthcare workers needed to consider. Accounts from the Tarai bring to the fore the impact of Nepal's changing population demographics. This section draws on people's experiences, but at a population level particularly considers the findings of the country's first national health survey carried out in 1965–66, which for the first time provided information from across the country.[3] The second part examines how Nepal's officials engaged with global smallpox policy and vice versa of how the new, small WHO smallpox unit in Geneva and the regional office in New Delhi interacted with a nation state such as Nepal.

Smallpox in Nepal

Throughout the 1960s smallpox remained widespread in many parts of the country. Even in the Kathmandu Valley, despite four years of the pilot project, vaccination coverage was still inadequate, and smallpox was still a diagnosis that healthcare personnel needed to consider. In 1965 Dr Hemang Dixit, who had returned from medical training at Charing Cross Hospital Medical School in London, was working in the busy paediatric department at Bir Hospital in central Kathmandu where he had to deal with a range of communicable diseases.[4] On one occasion a small Tibetan boy of around eighteen months was brought in. He had a few vesicles on his body and 'My first thought was the diagnosis of chicken pox.'[5] The child was brought back the next day much worse, and it was clear to Dixit that this was a case of smallpox. The child was sent immediately to the hospital's Infectious Diseases Unit further away at Teku. Fortunately, he recovered, but his refugee family had disappeared, and sadly the little boy was sent to a children's orphanage.

Protecting other patients, staff and family from a patient with smallpox was not easy. In September 1966, Dr Satnam Singh came to Nepal as the WHO Public Health Officer attached to the renamed Smallpox Eradication and Control of Other Communicable Diseases Project (Nepal 9). He provides glimpses into the unit at Teku and recounted how a seriously ill infant girl was admitted with smallpox and 'nursed in a cubicle opening into a ward where patients suffering from other diseases were laying'.[6] She died. The same evening, a one-year-old boy suffering from infantile diarrhoea was admitted with his mother, but the child's symptoms settled the next day, and they both left the hospital. Nine days later, the mother developed smallpox and three days after that her son. In his November 1966 monthly progress report to SEARO, Singh commented on the lack of 'suitable isolation facilities' at Teku and that he gave assistance 'in organizing, as a part of hospital services compulsory vaccination facilities for unprotected patients, attendants and visitors'.[7] Two weeks after the earlier incident, an infant was admitted into the unit – again with diarrhoea – and discharged two days later. The child was given a primary vaccination on his second day in the unit, but it did not 'take', and six days later he developed smallpox. Singh thought that the only possible exposure was another child admitted the day before the infant was discharged.

In his chapter on smallpox hospitals, Dixon acknowledged that 'Although it sounds easy, it is surprisingly difficult to provide single-room isolation accommodation clear of other patients, in the ordinary or general fever hospital ...'[8] Incomplete notification also made it 'impossible to assess the danger' when a patient was admitted.[9] Some institutions did not accept patients known to have smallpox, but in both of Singh's examples the reason for the child being brought to hospital was the very common infantile diarrhoea. Such an example of hospital (nosocomial) spread of the disease could happen anywhere in the world and not just in a country like Nepal with its limited facilities and resources.[10]

Under International Sanitary Regulations, all countries were supposed to notify WHO by telegram within twenty-four hours of receiving reports of cases of the five quarantinable diseases (smallpox, cholera, plague, yellow fever and typhus) and indicate the locality. Reporting of smallpox in all endemic countries, however, was 'seriously deficient'.[11] The poor quality and under-reporting from Nepal, therefore, were no exception; such data could represent a very incomplete picture of the real presence of the disease. At the beginning of 1966 four cases were notified from Nepal in the *Weekly Epidemiological Record* (WER) for Dharan and during early March another four cases.[12] Dharan was in Sunsari district, where a vaccination programme was underway. Situated on the edge of the Tarai, Dharan was about thirty miles from the border with India and a similar distance from the main town of Biratnagar. It was also a recruiting depot for Gurkha soldiers joining the British Army. In April 1966, Major Peter Pitt arrived in Nepal for two years as surgeon at the British Military Hospital (BMH) at Dharan. Opened in 1960, the hospital's prime role was to provide healthcare for the British at the camp and the Gurkha soldiers and their families, but surgeons were scarce, and Pitt treated patients from all over eastern Nepal. Smallpox was a problem in the area at the time – much more than was indicated by the small number of cases in the WER. 'My staff estimated that between 150 and 500 deaths occurred around Dharan from smallpox in the three months before my arrival at the B.M.H., and my predecessor had estimated that a thousand had died in this eastern part of Nepal in that same period.'[13] Pitt recalled that he was told not to go into the forest as there were lots of bodies left there during the epidemic. Overseas and local medical and nursing staff 'did lots of vaccinating – everyone did it'.[14]

In a second book Pitt described a more personal story but one that illustrated how differently smallpox was usually regarded and treated in different parts of the world. Pitt travelled from Britain where smallpox was not a major health concern into India where it was. In Britain, although injury was rare, concern about the safety risk of the vaccine was higher for smallpox than for the new, laboratory-developed vaccines.[15] The young family arrived in Calcutta where a paediatric doctor friend of his wife Anna wanted to know if their baby had been vaccinated. 'I explained that he was not yet three months and that the best authority I could find had advised us not to vaccinate him until nine months, as the risk of encephalitis (inflammation of the brain) and vaccinia might be more serious than the disease.'[16] Pitt wrote that they were told they had been given 'bad advice and that all babies in Calcutta are vaccinated in their first few weeks, this being an endemic area'.[17] He felt 'suitably chastened'. He and his wife had to keep the baby in the house. Pitt continued that when he arrived in Nepal, he was 'greeted by the same lecture' from the surgeon, Jim Arnott, whom he was replacing.

Research was an important part of the new global programme.[18] Although spending most of his time in the Kathmandu Valley, Singh in January, October and November 1967 spent three weeks in different parts of the Tarai. With assistance from Henderson, he wrote up his findings.[19] Prior to the recent introduction of case reporting, local newspapers were often the main source of information about smallpox deaths, although by the time of a death it was too late to stop the spread of infection. The number of newspapers had expanded considerably since 1950, although still did not reach many parts of the country. By visiting a few infected villages and making enquiries Singh 'easily' concluded that 'smallpox was widespread, that case fatality ratios were high and in many hamlets the disease stopped only after most of the susceptibles had developed smallpox. It was not uncommon for 4 to 5 members in a family to be taken ill with smallpox.'[20]

With the government of Nepal already committed to eradication and to expanding the pilot programme nationally, what other vaccination activities were happening elsewhere in the country? In many places, the answer was little. Of the forty-six cases that Singh observed in the Tarai, thirty-seven were under the age of fifteen years and none had been vaccinated or variolated. Of the nine adults, six had not been vaccinated and three had been variolated as children.[21] The most noteworthy vaccination initiative was that undertaken in the Sunsari and Morang districts of Kosi Zone which had an estimated population of 335,000 and where 113,016 vaccinations had been given by August 1966.[22] Between July and October, twenty-five vaccinators from the project were then sent four hundred kilometres into central Nepal to carry out a mass vaccination programme in the five districts of the Bagmati Zone – expanding out from the Kathmandu Valley.[23] In October the vaccinators were withdrawn as the programme was to be reorganised in line with the draft plan drawn up during Yarom's visit. Some vaccination activities occurred elsewhere and by other groups, but information is scarce. In Okhaldhunga, Amp Pipal and Tansen, the United Mission to Nepal (UMN) provided smallpox and other vaccinations as part of their maternal and child health (MCH) clinics and in the community.[24] Again illustrating that vaccination was widely accepted, it was noted that mothers appeared keen to bring their babies to the Women and Children's Welfare Clinic set up in the centre of Tansen, for vaccination, 'but very few mothers bring their babies for advice and health teaching'.[25]

Much of what is known about the wider picture of smallpox in Nepal in the mid-1960s comes from Nepal's first national health survey, which gathered information from across the country in 1965–66. The findings were published in 1969 and the book's authors hoped they would 'assist in comprehensive health planning'.[26] Dr Narayan Shah and Dr Robert Worth, who had been students together in the USA at Johns Hopkins University, School of Hygiene and Public Health, were very aware of the fractured and limited – if slowly expanding – state of knowledge and sources in Nepal. The need, they wrote, was for a 'concise, quantitative picture of the most important current health problems' which it was hoped would add 'a significant and orderly increment of knowledge to that already available' from the few published sources, unpublished data and 'in the store of practical experience being rapidly accumulated by Nepali physicians working in the increasing number of small hospitals and dispensaries being opened in the remote, but populous, areas of the country'.[27] All of the considerable sum of $250,000 required for such an undertaking came from public contributions in Hawaii – where Worth was based – and mainland USA.[28]

The experiences of carrying out the survey illustrated the still very real difficulties of working in Nepal at this time. In August 1963 the Ministry of Health and the Thomas A. Dooley Foundation in the USA signed a contract to undertake the survey.[29] In September 1964 the Foundation reached agreement with the School of Public Health of the University of Hawaii to develop and assist with the survey, to process and analyse the data, and with representatives from the Ministry of Health write up the final report. It was hoped to complete the survey in a year. The sample unit was a village.[30] Survey villages ranged in size from a population of 219 in the central mountains to 466 in the more populous eastern Tarai. A team would spend two weeks in each gathering household data and examining all the inhabitants. Staff training was held in Kathmandu and the survey got under way in August 1965. Although a film was made to show in villages 'to allay the suspicions and anxieties of individuals invited to participate', the survey was challenged more by 'prodigious transportation problems'.[31] By May 1966, eighteen of the selected twenty-four villages had been surveyed, but the monsoon was approaching making travel even more difficult. The remaining six villages were in the mountains. By this time, many in the team had other commitments and funding was exhausted, and so the plan was changed to survey an urban block of Kathmandu for comparison.[32]

Brief information was provided for each of the village sites. A standardised description included medical services and therefore provides valuable insight into the low level of Nepal's nationwide health services at this time (Table 7.1).[33] The WHO viewed the development of health services to be the key factor determining the level of vaccination in a country but the list highlights their lack in many parts of the country with a trend to services being more available in the southern Tarai and the Kathmandu area than the hills and mountains in the north.

The survey team collected data about smallpox based on the presence of scars from smallpox or from vaccination. The pattern was variable. The results showed a rather limited experience with smallpox in all three age groups being looked at (0–9 years, 10–29 years, 30+ years) in the central and eastern mountains, with a much wider range of experience in the western mountains (some villages with almost no experience, and some with heavy experience).[34] Given how little information exists about western Nepal, such comments are valuable. Worth and Shah referred to 'mountains', but the highest village surveyed was just over 2,300 metres (7,600 feet). No village was sampled in the high mountains of northern Nepal which includes the Mt Everest area, although we know from Khunde Hospital archives that no further cases of smallpox occurred after 1963.[35] The eastern Tarai also showed a wide range of experience.[36] The authors, however, cautioned that the presence of a 'vaccination' scar could have been produced by secondary bacterial infection rather than implying immunological protection.[37] Also, the sampling error could be quite large when only a few villages were visited.

Villagers were asked their age when they had their first vaccination, although 'these questions were not answered with enough completeness or precision to allow any rigorous analysis, particularly the questions about most recent vaccination'.[38] Adding to the difficulties, the Nepali calendar differs from the Gregorian calendar by fifty-seven years and operates on a July to June basis. Also, different ethnic groups may view age differently which had and

Table 7.1 'Modern' health services in the sample villages of the Nepal Health Survey

Western mountains:	
Bhawanipur	None locally
Bajura	A panchayat (local government) health office, but without supplies
Dandagau	None locally
Talichaur	Doctor nearby at Jumla
Central mountains:	
Lamatar	Health services in Kathmandu (13 km away), but no public transportation
Pardidhan	Health services at a nearby government health centre, usually staffed by a nurse; mission hospital with medical staff nearby in Pokhara
Piutar	None locally
Brahmin Dada	None locally
Eastern mountains:	
Debatar	None locally
Sakkejung (2 small villages)	None locally
Phulpaw	None locally
Eastern Tarai:	
Godar	None locally, but a health centre (often lacked medicines) one hour walk
Dulari	Hospital – one hour walk plus one hour by bus
Jhapa Bazar	None locally, but had a pharmacy
Ramnagar	None locally, but medicines could be bought in a bazaar 4.5 km away
Kathariea Tola	None locally

(*continued*)

Table 7.1 (Cont.)

Midwest Tarai:	
Kathauti-Annapurna	Small hospital and dispensary, plus several shops selling medicines nearby at Bhairawa
Far-west Tarai:	
Kailali	Small hospital and doctor available in Dhangari
Urban (Kathmandu):	
Inbaha	Private doctor's office in the neighbourhood; several hospitals and pharmacies available

Source: Worth and Shah, *Nepal Health Survey 1965–1966*, pp. 6–17.

continues to have implications for vaccination policy and practice. Among Sherpa of the Mt Everest area, a person was thought of as one year old when born and age was calculated based on a twelve-year cycle where each year had an animal sign. The authors noted a general difference in practice between the first vaccination in rural areas tending to be given between one and five years of age, but in Kathmandu in infancy; this most likely reflected the limited availability of services and health personnel in the former as well as economic barriers that travel entailed. Many more doctors in Nepal were in Kathmandu and so it is perhaps not surprising that vaccinations there tended to be done by doctors, while lay vaccinators were more active in rural areas and particularly in the Tarai.

The vaccination data for rural areas were 'disturbing' to the authors as the level of vaccinations for the large 0–9 years age group was low. This was considered 'very likely related to rather infrequent visits by the vaccinator, which allows the accumulation of a large number of unvaccinated children between visits, and allows the falling off of immunity of previously vaccinated adults'.[39] The only area found to have a satisfactory vaccination rate for this group was the eastern mountains, although the authors acknowledged the small number of villages sampled. None of these villages had any medical services, which was counter to prevailing ideas about vaccination levels and services. Unfortunately, no reasons were given. Worth and Shah concluded that the stage is therefore set for a continuation of sporadic epidemics introduced from across the border, with accompanying child mortality and interruption of the economic life of the village. It is generally accepted that good vaccination status (within three years), with live vaccine, of at least 85 per cent of the population will lead to permanent and complete control of the disease.[40]

Worth and Shah's recommendations considered smallpox alongside other health issues and diseases and as part of a broad and integrated health programme for Nepal. The authors identified a range of strategies, but they indicated that providing basic treatment services and immunisation against cholera and smallpox were the three that people most valued. While the research was undertaken in 1965–66, analysis and writing up continued afterwards. No mention was made, however, of the global smallpox programme or of Nepal's own developing programme, although they referred to the 'major' psychological effect of immunisation against smallpox and cholera in gaining the 'confidence' of people.[41]

A revised plan for smallpox

The Nepali government intended to expand its smallpox activities from the pilot areas in the Kathmandu Valley and prior to the discussions with WHO had begun to do so. While the WHO history of the organisation's second decade noted 'that an intensified and co-ordinated global effort, commencing in 1967, could eradicate the disease over a period of ten years', the new global programme was accompanied by 'increased awareness of the difficulties to be overcome' regarding its organisation and administration, and needing to relate implementation to the material and human resources of the countries concerned.[42] Scepticism about the programme and its likelihood of success was rife.

The WHO was to coordinate the 'global effort' with a small, designated unit at its headquarters in Geneva which would work to implement the programme through the various regional offices. In the new environment of the intensified programme Director Dr Donald (D. A.) Henderson and his unit would want to have much more involvement in a Region's response to smallpox and within each country. In his memoirs Henderson later wrote how he was 'struck by the disparity between the extravagant expectations and the smallpox unit's modest, three-room headquarters; its very small staff; its shoestring budget; and few other resources'.[43] Initially joining him were two other medical officers: Dr Stephen Falkland from the UK, and Dr Isao Arita from Japan. Falkland was on temporary loan but was experienced in international programmes, while Arita had been a WHO smallpox adviser in Liberia.[44] Dr Georgii Nikolaevskii from the USSR came in 1967.[45] For most of the programme's duration the Unit had a support staff of six, which comprised a technical officer, an administrative officer and four secretaries.[46] Henderson regarded John (Jock) Copland from the USA, who was administrative officer from 1966 to 1977, as key to navigating Geneva's 'tangled bureaucracy'.[47]

Henderson was aware that the six WHO regional offices were very independent and 'unaccustomed to working closely with headquarters staff or with each other'.[48] At a WHO regional level, the directors of the different offices varied significantly in their views about the wisdom of the new programme. The South-East Asia Region, noted the programme's official history, appeared 'frankly negative'.[49] This was not unrealistic in the case of Nepal in view of the many challenges to providing any services. From the Region's perspective, the smallpox situation in 1966 contrasted significantly with 1958 when WHO had no increase in resources in its regular budget and so had to rely on only providing technical assistance and advice.[50] In 1958 the Executive Board of the WHA recommended the setting up of a special account inviting voluntary contributions from WHA member states, but donor response was limited – although Nepal contributed despite its limited resources. Not surprisingly, the authors of the official history were critical.[51] Consequently, without additional funding, the Region's member states had had – not least for the obvious reason of having to pay for the greater part of smallpox activities – to consider smallpox from a national health perspective. India's smallpox programme was facing considerable financial pressure.[52]

With the new global intensified programme planned to commence in 1967 the remainder of 1966 was busy in preparation. In his annual report, Regional Director Mani began the section on communicable diseases with reference to the budget. In 1966 the proportion had dropped 'from 50% to about 40%, but estimates for

1967 have risen to nearly 50% again, mainly because of increased expenditure on the global smallpox eradication campaign'.[53] Mani was strongly in favour of strengthening basic health services rather than 'dramatic short bursts of gunfire' of mass campaigns. Only then – and with adequate supervision – could the Region's high morbidity from communicable disease be reduced. 'Let there be no mistake about this.'[54] In his overview of the smallpox situation in the Region the following year, Mani indicated that smallpox programmes were intensifying activity in all countries where the disease was still endemic.

In May 1966 the Regional Office sent a draft revised plan of operation to Nepal's government. Not receiving a response, SEARO in July announced that it would send a team of two consultants to review project progress and to assist 'in the further planning of this programme within the context of the global eradication programme in the next ten years'.[55] Yarom arrived in Nepal in early August and had meetings with the Minister of Health, the Director of Health Services, the Secretary of Health, departmental heads as well as WHO staff members discussing smallpox control and public health problems 'in great detail with mutual understanding'.[56] Yarom's draft report began with an introduction to the wider context of Nepal's health services and indicated that infrastructure and health personnel were increasing. Nevertheless, Nepal relied on outside assistance. Development funding provided two-thirds of Nepal's national budget, and in the case of the country's health budget it was nearer 80 per cent.[57] Such a high reliance made Nepal even more susceptible to changing priorities within the foreign aid environment.

The outcome of the various meetings was that – in Yarom's words – the 'responsible authorities decided on extending the smallpox control project to a country-wide eradication plan (within the context of [the] global Eradication Programme)' and they had asked him 'to assist in drawing up a detailed plan of action taking into account the general state of development of the country especially in relation to road communications, personnel capability and general progress plans in national health services'.[58] He noted, in what would remain a draft report, that no statistical information about smallpox in Nepal was available for 1965.[59] His list of the numbers of different types of health workers was evidence, however, of the slowly developing and changing workforce capacity, although still very small for a country with a population of around ten million people (Appendix 2). Nepal had 230 national registered medical practitioners, almost all in government services, with 154 medical students abroad, mostly in India. Of these, twelve to fifteen were expected to qualify annually and to return to Nepal. Other health staff were: eighty-six graduate nurses; fifty-one assistant nurse-midwives; ninety-six health assistants; sixteen senior auxiliary health workers; fifty-five auxiliary health workers; twenty-four sanitarians (environmental health); seven health educators; six laboratory assistants; six X-ray technicians; and forty compounders.[60]

The general principles of the plan were to be country-wide eradication of smallpox and to follow the new administrative division of the country into seven areas, each with two zones. Activities were to be separated – in line with language of the global programme – into three phases: preparatory; attack; and maintenance. He allowed for the 'slow development of supporting health services throughout the country'.[61] Further work was followed with senior health officials to define and select target areas that was cognisant of the present and future zonal administrative structure of the 3rd Five-Year national economic plan; zone population density; population movement; and the national malaria eradication programme. In practical terms, each year one of the seven areas would begin the attack phase. With this timeframe, the last area would complete this in 1975 and the first area would enter the maintenance phase in 1970. Yarom prepared an estimate for budgetary, personnel, vaccine, transport, and equipment requirements for the ensuing four years (1967–70) and again recommended the appointment of an experienced senior medical officer to be responsible for the programme. This was not a new recommendation.

In Geneva, Henderson's unit (HQ) expected to be able to exert considerable control over the global programme. In early October 1966, staff were in possession of Yarom's draft report, a report from Singh, and Mani's letter to Singh detailing the terms of reference of his role.[62] The communication from HQ back to the Regional Director suggested that Singh have access to Yarom's report as he prepared to intensify the Nepal programme. Also, HQ wanted 'in due course' to have samples of Singh's improved family records and reporting forms. Singh had also raised the question of appropriate medication to clean up skin infection, but HQ in their reply also considered that some septic skin infections should be regarded as contra-indications of smallpox vaccination.[63]

Yarom's report indicated that overall policy and planning of Nepal's programme would be retained at Directorate level in Kathmandu, but the aim was decentralisation by delegating powers to the new zonal units.[64] The first target areas were Bagmati and Kosi which would begin the attack phase in 1967. Each would have a zonal medical officer and senior supervisor, five district supervisors and ten vaccinators' supervisors. Supervisory staff would be drawn from existing staff as well as being recruited and trained locally and abroad. The number of vaccinators in each zone would vary 'depending on local conditions' such as terrain difficulty or the availability of 'sufficient' panchayat vaccinators.[65] This latter group could outnumber the government vaccinators by four to one and was expected to have a major influence. The Ministry of Health's acceptance of their wider use commented Yarom, 'is an important step towards a wide acceptance of the eradication programme'. Each zone was to have this personnel structure with staff recruited and trained during the preparatory phase. Annex 4 of Yarom's report also listed a health educator, administrative clerk, two drivers and a peon for each zonal unit.

Retaining the WHO project number of Nepal 9, the revised plan directly linked the new programme to previous smallpox activities.[66] While the project would 'expand a smallpox eradication programme starting from 1967 with the attack phase and ending this phase by the end of 1970', it was also clear that although it was a separate programme for smallpox and more advanced, it was one part of a broad attack on communicable disease. Another aim was to establish an epidemiological unit within the Directorate of Health Services 'for formulating control schemes and wherever possible the eradication of communicable diseases and to evaluate them periodically'.[67] The project would train local health officers in the 'newer epidemiological concepts to enable them to take their place in the efforts of the country to rid itself of endemic diseases'. To achieve these aims the Government requested the services of an international epidemiologist; Singh's presence in Nepal was part of this wider remit.[68] The Government was also to provide regular reports (assisted by WHO staff), and in line with broader WHO health policy 'giving particular emphasis to the integration of activities within the framework of the basic public health services of the country'.[69] The support from WHO was initially for two years but would be 'automatically extended until international assistance provided by WHO has ended'.[70] Everything pointed to a long term involvement from WHO.

Less than a month after signing, WHO short-term consultant Dr Krishan Murari Lal arrived in Nepal. As retired Deputy Director General of Health Services (Smallpox), Government of India, Lal was senior and experienced. His visit followed a regional seminar held in New Delhi (12–16 December) for the medical officers responsible for the different national programmes, but Nepal did not yet have a national project chief. Lal was to 'assist the Government in their planning for an eradication programme', but while he would allow for local conditions, he also had more pressing issues. He wanted to discuss with Nepal's health authorities whether 'speedier execution and intensification of the programme' outlined by Yarom in August was possible and whether 'some rephrasing of the priorities of the zones to be taken up for attack phase is called for'.[71] Lal looked at further progress of the existing programme. Within the project area, smallpox vaccinations were now to be given by a member of the maternal and child health centre staff rather than have an outside vaccinator visit. Vaccination clinics would also be held on a fixed day of the week at all hospitals and health centres – people needed to know so that they could organise their life to attend. Like Yarom, Lal was also aware of the activities and better results from Morang and Sunsari in Kosi Zone.

In section ten of his report in March, Lal outlined the difficulties – as he saw them – that had arisen regarding the implementation of the draft plan of operation: first, that at the national level a full-time medical officer responsible for the programme had not yet been appointed; second, no agreements had yet been made with the Home and Panchayat Ministry regarding use and payment of panchayat personnel for vaccination work; and, third, the challenges posed by the slow development of basic health services for launching systematically the attack phase.[72] Section eleven discussed his meeting on 22 December with the Director of Health Services and his staff when 'all the difficulties mentioned in Section 10 were brough[t] out in detail'. He had a final meeting on 26 December, which was also attended by SEARO's country representative, Dr Andre Malaterre.[73]

Lal's conclusions were forceful and damning. They are worth quoting in full to better convey the challenges ahead for all concerned.

(1) In the absence of leadership at the national level and of adequate supervision at the zonal level, it is difficult to visualize a systematic launching and execution of the attack phase of the programme in 1967 in two districts of Bagmati Zone and two districts of Kosi Zone, as envisaged in the draft plan of operation and agreed to by the Government.

(2) Unless a solution is found to the problem of making more attractive and worthwhile the posts of those officers who are responsible for the smallpox eradication programme, at both the national and the zonal level, so that continuity may be assured for a reasonable time, the project is likely to run at best as a control project, to drag on and ultimately to cost the Government more, as has been the experience so far in the project in Kathmandu Valley.

(3) In the light of experience gained so far in Kathmandu Valley, where it has not been possible to control smallpox even after operating the control project for nearly four and a half years, mostly owing to inadequate supervision and leadership at the national level, the apparent difficulties and problems arising from the launching of the country-wide eradication programme have to be realized by the Government and solutions found, if the goal of ridding the country of smallpox is to be achieved within the agreed time schedule.[74]

The situation looked very unpromising for the start of the intensified programme in Nepal. Nevertheless, important progress from Nepal's perspective had been made since the 22 December meeting. As the organisers of the campaign in Sunsari and Morang districts had well understood, a solution to the question of who paid the panchayat vaccinators was extremely important. The Director of Health Services informed Lal that 'a decision had been taken to pay the special allowance to panchayat vaccinators for vaccination work from the health budget and not out of panchayat funds'.[75] Details were still to be worked out, but the budget would be reworked and adjusted 'within the existing ceiling for the smallpox control programme under the National Five-Year Plan'. The panchayat vaccinators would work under the supervisory technical control of health department personnel.

A new plan was drawn up. It was solely for a smallpox eradication project and had a new but short-lived project number – Nepal 20. It had the same template as the earlier revised plan (Nepal 9) and some of the same wording, but whereas the revised plan conveyed a more cautious sense of scaling up and expansion within the Nepali context, the tone and language of the new project plan was direct. It explicitly stated as its objective that 'The Government, with assistance from WHO, has a fundamental aim and <u>as a part of global programme</u> to eradicate smallpox from the Kingdom of Nepal by the vaccination of the entire population within seven years (attack phase).'[76] The underlining was in the text and creates the impression that only now was the Government serious about eradication. Yet the revised plan for Nepal had stated the expansion of the eradication programme was to cover the whole country and indeed with the attack phase ending in four years rather than seven.[77] The latter target of seven years was a more realistic assessment of the situation. The revised plan had also indicated that a detailed plan of action would be drawn up and 'will have to take into account the specific condition of the country and to be phased according to the possibilities and development of health services in the country'.[78] The equivalent section in Nepal's new plan accelerated the process.[79] One objective of the new plan was to introduce legislation banning variolation throughout the country although the 1964 law already prohibited vaccinators from using 'medicines that produced smallpox'.[80]

The operational structure followed that of the global programme with three phases: preparatory, attack and maintenance (Table 7.2). In general, during the first three quarters of a year the preparatory phase was to take place so that the attack phase could be launched in the last quarter. 'Religious beliefs and taboos', it was noted, 'stand in the way of acceptance of vaccination, particularly amongst the section of the population known as "Newars". Their resistance to vaccination is more in evidence in urban areas than in rural areas.'[81] The situation among the Newar, as Adiga had made clear, was more complex than Lal suggests.[82] Nevertheless, as had become well recognised, the colder winter months of the last quarter of the year was the time when vaccination was most acceptable to the general population.[83] The attack phase was to last about two years in each area, after which if successful the Government would continue with a four-year maintenance phase.[84] Although mentioned in a separate section, monitoring of the situation (surveillance) to generate information for the programme was to be started during the preparatory phase and 'intensified' throughout.[85]

Table 7.2 Preparatory, attack and maintenance phases in Nepal's plan to eradicate smallpox

Preparatory (first three-quarters of the year)

- Department of Health Services to instruct zone to prioritise smallpox eradication – to plan training and supervise activities under guidance of zonal medical officer
- Detailed briefing of zonal medical and health officer
- Two weeks' training of zonal sanitarian at the SEP HQ in Kathmandu
- Establish stations where smallpox field staff to operate, based on local situation
- Determine places to store vaccine under refrigeration to enable distribution to vaccinators in the field
- Ensure transport is available for the SEP
- Organise and carry out intensive health education particularly through different levels of panchayat institutions
- In third quarter – recruit and train sufficient temporary vaccinators, long-term vaccinators, and supervisors to complete attack phase in about two years (long-term staff to continue for maintenance phase and then be absorbed into respective zonal health services)

Attack (initiate in fourth quarter)

- Vaccinate population according to plan schedule; vaccinators to record daily work in family cards and submit weekly returns indicating volume of work done and amount of vaccine used; immediate supervisors to periodically check and report on 'take' rates of each vaccinator; on completion in a locality supervisor to report on immunological coverage achieved
- To investigate every locality where inadequate immunological coverage (less than 80 per cent of every section of the population of all ages) and carry out 'mopping up'
- Ensure participation of community leaders and all zonal health workers, including NMEP (National Malaria Eradication Programme) field workers, in early case reporting
- Smallpox supervisory staff to carry out case investigation and containment

(*continued*)

Table 7.2 (Cont.)

Maintenance

- To begin when successful vaccination coverage of 80% of total population (all sections, all ages) achieved; independent assessment to confirm coverage and smallpox free status
- Requirements
o Vaccinate all new-borns
o Revaccination within 3–5 years after last successful vaccination
o Vaccination of all immigrants and 'floating' population
o Maintenance of nearly 100 per cent immunological coverage of population of districts bordering adjoining countries, especially where smallpox endemic
o Surveillance of cases, epidemiological investigation and rapid application of control measures

Source: Adapted from the plan of operation 1967, pp. 5–8.

Nepal is not a large country, but the planned phasing of the programme nationwide was ambitious. Lal had reservations, but the agreed plan indicated that the attack phase would be launched in 1967 not in two but four zones – Bagmati, Kosi, Narayani and Bheri (Map 1). In May 1967, the state owned and operated newspaper *Gorkhapatra* announced that WHO and UNICEF 'were reported to have to have supplied a total of 800,000 doses of small-pox vaccine to Nepal to enable her to launch a Small-pox Eradication Program' in the Bagmati and Kosi zones.[86] In the last quarter of 1968 the attack phase would begin in Janakpur and Lumbini; in 1969 in Sagarmatha and Gandaki; in 1970 in Mechi and Rapti; in 1971 in Dhaulagiri and Seti and in 1972 Karnali and Mahakali. By 1974 the whole of Nepal would be in the maintenance phase. Although this was the zonal schedule, only some districts in each zone were identified for launching the programme. In 1967 the programme would commence in fifteen of the country's seventy-five districts. For areas not yet in the attack phase and following 'encouraging results' in Morang and Sunsari in 1965 and 1966, vaccination – where feasible – was to be carried out as early as possible using panchayat personnel and resources under the leadership of local medical officers.

We know little, however, about vaccination activities outside the formal SEP.

Henderson was unhappy with the plan for Nepal and communicated to Mani his concerns about the seven-year length for the programme. Technically, he thought it 'considerably less satisfactory' than the plan for Afghanistan, although he did not explain why.[87] He acknowledged that there were 'real difficulties' in implementing a plan in a shorter time but wondered if with 'additional external resources' it might be possible to achieve the goal in a shorter period. He also suggested that

> Perhaps it might be appropriate to consider the first two years to be essentially pilot projects, if you will, with some form of written understanding that there would be a complete reevaluation of the programme at the end of this time to determine the subsequent course of action.

Despite the critical reports on the situation in Nepal, a memorandum in March 1967 from Mani to Candau, WHO Director-General, who had held 'personal discussions' with the Regional Directors in Geneva in February, discussed the feasibility of conducting smallpox eradication programmes in the region. Mani was thinking particularly of Afghanistan and Nepal and indicated his preference for the latter. Mani outlined the many difficulties in Afghanistan at length such as insufficient resources, undeveloped health services, poor economic situation, inaccessibility of the female population to male vaccinators and felt that 'to proceed with the launching of the eradication programme will be a waste of effort and money'.[88] The Afghan government had not asked for the programme and initially it requested all the funding from WHO. In contrast Mani only briefly mentioned that in Nepal an eradication programme had begun in two provinces and would be gradually extended. The attack phase 'will last longer than is usually accepted' but 'we have some indications that an immediate and successful maintenance phase could be organised in the zones covered'.[89] The Regional Office would keep a close eye and hoped improvements would be possible. They would also investigate the possibility of local subsidies as suggested earlier by the Director-General in October 1966. Illustrating the multiple voices and levels of operation within WHO at headquarters and regional level, the plan to eradicate smallpox from Nepal was to proceed despite Henderson's reservations.

Conclusion

Smallpox in Nepal was widespread in 1967 when the worldwide smallpox programme shifted gear to a global intensified smallpox eradication programme directed at countries where the disease remained endemic. Smallpox was one of many communicable diseases facing Nepal's population and for clinicians it was a diagnosis they needed to consider when they saw a patient. At a population level a first national health survey revealed a variable pattern of smallpox throughout the country and that vaccination levels were generally low. Although health services and workforce capacity were slowly developing, the survey village sample units also highlighted the still very limited health infrastructure throughout most of the country. Practical difficulties in carrying out the survey illustrated the problems any nationwide programme would have to face.

The years between the pilot project with its aim to begin to control smallpox and the eradication plan in 1967 were transitional, moving from more patchwork responses by different groups to planning and developing a nationwide programme that aligned with both the global goal and Nepal's national development. At the forefront of people's thinking were the challenges and what needed to be done, but underpinning this caution was increasing buy-in to the possibility of success. The pilot project had not achieved control of smallpox in the Kathmandu Valley, but both Nepal and WHO were aware of the initiative in the Morang and Sunsari districts that demonstrated what might be possible. These experiences informed the planning in 1966 and 1967, as did the knowledge of people's preferences for vaccination during the colder winter months. Community support would be essential if the new plan was to succeed. Its development also revealed different voices within WHO at HQ and between HQ and SEARO.

Notes

1 WHO, *The Second Ten Years*, p. 108.
2 Report on health and health administration in Nepal 1969, p. 62.
3 Robert M. Worth, and Narayan K. Shah, *Nepal Health Survey 1965–1966* (Honolulu, HI: University of Hawaii Press, 1969).
4 Hemang Dixit, *My 2 Innings*, 2nd edn (Kathmandu: Makalu Publication House, 2009), p. 73.

5 Hemang Dixit, personal written communication, May 2017.
6 Singh, 'Some aspects of the epidemiology of smallpox in Nepal', 132. Sanitarian T. O. Crisp finished in December 1965 but had not been replaced.
7 SEA/WHO, File 828, Box 210, Monthly progress report, November 1966.
8 Dixon, *Smallpox*, p. 370.
9 *Ibid.*, p. 371.
10 P. F. Wehrle, J. Posch, K. H. Richter and D. A. Henderson, 'An airborne outbreak of smallpox in a German hospital and its significance with respect to other recent outbreaks in Europe', *Bulletin of the World Health Organization*, 43:5 (1970), 669–79.
11 Fenner et al., *Smallpox and Its Eradication*, p. 475.
12 *WER*, 41:1 (7 January 1966), p. 8 and *WER*, 41:10 (11 March 1966), p. 126. No deaths were listed.
13 Peter Pitt, *Surgeon in Nepal* (London: John Murray, 1970), p. 41.
14 Major Peter Pitt, interview with author, Lavenham, April 2015.
15 Millward, *Vaccinating Britain*, p. 78.
16 Peter Pitt, *The Scalpel and the Kukri: A Surgeon & his family's adventures among the Gurkhas* (Chippenham: Peter Pitt, 2005), p. 22. Vaccinia is a complication of vaccination caused by the vaccinia virus. It occurs six to nine days after vaccination and is characterised by a generalised eruption of skin lesions.
17 Pitt, *The Scalpel and the Kukri*, p. 22.
18 Fenner et al., *Smallpox and Its Eradication*, pp. 478–9.
19 SEA/WHO, File 828, Box 210, Letter from Henderson to Singh, 28 January 1969. Other operatives talk of Henderson's 'empowerment' and support of people working at the local level in the global programme. Conversation with Robert Steinglass who went to Ethiopia, 15 June 2021.
20 Singh, 'Some aspects of the epidemiology of smallpox in Nepal', 133.
21 *Ibid.*
22 Yarom, Draft report on a visit to Nepal 1966, p. 9; UN Digital Library Nepal, SEA/Smallpox/13, 27 March 1967, Dr K. M. Lal, WHO short-term consultant, Assignment report on Smallpox Eradication Programme in Nepal (WHO Project: SEARO 136), 17–26 December 1966, pp. 4–5. https://un.info.np/Net/NeoDocs/View/3614.
23 SEA/Smallpox/13 Lal, Assignment report on Smallpox Eradication Programme in Nepal 1966, p. 5.
24 UMN RG212, Box 78, H020701/0002, 0003, 0005, UMN/HSB evaluation study, December 1985, Historical notes.
25 UMN RG212, Box 78, H020701/0005, UMN/HSB evaluation study, December 1985, Historical notes of Tansen Hospital and Palpa Community Health Program.

26　Worth and Shah, *Nepal Health Survey 1965–1966*, p. 1.
27　*Ibid.*, pp. 1–2.
28　*Ibid.*, p. v. Fundraising was led by Dr Verne Chaney, President of the Dooley Foundation.
29　*Ibid.*, p. 2.
30　*Ibid.* It was estimated that the survey would sample approximately 1 in 1,500 Nepalis.
31　*Ibid.*, p. 3.
32　*Ibid.*, p. 4.
33　*Ibid.*, pp. 6–16.
34　*Ibid.*, p. 71.
35　Khunde Hospital, Annual Reports 1967–83.
36　Worth and Shah, *Nepal Health Survey 1965–1966*, pp. 70–1.
37　*Ibid.*, pp. 69–70.
38　*Ibid.*, p. 70.
39　*Ibid.*, p. 71.
40　*Ibid.* The authors did not explain why they chose 85 per cent, which was neither the more often quoted level of 80 per cent nor the higher 90–100 per cent suggested for more densely populated areas.
41　*Ibid.*, p. 115.
42　WHO, *The Second Ten Years*, pp. 108 and 111; Fenner et al., *Smallpox and Its Eradication*, p. 418. The timeframe goal was omitted from the formal resolution.
43　Henderson, *Smallpox: The Death of a Disease*, pp. 79–80.
44　Arita, *The Smallpox Eradication Saga*.
45　Marennikova, *How It Was*, p. 256.
46　Fenner et al., *Smallpox and Its Eradication*, p. 431.
47　Henderson, *Smallpox: The Death of a Disease*, pp. 82–4.
48　*Ibid.*, p. 77.
49　Fenner et al., *Smallpox and Its Eradication*, p. 418.
50　WHO Regional Office for South-East Asia, *Collaboration in Health Development in South-East Asia, 1948–1988: Fortieth Anniversary Volume* (New Delhi: WHO Regional Office for South-East Asia, 1992), p. 280.
51　EB22.R12. Fenner et al., *Smallpox and Its Eradication*, pp. 367 and 418.
52　Sanjoy Bhattacharya, 'WHO-led or WHO-managed? Re-assessing the Smallpox Eradication Program in India, 1960–1980', in Alison Bashford (ed.), *Medicine at the Border: Disease, Globalization and Security, 1850 to the Present* (Basingstoke and New York: Palgrave Macmillan, 2006), pp. 60–75.
53　World Health Organization, Regional Office for South-East Asia. (1967). SEA/RC20/2 – The work of WHO in the South-East Asia

Region: Report of the Regional Director 1 August 1966–1 July 1967, p. 3. WHO Regional Office for South-East Asia https://apps.who.int/iris/handle/10665/130463.
54 WHO SEARO, Report of the Regional Director, 1 August 1966–1 August 1967, p. 3.
55 SEA/WHO, File 828, Box 210, C. Mani, Regional Director, to Ministry of Foreign Affairs, Kathmandu, 22 July 1966. The proposed second consultant Dr Karunaratne (formerly Director of Health Services, Ceylon) instead went to Afghanistan. Karunaratne would succeed Mani as Regional Director in 1968.
56 Yarom, Draft report on a visit to Nepal 1966, p. 9.
57 *Ibid.*, p. 4.
58 *Ibid.*, pp. 9–10.
59 *Ibid.*, p. 7.
60 *Ibid.*, p. 5.
61 *Ibid.*, pp. 10–11.
62 SEA/WHO, File SPX-1, Box 544, C. Mani, Regional Director, to Dr Satnam Singh, WHO Public Health Officer, Kathmandu, 1 September 1966.
63 *Ibid.*, Chief SE/HQ to Regional director, SEARO, 7 October 1966.
64 Yarom, Draft report on a visit to Nepal 1966, p. 7.
65 *Ibid.*, p. 11.
66 SEA/WHO, File 447, Box 185, Smallpox Eradication and Control of Other Communicable Diseases, Nepal. Project No.: WHO – Nepal 9, Revised plan of operation for Smallpox Eradication and Control of Other Communicable Diseases, Nepal (Previous title: Smallpox Control Pilot Project), p. 1.
67 *Ibid.*, p. 2.
68 *Ibid.*, p. 5.
69 *Ibid.*, p. 8.
70 *Ibid.*, p. 5.
71 SEA/Smallpox/13, Lal, Assignment report on Smallpox Eradication Programme in Nepal 1966, p. 1
72 *Ibid.*, pp. 10–11.
73 *Ibid.*, pp. 11–15.
74 *Ibid.*, p. 15.
75 *Ibid.*, p. 13.
76 SEA/WHO, File 828, Box 210, SEA-67/670, Plan of operation for smallpox eradication, Nepal, Smallpox Eradication Project Nepal 20, p. 3.
77 Revised plan of operation 1966, pp. 2–3.
78 *Ibid.*, p. 4.
79 Plan of operation 1967.

80 Section 12, Law enacted to provide for vaccination for the prevention of smallpox among children (Smallpox Control Act); Law No.27 of 2020 B.S. (28 February 1964). Published in Nepal Gazette Vol. 13 No. 29 (Extraordinary) of Falgun 16, 2020 B.S. The Smallpox Control Rules, 2023 B.S. (1967) were published in the Nepal Gazette in 1968. Dixit, *The Quest for Health* (1995), p. 206.
81 Plan of operation 1967, p. 3.
82 See Chapter 6.
83 Plan of operation 1967, p. 3.
84 *Ibid.*, p. 5, Annex 2.
85 *Ibid.*, p. 9.
86 Nepal Press Digest, vol. 11, Other international relations, 14 May 1967, p. 151.
87 SEA/WHO, File 828, Box 210, Nepal 20, Chief, SE/HQ to Regional Director SEARO and RA/CD, 24 February 1967.
88 SEA/WHO, File SPX-1, Box 544, Regional Director to Director General, 16 March 1967.
89 *Ibid.*

8

Expanding nationwide

Although the Government did not sign its new operational plan until 1 October 1967, expansion of the Smallpox Eradication Project (SEP) had already begun as the designated districts in the initial four zones prepared to enter the attack phase. In Kosi Zone, the work continued in Morang and Sunsari districts and showed what was possible under their local 'inspiring leadership'.[1] By May 1967 the panchayat (community) vaccinators had completed 210,000 vaccinations, with a confirmed biological coverage of more than 90 per cent of the population. Government vaccinators were appointed to mop up and complete vaccination of the remaining population. Nevertheless, the first few years of the overall SEP in Nepal were characterised by continuing references in visiting WHO consultant reports and a joint Government/WHO project evaluation in late 1969 to the problems and need for improvement. Nevertheless, the assessment team also acknowledged the 'substantial progress'.[2] The SEP had expanded into more districts, an administrative structure was set up to implement the programme, vaccine was secured, stored and distributed, staff were recruited and trained, reporting increased and information about cases began to appear that could be used within the country and also for the WHO Regional Office in New Delhi and HQ in Geneva. By 1972–73 all of Nepal's seventy-five districts were incorporated into the project.

This chapter examines how Nepal's SEP expanded to become the country's first nationwide health programme. The first section examines its decentralised structure. The project operated from a national plan and had a national headquarters in Kathmandu, but at the centre of the gradual planned nationwide expansion was decentralisation of its administrative structure to the zonal and district level which aligned with the political and administrative changes occurring in Nepal. Although districts were grouped into zones, the district remained the key administrative unit of the smallpox programme. Central to Nepal's success with smallpox were the district supervisors. The second part of the chapter looks more widely at the project which immediately faced financial and logistical challenges. Additional financial support from WHO enabled Nepal to meet the plan's targeted expansion into more zones and more districts. (The change in strategy in 1971 to emphasising surveillance and containment rather than mass vaccination is discussed in Chapter 9.)

The 'vital element'

In the official history, Henderson identified the lessons and benefits of the successful global programme and acknowledged the challenges for his small central unit in Geneva.

> Multinational, cooperative health programmes are inevitably difficult to manage, given the realities of national sovereignty and the intrinsic problems of international organizations. The smallpox eradication programme could not operate as a monolithic structure, like a military command; rather it was obliged to function in a collegial structure of many independent national programmes, each with its own administrative traditions and socio-cultural patterns, and utilizing resources from many different sources.[3]

The WHO was the 'coordinating organization' but had limited resources to support its work; its only authority over national programmes was 'moral suasion'. A 'hierarchical structure of international and national staff was not possible'.[4] For multiple reasons, therefore, the management and implementation of the global smallpox programme had to decentralise. That decentralisation began within WHO with the regional offices having 'a substantial degree of autonomy'.

Decentralisation is an important theme in health management; its organisation in any given country is strongly influenced by a particular government's structure. The two tend to be considered in isolation.[5] As but one function of government, only passing reference may be given in public administration literature to health while the literature concerning health services often does not give due attention to the wider context. Smallpox in Nepal illustrates how health should be considered an important part of public administration and how the wider context influenced the implementation of a health programme. Throughout the years of the global smallpox programme – both before and after 1967 – Nepal continued to experience ongoing major political and administrative changes. Signalled in the country's new 1962 constitution, King Mahendra's administrative reorganisation in 1965 divided the country into fourteen zones and seventy-five districts with the aim of fostering the country's much needed economic development. The smallpox plan sat within this overall national restructuring and development policy and its implementation throughout needed to align with wider government policies and practices.

While Henderson was operationalising the smallpox programme to work within the regionalised WHO structure, the different member states faced their own challenges. In Nepal, 'Because of the difficulties of travel, responsible district supervisors proved to be the vital element in the programme' wrote Henderson in the official history.[6] In 1977, Shrestha, Robinson and Friedman's analysis also commented that 'The district supervisors have always been seen as the keystones of the surveillance-containment programme and responsibility has been largely decentralised to them.'[7] Both accounts particularly referred to the period after 1971, although prior to 1971 each district gradually established a smallpox project office. The structure varied around the country. In forty-five districts, which were all in the Tarai or central hills, a district supervisor was in charge. In those without, which included all the mountain areas, seventeen had an assistant supervisor and seven a senior vaccinator, but a district supervisor from a neighbouring district 'directed' them.[8] The remaining six districts, of which five were in the Tarai and one in the central hills, came under the integrated health services trial project where multipurpose health workers were used.[9] Shrestha, Robinson and Friedman continued that 'The data on the quality of surveillance and containment described later are justification for the policy. Where the figures are poor so is the district supervision, and the most efficiently run districts are those with the best district supervisors.'[10]

Although the concept of districts was not new in Nepal, the division into seventy-five was more than double the previous system. Whelpton has commented that the new districts were 'not usually naturally economic or cultural units', but in an earlier study Agrawal noted that the new boundaries 'usually coincided' with the older *thum* administrative subdivisions.[11] 'Thus, in this major administrative change in modern Nepal, we may clearly discern the continuity of the traditional moorings as well as the retention of the old political divisions.' The two processes of zonal and district development and expansion of the smallpox project were linked; and could both enable but also constrain health service administration. Director of Health Services Joshi (Y. R.) informed Lal at their final meeting on 26 December 1966 that the assistant medical officers who would have responsibility for public health activities – including smallpox eradication – were sanctioned under the country's development programme and as such were only temporary postings. Present government policy was not to give special allowances to try and make these positions more appealing 'as that would create complications in the case of personnel posted to other departments'.[12] Such government jobs were, however, difficult to get and people did not want to lose them.

In 1967, Nepal was part way through its Third Five Year Plan (1965–70), but although smallpox eradication was a global programme and a priority for WHO it was not a national priority in Nepal. Staff at SEARO – and especially those who visited or were posted to Nepal – had a better understanding of the situation than those in Geneva. Not only were there pressures from within the country on Nepal's development, but the Third Plan was also characterised by conflict between Nepal's planners and the various and increasing number of foreign donors – whether states or agencies – who came to Nepal with their own agendas. Nepal, wrote Siller and Yadav, needed the funding and technical expertise with project preparation and programme design, but from the Third Plan onwards there was a 'constant effort to find a means of channelling foreign aid into a strategy of development that fitted Nepal's position as an agricultural, land-locked country'.[13] The number of staff in the Planning Ministry was expanding and, from the studies and publications undertaken, demonstrated that they were 'learning the mechanics of planning', but the 'weakness of the planning effort lay in trying to do too much too soon'.[14]

The Smallpox Control Pilot Project (1962–65) had covered three densely populated Kathmandu Valley districts of Bagmati zone but under the new plan all eight districts were included in 1967. It also scheduled the expansion of the SEP into further zones, although initially only into some districts in each. The early focus was on increasing coverage in the Tarai where smallpox was common. Two districts in Kosi, two in Bheri and three in Narayani zones were brought into the programme in 1967 with the remaining districts in each zone joining in 1968.[15] In May 1968, visiting WHO medical officer Dr Louis Gremliza reported that zonal health offices had been established in the three new zones.[16] These offices were headed by a zonal medical officer of health who was responsible for family planning, communicable diseases, tuberculosis and maternal and child health services. 'Effective field supervision' for the smallpox project, noted the Department of Health Services annual report, was done by the senior sanitarian or supervisor.[17] In Bagmati, the zonal smallpox office was located in the SEP's national headquarters 'and therefore functions under the immediate supervision of the medical officer in charge of the programme'.[18] In July 1968 the next round of expansion occurred and three districts in each of two further zones, Lumbini and Janakpur, entered the attack phase.

As the 1977 analysis noted, a diagram of the organisational structure could show the chain of command 'but it does not indicate the problems inherent in implementing this command'.[19] Continuing with the familiar theme of Nepal's challenges, 'Communication in much of Nepal is slow and difficult, but the nature of smallpox transmission is such that decisions need to be made and acted upon quickly.' Relying on people travelling out from the centre could not be the way forward. Reasons varied but 'It has often proved impossible to move more senior staff into a district for up to a week after their presence has been requested, and the burden of all the decisions during this time has had to be taken by the district supervisors.'[20] In a similar vein, Shrestha (P. N.) recounted in a presentation on the development of a reporting system in Nepal that

> in certain districts, messages sent from an affected village by any mode may take as long as a week or more to reach the district headquarters. Reports sent by post from certain district headquarters may take about a month to reach the national headquarters, the average for all the districts being about 2 weeks. Delays in receiving the reports are inevitable.[21]

While multiple references in this book to Nepal's communication challenges may seem repetitive, this was everyday life for people living and working in Nepal; it occupied such a central place in their thinking and planning and should not be underestimated. Stiller and Yadav discussed how in the earlier Rana period the terrain and communications 'had a direct influence on district administration in Nepal'.[22] Central administration learned how to work around these challenges. Now, in the new but fluid political environment of the 1960s the SEP would have to do likewise as many of the same challenges remained.

Good district supervision for the smallpox programme took time to develop. Initially it was hard to get qualified people for the programme. Nepali graduates tried for the government's gazetted posts which had better prospects. Senior positions in the SEP and zonal officers were gazetted and so bound by the rules and regulations of the Public Service Commission, but the district positions were non-gazetted and so could be appointed by the SEP. This gave flexibility. It also maintained the new zonal-district hierarchy.[23] Training of staff to equip them with the knowledge and skills to take on their new roles became an important part of the SEP. During the operation of the pilot project the issue of poor and inadequate supervision was repeatedly mentioned in WHO reports. It was still an issue for the SEP where the bulk of the work in the field was done by temporary vaccinators who were supervised by the permanent or senior vaccinators who also carried out primary and revaccinations 'as far as time permits'.[24] At the district office, the supervisor was supported by assistant supervisors who were responsible for supervising the senior vaccinators. Gremliza reported that 'In many instances it was found that the work done by some assistant supervisors was inadequate. Also, it appeared that they were not sufficiently well trained.'[25]

Senior staff were trained in Kathmandu, while district staff trained the senior (who were permanent) and temporary vaccinators.[26] In September and October 1969, WHO supported the provision of a refresher course in Kathmandu for SEP supervisors.[27] The sixty-two participants, who represented the majority of the supervisory staff, were divided into three groups and included senior supervisors from the central and zonal level of administration and district supervisors and assistant supervisors within the six zones.

The course was held at the Nursing School at Bir Hospital and included lectures on the epidemiology of smallpox, programming of vaccinations, containment activities and training in scar survey methodology and outbreak control. Field training was carried out in various villages in the Kathmandu Valley. During the first day a preliminary test was held to assess participants' level of knowledge and gaps. Another test was held at the end of the course. Analysis of the results found that questions relating to clinical features of smallpox, vaccination techniques, determination of population coverage 'were answered rather satisfactorily' and that in the preliminary test questions about the epidemiology of smallpox and outbreak containment activities 'were poorly answered'.[28] WHO medical officers provided most of the teaching but 'particular thanks' was given to Mr Ram Govind from the national smallpox unit. He taught reporting and statistics but had also provided translations for the participants of the written English materials and 'acted most successfully as interpreter'.[29] At WHO and Ministry level the SEP was run in English, but Nepali staff who ran it in the field worked in Nepali.[30]

In his subsequent report, the lead WHO trainer Dr Andrzej Oles recommended that supervision at all levels in the Nepal programme needed further development. Supervisors were to have an active role in vaccination activities and leadership in surveillance and containment of outbreaks. 'There should be an accepted rule that all supervisory staff should spend half their time in active field work – which would enable them to give systematic guidance and support to subordinate workers.'[31] Just over a month later, a joint Government of Nepal and WHO assessment team conducted an evaluation of the first three years of the SEP. Membership for the Government was: Dr Narayan Keshary Shah, Deputy Director, Medical Services; Shrestha (P. N.), recently appointed as national head of the SEP; and Dr Bainateya Nanda Vaidya, Medical Officer, Lumbini Zonal Hospital. For WHO the three members were: Dr Mahendra Singh and Dr Bahrawi Wongsokusomo, WHO consultants from SEARO, New Delhi; and Dr Paul Wehrle from the Smallpox Eradication Unit, Geneva.[32] Their report likewise recommended that 'improved supervision, with a more systematic approach towards vaccination coverage, must be developed' 'if further gains are to be made'.[33] It noted that 'The lack of supervision and of effective discipline over the vaccinators was the most critical deficiency in the present programme. Improper vaccination techniques, incomplete and erratic coverage of the population, ill-defined assignments and low vaccinator productivity required urgent attention.'[34]

Part of the assessment team's brief was to review how the SEP was working at the zonal level. Members of the team split into three pairs who each assessed the work in two zones. They found that because of 'limitations of personnel and resources in the zones' their organisational structures differed, but that 'In general, the activities of zonal programmes were essentially in accordance with the plan of operation and with SEP HQ schedules'.[35] The Department of Health Services annual report for 1970–71 expressed a similar view. 'The policies, plan and method of operation have already been described in the previous report and there had been no change.'[36] The programme was following the schedule outlined in the plan of operation, but there were problems and shortcomings. In Janakpur zone the SEP office was in Janakpur but had been moved and integrated into the zonal health office which opened in Jaleswar on the border with India. As in other zones, a recently posted senior sanitarian had responsibility for the SEP. Such changes were beyond the control of the SEP and contributed to a range of problems. Records 'had not been well maintained: for example, none could be found concerning a smallpox outbreak in Itharwa village (Mahotary District) which occurred in early December 1968'.[37] In Lumbini zone a senior supervisor was responsible for the SEP. He was based in the zonal hospital but appeared to have little 'regular communication' with the zonal medical officer.

The development of the district level structure similarly revealed a variable and evolving situation as the SEP expanded. In Narayani zone, two of the districts (Bara and Rauthat) had full-time district supervisors, each assisted by two assistant supervisors. The remaining three districts (Makwanpur, Parsa and Chitwan) had no district supervisors and the assistant supervisors were responsible for implementing the project. The SEP was now operating in ten zones involving fifty districts – two-thirds of the country's total. Each year it was meeting its target. In 1969–70 Gandaki and Sagarmatha zones entered the mass vaccination attack phase and in 1970–71 Mechi and Rapti zones. In Mechi two of the four districts were initially brought in, but still needed a senior supervisor. In Rapti the project began in two of its five districts. During the year a further three of the seven districts in both Sagarmatha and Gandaki zones were added. By this time all districts were covered in the other six zones. The quarterly field report filed in December 1970 by Shrestha and Sathianathan, who had arrived at the project in October as the counterpart WHO medical officer, illustrated the structure being made to work. It detailed, for example, their field visits to districts in the Bagmati and Lumbini zones. Elsewhere, 'One member of HQ staff (Health Educator) visited Mechi Zone to initiate the smallpox eradication [P]rogramme in 2 districts and another member of HQ staff (Statistician) visited Rapti Zone to initiate the programme in 2 districts'.[38]

In late 1970, Oles could again report that 'The organizational pattern of the smallpox eradication programme in Nepal is at present adequately established at central, zonal and district levels.'[39] Two further refresher courses, similar in content to those in 1969 and supported by WHO were run in 1970.[40] A total of forty participants, including five from Gandaki and three from Sagarmatha, came from seven of the eight zones.[41] Of the twenty-four participants in the second course, sixteen were newly recruited assistant supervisors not yet assigned to districts for the upcoming 1970–71 attack phase for Mechi and Rapti or to fill existing vacancies in other zones where the programme was in operation.[42] When developing the programme, project staff in Nepal had given priority to the districts where zonal health offices were established and to the Tarai districts; zones in the far-west of the country were yet to be included.[43] In December 1971 reports of suspected smallpox cases began coming into the newly established SEP office in Kailali district in Seti zone. Led by District Supervisor Hira Prasad Tiwari, all reports were investigated revealing 'a major endemic focus' in the district.[44] This plus the fact that the remaining seventeen hill districts were 'comparatively sparsely populated' led to a change in plan and the decision to include all seventy-five districts in the 1972–73 financial year rather than over three years.[45] The SEP was now nationwide, with a decentralised structure that if variable in practice, could be built on. Tiwari's work in Kailali district demonstrated the value of effective district supervision.[46]

A national health programme

The plan's objective was to 'eradicate smallpox from the Kingdom of Nepal by the vaccination of the entire population within seven years'.[47] By any stretch of the imagination it was a huge ask. Nevertheless, this was the government's – 'with assistance from WHO' – 'fundamental aim'. If the SEP was to be successful throughout Nepal, it would have to adapt – like the health survey – to Nepal's demographic structure. While smallpox was most common in the densely populated areas of the Kathmandu Valley and the Tarai, outbreaks could occur anywhere. Nepal had a total estimated population of 10.5 million of which 89 per cent lived in villages and towns of less than 2,000 inhabitants with 73 per cent living in 27,500 villages of less than 1000 people with an average population of 225.[48]

Any project needed to be financed, but the international economic environment was uncertain. Even before the plan was signed, its implementation faced an unexpected hurdle when the national budget for the year beginning mid-July 1967 was announced. 'It was expected all along by the Department of Health Services', wrote Singh to Dr Bozidar Ignjatovic, SEARO Regional Adviser in Communicable Diseases, 'that nearly 0.8 million rupees requested for smallpox eradication programme for the coming FY would be sanctioned'.[49] Unfortunately 'last stage cuts' in the budget included the smallpox programme and 'Only Rs 0.547 million have been sanctioned'. This had serious implications for rolling out the attack phase. While the Director of Health Services, Dr Gauri S. L. Das, would try to get the budget restored, the project would require significant changes. Singh requested comments and advice. With the lower budget, only seven of the earlier planned fifteen districts would be able to enter the attack phase. From his epidemiological perspective, Singh in order 'to achieve faster reduction in smallpox incidence in the country', proposed 'thinly' covering all the Tarai districts plus continuing with 'mopping up' in the three districts of the Kathmandu Valley. This approach 'is one of smallpox control in areas densely populated and at high risk'. 'To the best of our knowledge, Government's long-term commitment of resources to a time-limit SE programme may not be likely'.

In his reply to Singh, which was also sent to Geneva with a copy of Singh's letter, Ignjatovic commented on the 'disappointing state of affairs of the progress of the smallpox eradication programme in Nepal'.[50] A copy of the letter also went to the WHO country representative (WR) in Nepal, Dr G. J. Stott, with Ignjatovic saying that he was keen to have official comments on the smallpox project from the Government 'at the earliest'. He also instructed the WR to contact government authorities and convey the message that in view of the resolution at the Twentieth World Health Assembly (WHA20.15)

> WHO could favourably consider any request from Government for a major finan[cial] assistance to a smallpox eradication programme in Nepal – for instance, payment of allowances/salaries to temporary vaccinators or fuel for vehicles, in addition to supplies and equipment. But this assistance however will only be in the context of a smallpox eradication programme in Nepal.

This message was then conveyed to Singh in letters in August.[51] Ignjatovic also raised the question of irregular kerosene supplies for the refrigerators. If this was related to the budgetary constraints 'WHO might consider, if requested by the Government, financial assistance to cover the cost of kerosene supplies for the refrigerators being used to store the smallpox vaccine'.[52]

In a letter dated 24 October 1967 to Nepal's Ministry of Foreign Affairs, SEARO Director Mani accepted the request from Nepal for assistance of Rs 41,700 (US$ 5,472) per month for the next year for salaries and field allowances for national staff, fuel for six vehicles and 'other miscellaneous expenses'.[53] The finance was provided as a 'special case' with the stipulation the Government started the activities in the four zones according to the agreed plan, tried to get money for subsequent years, provided full details about the categories of workers being paid and how much. This agreement formed the second addendum to the revised plan concluded in 1966 with the amended plan concluded in October 1967 carrying the title 'Smallpox Eradication Project, Nepal (Nepal-0020)' being the first addendum. In November, Ignjatovic visited Nepal, noting in his report the Director of Health Services' concern 'as to how to obtain better results in the programme to match WHO assistance' and his own doubts 'whether adequate national funds would be available for smallpox eradication in the years to come'.[54] The amount of funding required for smallpox was small in comparison to the malaria programme, which was considered part of Nepal's plan for socio-economic development. In the estimates for 1969–70 it consumed over 40 per cent of the total health budget at Rs 17,040,000.[55]

Nevertheless, the SEP expanded as scheduled. Further addenda detailing additional financial support were added in subsequent years as the project incorporated new zones. Except at the start of the intensified programme, the Nepali government mostly matched the funding for the eradication of smallpox (Appendix 3).[56] The SEP received an important boost on 25 March 1968 when King Mahendra proclaimed through a royal decree that the smallpox pilot project would become a smallpox eradication project.[57] Since the King was the centre of political and administrative power in Nepal, royal support ensured firm government support for the project.

The SEP, with its national office in Kalimati, was situated within the Communicable Disease section of the Ministry of Health Directorate of Health Services alongside the malaria, tuberculosis and leprosy projects.[58] It operated under a project medical officer and was headed by the Assistant Director Communicable Diseases Division. Dr A. Prajapati was appointed to lead the project in 1967. The SEP was also a development budget project for the Department of Health Services rather than coming out of its regular budget.[59] When the smallpox programme assessment team visited at the end of 1969, they noted that the 'project in charge' – as the medical officer position was referred to – was responsible for programme planning and implementation; importantly, he had a budget and the authority to commit the funds.[60] It was independent of other projects under the Department, which gave it flexibility to respond to challenges; its personnel only carried out smallpox work. As Shrestha, Robinson and Friedman later emphasised, 'It is important to realize that the basic health services – district medical officers, hospitals, etc. – have no responsibility to smallpox eradication beyond reporting any cases of which they happen to be informed.'[61]

For a vaccination programme to be successful, it needed – as discussed in Chapter 6 – an assured supply of good quality vaccine and logistical provision that would enable the vaccine to reach the intended recipients. Between February and May 1968, the programme received 752,000 doses of freeze-dried vaccine from WHO and the USSR. Intensified activity during May had resulted in vaccine shortage and WHO supplying 200,000 doses on an emergency basis.[62] At this stage 'locally purchased' needles were being used. 'Simple' needles, wrote Gremliza, were resulting in vaccine wastage which could be reduced if bifurcated needles, which could be supplied by the WHO, were to be used.[63] The bifurcated needle was dipped directly into the ampoule and held a droplet of vaccine between the fork sufficient for vaccination. With the expected increase in the numbers of vaccinations, Gremliza thought that pressure on vaccine supplies would increase. While potentially valuable, bifurcated needles were considered too costly for a mass campaign, but 'modifications of this device are being studied'.[64] When the assessment team visited in late 1969 these new needles had just been introduced and were being used with the multiple puncture method of vaccination.[65]

In practice, vaccine supply to Nepal was less the issue; the real logistical challenge was storage – in Kathmandu, in the districts, and then to vaccinators in the field. Although freeze-dried vaccine was more heat stable, it still required proper storage below 10 degrees. 'Vaccinators have to be repeatedly instructed', wrote Gremliza, 'not to allow the vaccine to remain outside cold storage conditions for more than two weeks'.[66] The problem was the refrigerators – or rather their lack or not being in working condition. On the basis of a storage capacity of 50,000 doses of vaccine per refrigerator, storage facilities across five districts in the first four zones in the SEP had been arranged based on eleven refrigerators.[67] Other storage capacity existed in hospitals and health centres, but 'little is known about the exact capacity of these facilities except that it is reported that many refrigerators are out of operation' and 'Certainly, these limited storage facilities will create difficulties when larger consignments of vaccine arrive in Nepal.'[68]

The numbers of electric and kerosene operated refrigerators increased significantly but problems continued. The assessment team found in 1969 that the refrigerators in the zonal offices and HQ in Kathmandu were in operation and that a member of staff was on a three-month fellowship for training in maintenance, but those in three of the twelve district offices visited were not functioning 'and large supplies of vaccine were found in some of these refrigerators'.[69] On his visit to Kapilvastu district in Lumbini zone in the Tarai, Oles described how:

> The last shipment from the zonal office had taken place in December 1968. The vaccine was kept in a refrigerator (at the nearby dispensary), which unfortunately, had gone out of order some time during May 1969, and since then up to the time of the writer's visit, the vaccine has been kept at room temperature and distributed among vaccinators. Authorities at the higher échelons (zonal and national levels) were not informed about this fact. At the time of the visit, the stock of this vaccine was about 5 000 doses.[70]

This meant that throughout the heat of the summer months from May to September no refrigeration for the vaccine was available in the district. The effectiveness of any vaccination carried out during this time is not known.

Maintenance problems and delays also applied to vehicles used to transport supplies and personnel. A zonal office tended to have a vehicle, district supervisors where possible used motorcycles and vaccinators bicycles. In two of the six zones in 1969 'the drivers were not competent to manage motor vehicles' and had been involved in accidents. The vehicles were being repaired, but some of this work had to be done in India and 'Because of vehicle import restrictions in India, both travel and access to repair facilities have presented problems.'[71] In the flatter Tarai, motorcycles and bicycles were useful but 'walking is the only feasible method of transport in much of the hill and mountain region'. At the best of times road conditions were hard on vehicles, but transportation was further challenged during the monsoon months between June and September when roads were often impassable. Also, some WHO supplies were not appropriate for conditions in Nepal. 'Vehicle battery-powered microphones for field use are of no value in this programme' noted the assessment team.[72] Nepal had few vehicles and much of the country was inaccessible to vehicles. The report suggested that the microphones should be returned to WHO for reallocation to somewhere where they could be used.

In January 1968, Dr R. Wasito (from Japan) became the WHO Public Health Officer replacing Singh who had left Nepal the previous November and moved to Afghanistan. Staff in Geneva were impressed with Wasito's early activities, which 'suggests that new life has been breathed into the Nepal programme'.[73] They had also received communication from the Ministry of Health and Welfare of Japan that it was willing to 'provide vaccine to the limit of approximately 3 million doses per year to Nepal under the general terms of reference of the Colombo Plan'.[74] In March 1969 Henderson communicated with the new SEARO Director, Dr V. T. Hevat Guneratne, following Wasito's February report, that 'The man is quite unbelievable. My regret is that we do not have about 20 of him.'[75] In May, however, Henderson wrote to Guneratne that he had received a copy of the draft notes of Dr Jacobus Keja's visit to Nepal.

> Clearly the lesson to be learned is that a project is best judged in the field by direct appraisal ... I had thought the situation was generally better than the sorry state of affairs portrayed. I hope this serves as a stimulus to better performance on the part of all concerned but I had thought Dr Wasito was in better touch with things than evidently he is.[76]

Henderson also drew on his other connections to assist him. He had his reservations about the comprehensive health workers who were envisaged as having a key role in an integrated health service. In March 1967 he received a copy of the first malaria evaluation report from his CDC colleague, Dr Robert L. Kaiser.[77] In a personal note Henderson asked him about how malaria workers could 'effectively' play a part in the smallpox programme:

> There is a problem in assigning a lowly worker too many tasks. On the other hand, there is a personnel problem in many of these countries. Could the Malaria surveillance workers carry out smallpox case surveillance? Can they efficiently carry out vaccination activities?
>
> Your personal thoughts and comments on these matters would be of real help to me.[78]

Kaiser's reply is not in the file, but a further letter from Henderson a month later outlined the general view, following a meeting in Alexandria that had discussed the potential relationships between the two programmes, that 'Although it would seem logical that both eventually emerge in a multi-disease-oriented set-up, I believe we were quite unanimously of the view that we should not be too precipitous in encouraging this.'[79] He thought the malaria surveillance workers could act as smallpox surveillance workers. To require them to vaccinate would be 'heroic'. The pilot in Pakistan 'contrary to your reports' was experiencing logistics problems as the number of vaccinations was fewer than planned for. For an eradication programme to be effective, Henderson believed:

> there must be rigorous supervision of a type that is difficult to obtain when several diseases are attacked simultaneously by the same group ... I fear that the theoreticians, however, are stampeding the multiple oriented basic health worker concept without a full comprehension of the intrinsic problems of the field.[80]

The SEP's goal was 'Total coverage of the population with systematic vaccination'.[81] During the first four months of 1968, SEP vaccinators carried out 188,623 primary vaccinations and 568,199 revaccinations in the fifteen districts of the programme, covering an estimated 2,278,412 people or approximately 23 per cent of Nepal's total population.[82] Gremliza felt that to achieve 'a more effective implementation of the programme' some adjustment should be made to 'suit the particular ecological features of the country' relating to its geography and density of population.[83] He suggested viewing Nepal horizontally rather than the north–south division in many zones. By making use of the 'excellent Kathmandu-Birgunj highway', work should proceed systematically eastwards and westwards from Birgunj.[84] The east–west highway that was under construction would gradually help communication in the Tarai. He also questioned the need for vaccination activities in the mountain areas to the north other than for emergency purposes. The assessment team later noted that of the 357 cases of smallpox reported since 1 January 1968, only one was located north of the Tarai in Syanja (Syangja), to the southwest of Pokhara.[85]

A key feature of the intensified global programme after 1967 was its emphasis on surveillance and containment. This relied on good reporting of cases. In Nepal, legislation passed in 1964 required the notification of cases of smallpox but, as already identified, reporting was 'irregular and incomplete'.[86] Similarly, the system for reporting other communicable diseases throughout the country was 'very patchy'.[87] In the pilot project area, case reporting was carried out by project staff assisted by local health centres and panchayat institutions and this had 'considerably improved' the reporting. This system was to be used as the SEP expanded.

Improving the situation also required sound record-keeping. This was an important feature of the pilot project and was regularly commented on in the WHO field visit reports. Literacy levels were improving but were still low and methods of communication limited. Although detailed records for tax purposes had been kept for a long time, the kind of record-keeping and timeliness envisaged by those devising the global smallpox programme was different. The arrival of Singh in September 1966 led, after a three week pre-testing in a rural area of the Kathmandu Valley and staff training, to the introduction of a simpler but more informative family record form; a new form for evaluating both vaccination technique and vaccine potency; a form to see easily the immunity status of a community; and a revised and simplified weekly return for each vaccinator of work done and how much vaccine used each day.[88] Under the 1966 revised plan, the Government was to provide the 'necessary telephone, telegraph and postal communications', but in 1966 in much of Nepal these did not exist or would be regarded as inadequate from an international reporting perspective.[89] Foreign organisations and their personnel had struggled for many years in this environment.

Better reporting provided useful information for health authorities. It became possible, for example, to see the importance of internal and external migration in the spread of smallpox in Nepal. Hillary's account had earlier traced people's movements that led to the 1963 outbreak of smallpox in the Mt Everest area. In that example, smallpox was present in the capital Kathmandu, but smallpox could also be brought in from outside Nepal and then spread along communication routes and through people's networks. Having the epidemiologist's interest in method of transmission, Singh documented two examples of how smallpox was introduced into villages. In one, a minstrel group worked on both sides of the India–Nepal border and in another a beggar family who annually walked from the mountains in the north to the plains each winter were the sources of the infection. In the Tarai, roads were being built. Singh noted a case where a man was infected travelling on a bus which was carrying '4 to 5' people in the vesicular phase of smallpox on their way home having been denied admission to a large hospital. 'He sat so close to one of them that he was smeared with the discharge from the skin lesions.'[90] On another occasion a woman, who was in an earlier stage of the illness and became the index case for an outbreak in Kathmandu of twelve cases, travelled for eight hours by bus from Birganj, which was near the border. A few of the people who had travelled on the bus were traced and kept under surveillance, but none of the subsequent cases notified could be traced to contact on that particular bus.

While the Tarai and the Kathmandu Valley were the most densely populated parts of Nepal, half of the population was spread across the hills and small valleys. Worth and Shah concluded from their survey that the low immunisation coverage meant that the 'stage is therefore set for a continuation of sporadic epidemics'.[91] Mountain areas were the most sparsely populated and Singh – like Gremliza – thought that 'Mountain communities may not need total vaccination coverage'.[92] Singh recounted that it was 'customary' for people to travel south to the plains of Nepal and adjoining Indian states almost every winter in search of labour or merchandise and reported that 'accounts given by the few [m]edical officers posted in such areas leave no doubt that persons returning from the plains carry the disease back and spread it among the mountain settlements'.[93] Singh's 'mountains' were more truly the hill regions as he described how a project supervisor 'was sent to the mountain villages of Sindhu Pal Chok district lying northeast of Kathmandu Valley' where in May 1967 he discovered thirty-nine cases of whom thirteen had died. The outbreak was said to have started in early February by an itinerant tailor who travelled from the Tarai in search of business.

After three years of the SEP's steady expansion, the joint Government/WHO assessment team concluded at the end of 1969 that smallpox eradication was now strongly supported by the Government and the people – although the latter 'to a lesser extent'.[94] This they thought was due to people not seeing smallpox 'as a dramatic threat requiring immediate action, like a cholera outbreak' and lacking the community visibility of malaria and tuberculosis which had high incidence rates. The Directorate of Health Services' 1969 report was less enthusiastic:

Expanding nationwide 211

It will be apparent that the smallpox eradication programme is an example of another single disease eradication project which must be integrated, inevitably, with the basic health services, when these services become strong enough to absorb the additional load. At the present time, as will be seen later, the basic health services have a very heavy clinical case load and public health measures are hampered by lack of staff, a limited budget for transportation, poor communications and a lack of real interest in public health on the part of the public.[95]

For many Nepalis, the SEP at the end of the 1960s was still not operational where they lived.

Vaccination was encouraged in other parts of the country, but little information exists. Non-SEP institutions during the first four months of 1968 reported 15,377 vaccinations which represented only 2 per cent of the total vaccinations carried out, but panchayat vaccinators who 'are at present working on a country-wide basis seem to perform a substantial portion of the vaccinations in those zones and districts which are not yet covered by the NSEP [National Smallpox Eradication Programme]'.[96] Gremliza based this conclusion on observations he made in the Palung area of Makwanpur district (Narayani zone) 'where 54% of the individuals within the age-group 0–14 years had been vaccinated, and it was found that this had been accomplished without any centrally organized vaccination campaign'. Also, 'investigations revealed that the panchayat vaccinators are supplied with the necessary vaccine by the NSEP Headquarters in Kathmandu'. Other non-government groups providing healthcare services were also carrying out vaccination activities. A 1969 report from the International Nepal Fellowship Sikha dispensary in central Nepal noted that 'there was an opportunity to do a tour of Giramdi, Histang Aulo and Rima where we did over 1,000 B.C.Gs. We are now going to do smallpox vaccinations there.'[97] This is the first reference in these reports to smallpox vaccinations being given in a non-epidemic situation, but no mention was made of the SEP. In the Mt Everest region, archives from Khunde Hospital also do not mention the global programme.

The assessment team's report also noted the usual challenges – 'problems of terrain, the barrier of illiteracy, staffing difficulties and those of vaccine storage and distribution'.[98] It made a long list of recommendations, but in terms of actual modifications to the plan there were only three suggestions: that in the Tarai vaccinators should be assigned according to geographic area; that there seemed to be 'little merit' in assigning vaccinators to mountainous regions where the sparse population did not favour transmission and supervision was difficult; and increased attention should be given to immunising people crossing the border.[99] Nevertheless, the report also concluded that by the end of 1969 it was:

> apparent that the attack phase of the programme has made substantial progress by way of establishing a reasonably staffed organization at the centre and at the periphery, viz., at both zonal and district levels. Rapid strides too have been made to improve the case reporting, which was practically non-existent before 1965. The significance of incidence data and their geographical distribution, break-up in age groups, and sex and vaccination status is being realized. Similarly, a nucleus for health education and publicity measures to enhance the voluntary acceptance of vaccination has been created.[100]

This was a much more positive assessment than in the past.

Conclusion

In 1967, smallpox was still widespread throughout Nepal, but by the end of the decade Nepal's Smallpox Eradication Project staff were increasingly focused on the south to the Tarai and the open border with India. If the middle of the 1960s was a time of transition from the fragmented and local responses to outbreaks of the disease as in 1963, the first few years of the implementation of the intensified programme in the latter part of the decade were a time of gradual but sustained expansion nationwide. Challenges were many and familiar, but after three years the joint Government and WHO assessment team could both acknowledge progress as well as the need for further improvement.

No health programme in Nepal had yet reached nationwide coverage. Key to achieving this was the establishment of a structure that could meet the plan's annual expansion targets. Nepal met these with the WHO providing additional financial support – especially for training and coordinating vaccine supply. The SEP was set up and run separately from other health services but also had

Expanding nationwide 213

to operate within the wider context of administrative and political restructuring within Nepal and the development of a zonal and district system. The district for a long time had been the key administrative unit; it was a familiar concept. While strong leadership of the SEP at the centre was much needed, it would be the district structure that in Nepal set up the country's success. In line with the global programme, the smallpox plan's strategy was mass vaccination of the entire population. Surveillance was supposed to be developed from the start, but until the people and the means to do this were in place it neither would nor could happen. The foundations were in place when the SEP finally incorporated all of Nepal's seventy-five districts in 1972–73.

Notes

1 SEA/WHO, File SEARO 30, Box 211, Smallpox Eradication & Epidemiological Advisory Team, Quarterly field report, Second quarter 1967, 1 July 1967.
2 SEA/WHO, File 658, Box 220, SEA/Smallpox/36, 9 March 1970, Report on an assessment of the Smallpox Eradication Programme, Nepal (WHO Project: Nepal 009) by a joint Government of Nepal/WHO assessment team, 20 November–16 December 1969, p. 11.
3 Fenner et al., *Smallpox and Its Eradication*, p. 1355.
4 *Ibid.*
5 Anne Mills, J. Patrick Vaughan, Duane L. Smith and Iraj Tabibzadeh, *Health System Decentralization: Concepts, Issues and Country Experience* (Geneva: World Health Organization, 1990), p. 11.
6 Fenner et al., *Smallpox and Its Eradication*, p. 796. Henderson was the chapter's primary author.
7 SME/77.1, Shrestha, Robinson and Friedman, *The Nepal Smallpox Eradication Programme*, p. 14.
8 *Ibid.*
9 Judith Justice, *Policies, Plans, & People: Foreign Aid and Health Development* (Kathmandu: Mandala in association with University of California Press, 1989), p. 52.
10 SME/77.1, Shrestha, Robinson and Friedman, *The Nepal Smallpox Eradication Programme*, p. 14.
11 Whelpton, *A History of Nepal*, p. 126; Agrawal, *The Administrative System of Nepal*, pp. 2–3. Agrawal began his research while he was in Nepal from 1963 to 1965 as part of the Colombo Plan Technical

Assistance Programme under the Indian Aid Mission and was attached to the Department of Political Science, Tribhuvan University; Hitchcock, 'Some effects of recent change in rural Nepal'.
12 SEA/Smallpox/13, Lal, Assignment report on Smallpox Eradication Programme in Nepal 1966, p. 14.
13 Stiller and Yadav, *Planning for People*, p. 180.
14 *Ibid.*, p. 178.
15 SEA/WHO, File 658, Box 220, His Majesty's Government Ministry of Health, Department of Health Services, Smallpox Eradication Project Nepal, annual report fiscal year 2027/28 (1970/71), pp. 5–8.
16 SEA/Smallpox/23 Rev.1 3 September 1968, Dr F. G. L. Gremliza, WHO Medical Officer (WHO Project: SEARO 30), Smallpox Eradication and Epidemiological Advisory Team, Report on a visit to the programme for Smallpox Eradication and Control of Other Communicable Diseases, Nepal (WHO Project: Nepal 9), 6–16 May 1968.
17 SEA/WHO, File 658, Box 220, HMG, annual report 1970/71, p. 2.
18 *Ibid.*
19 SME/77.1, Shrestha, Robinson and Friedman, *The Nepal Smallpox Eradication Programme*, p. 14.
20 *Ibid.*
21 SE/WP/72.13, Inter-country seminar on surveillance in smallpox eradication, New Delhi, 30 October–2 November 1972, P. N. Shrestha, 'Development of reporting system in Nepal'.
22 See Chapter 3. Stiller and Yadav, *Planning for People*, p. 13.
23 Dr Benu Karki, email communication with author, 15 September 2021.
24 SEA/Smallpox/23 Rev.1, Gremliza, Report on a visit 1968, p. 6.
25 *Ibid.*, p. 8.
26 SEA/WHO, File 438, Box 211, WHO SEARO, Quarterly field report, fourth quarter 1970, Nepal 9, p. 3.
27 SEA/WHO, File 827, Box 211, SEA/Smallpox/37 15 June 1970, Dr A. J. Oles, Medical Officer, Smallpox Eradication and Epidemiological Advisory Team, Report on a visit to Nepal (WHO Project: SEARO 30), 29 September–17 October 1969. Kathmandu hosted the twenty-second Regional Committee session 29 September–5 October 1969.
28 SEA/Smallpox/37, Oles, Report on a visit to Nepal 1969, p. 1.
29 *Ibid.*, p. 3.
30 Jay Friedman, WHO Technical Officer (1972–77), telephone interview with author, 3 July 2014.
31 SEA/Smallpox/37, Oles, Report on a visit to Nepal 1969, p. 10.
32 SEA/Smallpox/36, Assessment of the Smallpox Eradication Programme, Nepal 1969, p. 2.

33 *Ibid.*, p. 11.
34 *Ibid.*, p. 6.
35 *Ibid.*, p. 3.
36 SEA/WHO, File 658, Box 220, HMG, annual report 1970/71, p. 1.
37 SEA/Smallpox/36, Assessment of the Smallpox Eradication Programme, Nepal 1969, p. 3.
38 SEA/WHO, File 438, Box 211, WHO SEARO, Quarterly field report, fourth quarter 1970, Nepal 9, p. 2.
39 SEA/WHO, File 658, Box 220, SEA/Smallpox/47 15 January 1971, Corr.1. 4 June 1971, Dr A. J. Oles, WHO Medical Officer, Report on a visit to Smallpox Eradication Programme in Nepal (WHO Project: Nepal 9) 21–30 October 1970, p. 5.
40 SEA/Smallpox/47 Corr.1, Oles, Report on a visit 1970.
41 No reason was given but none came from Bheri.
42 SEA/Smallpox/47 Corr.1, Oles, Report on a visit 1970, Annex 1.
43 SE/WP/72.12, Inter-country seminar on surveillance in smallpox eradication, P. N. Shrestha, 'Present status and future plans for the Smallpox Eradication Programme in Nepal', p. 2.
44 SE/WP/72.13, Shrestha, 'Development of reporting system in Nepal', p. 4.
45 SE/WP/72.12, Shrestha, 'Present status and future plans', p. 2.
46 Tiwari was awarded a WHO fellowship trip to India and Afghanistan. Jay Friedman, Trekking for smallpox in Nepal 20 March–1 April 1973. www.zero-pox.info/narratives/friedman_nepal.pdf.
47 Plan of operation 1967, p. 3.
48 *Ibid.*, p. 2.
49 SEA/WHO, File 828, Box 210, Singh to Dr B. Ignjatovic, Regional Adviser on Communicable Disease, SEARO, 17 July 1967.
50 *Ibid.*, Ignjatovic to Singh, 26 July 1967. Although the plan is referred to as Nepal 20, Singh's position in Nepal was as part of Nepal Project 9 where smallpox was part of the wider communicable disease remit.
51 *Ibid.*, Ignjatovic to Singh, 14 and 21 August 1967.
52 *Ibid.*, Ignjatovic to Singh, 14 August 1967.
53 *Ibid.*, 24 October 1967.
54 SEA/CD/14, Ignjatovic, Report on a visit to Nepal 1967, p. 1.
55 Report on health and health administration in Nepal 1969, p. 12.
56 Nepal's economy was under pressure with a major currency devaluation in December 1967 and rising domestic inflation. Peter Svalheim (trans. Katherine M. Parent), *Power for Nepal: Odd Hoftun & the History of Hydropower Development* (Kathmandu: Martin Chautari, 2015), p. 157.
57 SEA/Smallpox/23 Rev.1, Gremliza, Report on a visit 1968, p. 2.

58 SEA/WHO, File 438, Box 211, WHO Inter-regional seminar on smallpox eradication, Bangkok, 11–16 December 1967, Table 4, Questionnaire – Status of smallpox eradication activities – Nepal.
59 SEA/Smallpox/75 27 October 1976 Restricted, M. Sathianathan, WHO Medical Officer, Smallpox Eradication Nepal: Assignment report, October 1970–April 1976, WHO project NEP SME 001, p. 2.
60 SEA/Smallpox/36, Assessment of the Smallpox Eradication Programme, Nepal 1969, p. 2.
61 SME/77.1, Shrestha, Robinson and Friedman, *The Nepal Smallpox Eradication Programme*, p. 12. Underlining in original.
62 SEA/Smallpox/23 Rev.1, Gremliza, Report on a visit 1968, pp. 3–4.
63 *Ibid.*, p. 12.
64 WHO, Handbook for smallpox eradication programmes in endemic areas, 3.1.4 Devices for multiple pressure and scratch vaccination, p. III-11 https://apps.who.int/iris/handle/10665/67940 (accessed 31 July 2019).
65 SEA/Smallpox/36, Assessment of the Smallpox Eradication Programme, Nepal 1969, p. 6.
66 SEA/Smallpox/23 Rev.1, Gremliza, Report on a visit 1968, p. 12.
67 *Ibid.*, p. 4.
68 *Ibid.*
69 SEA/Smallpox/36, Assessment of the Smallpox Eradication Programme, Nepal 1969, pp. 6–7. The earliest expiry date in the Kathmandu fridges was 25 December 1970.
70 SEA/Smallpox/37, Oles, Report on a visit to Nepal 1969, p. 5.
71 SEA/Smallpox/36, Assessment of the Smallpox Eradication Programme, Nepal 1969, pp. 6–7.
72 *Ibid.*, p. 7.
73 SEA/WHO, File 828, Box 210, Chief, SE/HQ to Regional Director, SEARO, 30 May 1968.
74 *Ibid.*, Chief, SE/HQ to Regional Director, SEARO, 25 April 1968.
75 *Ibid.*, Chief, SE/HQ to Regional Director, SEARO, 18 March 1969. Guneratne was President of the Twentieth WHA in 1967 which adopted Resolution WHA20.15 to strengthen efforts to achieve eradication.
76 *Ibid.*, Chief, SE/HQ to Regional Director, SEARO, 6 May 1969.
77 *Ibid.*, Robert L. Kaiser to D. A. Henderson, 20 March 1967.
78 *Ibid.*, D. A. Henderson to Robert L. Kaiser, 5 April 1967.
79 *Ibid.*, Henderson to Kaiser, 3 May 1967.
80 *Ibid.*
81 Plan of operation 1967, p. 4.
82 SEA/Smallpox/23 Rev.1, Gremliza, Report on a visit 1968, pp. 3, 6.

83 *Ibid.*, p. 9.
84 *Ibid.*, p. 10.
85 SEA/Smallpox/36, Assessment of the Smallpox Eradication Programme, Nepal 1969, p. 7.
86 Yarom, Draft report on a visit to Nepal 1966, p. 6.
87 SEA/Smallpox/13, Lal, Assignment report on Smallpox Eradication Programme in Nepal 1966, p. 6.
88 *Ibid.*, p. 5.
89 Revised plan of operation 1966, p. 8.
90 Singh, 'Some aspects of the epidemiology of smallpox in Nepal', 133.
91 Worth and Shah, *Nepal Health Survey 1965–1966*, p. 71.
92 Singh, 'Some aspects of the epidemiology of smallpox in Nepal', 134.
93 *Ibid.*
94 SEA/Smallpox/36, Assessment of the Smallpox Eradication Programme, Nepal 1969, p. 11.
95 Report on health and health administration in Nepal 1969, p. 64.
96 SEA/Smallpox/23 Rev.1, Gremliza, Report on a visit 1968, p. 7.
97 International Nepal Fellowship RG214, Box 4, AO30101/0010/000, Sikha report 1969.
98 SEA/Smallpox/36, Assessment of the Smallpox Eradication Programme, Nepal 1969, p. 11.
99 *Ibid.*, p. 12.
100 *Ibid.*, p. 11.

9

Success

> I believe we have every reason to argue, based on four years of experience in many countries with difficult conditions, that eradication is a feasible concept, that mass vaccination in Nepal is highly desirable but must be and can be made far more effective than at present and that surveillance, at nil level now, must be and can be appreciably strengthened. If this is done and assuming continued progress in India, there is no reason why eradication cannot be achieved in a matter of 4 to 5 years – perhaps less.[1]

In Geneva, Henderson was unimpressed with the situation in Nepal at the end of 1970 and was frustrated with the WHO's country representative who supported the 'outmoded concept of vaccination of all'.[2] Although the official history noted that the programmes in Nepal and Afghanistan were 'progressing well', Henderson considered the programme in Nepal to be 'unsatisfactory' and 'one of the worst we have'.[3] He would continue to have his concerns, but from March 1973 Nepal was classified as 'non-endemic'.[4] The last case of smallpox in Nepal was on 6 April 1975 and on 24 May 1975 Nepal officially became free of the disease.[5] On 13 April 1977, the Nepali New Year, the report of the International Commission for the Assessment of Smallpox Eradication in Nepal declared that smallpox was eradicated from Nepal.[6]

This chapter explores how success was achieved and then maintained. It argues that although the strategy changed to emphasise surveillance and containment, implementation was enabled by the decentralised district structure, which helped circumvent topographical and communication challenges, and by the reorganisation of the vaccination schedule. Mass vaccination remained an important and complementary component but shifted to a time-limited annual campaign carried out around Nepali people's preference for vaccination during the winter. The official history records that globally 1971 and 1972 were:

> years of transition between the remarkably successful period 1967–1970—when smallpox was successfully eliminated from large areas of the world with few resources—and the succeeding years, 1973–1977, when ever larger resources and more heroic measures were required to stop transmission in the few remaining endemic countries. In some parts of the world remarkable progress was made during 1971 ... [7]

In Asia, Nepal – along with Afghanistan and Indonesia – was one of those countries. A field assessment carried out in 1975 by WHO epidemiologist Dr Alberto Monnier concluded that Nepal's smallpox programme had been effective and that since 1972 was 'roughly' one of the cheapest programmes in the world.[8]

The first part of the chapter discusses how Nepal reached non-endemic status and examines the change in vaccination strategy in mid-1971. While WHO pushed surveillance and containment from the top, it could only work if the situation existed on the ground to implement it. In Nepal, decentralisation with effective district supervisors could provide this. Improved surveillance and reporting were accompanied by a large increase in the number of vaccinations undertaken during the winter. The second section looks at 1973–75. The dominating concern was the importation of cases from outside Nepal and preventing local spread. While this was the pattern in 1973, local spread became an issue in 1974 in response to the epidemic in Bihar and threatened Nepal's 'non-endemic' status. The final part examines how 'Target Zero' or 'zeropox' was maintained – as the global programme's final stage was referred to – resulting in smallpox being declared eradicated from Nepal.

A change in strategy

In 1970, eighteen countries reported endemic cases of smallpox but most of the global total of 33,663 cases were in Asia; India reported 12,773 cases and Indonesia 10,081.[9] Nepal reported 76 cases (Appendix 1). In early December, WHO held an inter-regional seminar in New Delhi to bring together key people involved in implementing the global programme in Asia. Participants were to 'discuss and compare their experiences' and 'learn various approaches' used elsewhere in the world where surveillance rather than mass vaccination was the 'dominant element'. As the preface to the seminar documentation noted, 'This change in strategy, perhaps more than any other single factor, was felt to have played the principal role in the unexpectedly rapid progress in the programme to date.'[10] In 1971 Ethiopia became the first country in the world to start its programme 'from day one' with the strategy of surveillance and containment and never used mass vaccination.[11]

Henderson summarised the status of the global programme, saying that 'I should be less than frank if I did not note regretfully that our principal disappointment this year has been the lack of progress thus far made by India in respect to improved reporting.'[12] Bhattacharya has discussed Henderson's frustrations and highlights divisions of opinion within WHO SEARO, but the situation in India also influenced Henderson's perception of the programme in Nepal because of the long, shared and largely open border which enabled people to move freely in either direction.[13] Oles, from the regional Smallpox Eradication and Epidemiological Advisory Team, provided the meeting with a South-East Asia summary but also had recent first-hand knowledge from Nepal. He attributed the under-reporting to the familiar explanation of lack of basic health services, difficult communications and superstitious beliefs.[14] These were not problems that could be fixed quickly or easily. The situation meant that Nepal had to confront the issue of smallpox from two perspectives: handling local cases and outbreaks but also being able to deal with those originating from another sovereign country.

Reporting must have been improving in Nepal as Oles found the geographical distribution of cases 'of interest' because in recent years 99 per cent of cases were in the Tarai bordering the Indian states of Bihar and Uttar Pradesh where 'the implementation of the NSEP is still far from successful, and as various mobile segments of the population, i.e. migrants, labourers and pilgrims, can cross the border unchecked, smallpox cases are readily imported into Nepal'.[15] At the start of the intensified programme officials would have had no idea of the number of cases of smallpox or their location. Project chief Shrestha (P. N.) spoke further on the issue and indeed made the comment that 'It is worth mentioning here that people have generally become more aware of the programme and that case reporting has definitely improved.'[16] He believed that the issue of border transmission could be handled best with close cooperation 'at the local level' rather than at a regional or HQ level.

Shrestha's appointment in 1969 as national project chief was one of two key senior positions. Born in 1939 in Kathmandu, he had studied medicine at Amritsar in India between 1956 and 1961. On his return, Shrestha worked as a medical officer in various clinical posts before becoming Assistant Director, Community Health in 1966. In 1969 he gained his Master of Public Health from Harvard School of Public Health in the USA.[17] In 1972 the King awarded him the Gorkha Dakshin Bahu, the second highest civilian honour.[18] The other key senior appointment was his WHO counterpart, Sathianathan, who arrived in Nepal in October 1970 and like Shrestha was based at the project headquarters in Kalimati. From 1965 Sathianathan had been WHO Public Health Officer in the small Republic of Maldives.[19] Informally known as 'Sathi', he was 'gentle', well-liked and respected by all.[20] Later in his assignment report Sathianathan attributed part of the SEP's success to the continuity in these senior positions.[21] Sathianathan was in Nepal until 1976 and Shrestha remained in charge until 1977. Such lengthy involvement at this level was unusual for Nepali personnel. Between them they navigated the project through the organisational pathways, hierarchies and personnel of the government of Nepal and the WHO.

In 1971 the SEP's vaccination programme was reorganised. Although in his later assignment report Sathianathan listed first the 'shift in the emphasis from vaccination to surveillance-containment' in factors contributing to the programme's success in Nepal, the change in strategy in 1971 related to vaccination and when it was carried out rather than surveillance-containment.[22] Limiting vaccination to certain months of the year, freed staff time for surveillance. Previously, when a district was brought into the programme, temporary vaccinators were used for three months and after that the senior vaccinators carried out routine vaccinations throughout the year. A senior vaccinator was assigned a number of panchayats and in each panchayat had to maintain a household register of families. 'However', Shrestha explained at an inter-country seminar on surveillance held in New Delhi towards the end of 1972, experience showed that household registers were cumbersome and were not maintained properly by the vaccinators and hence could not be utilised. Further, it was found that people accepted vaccinations only during the winter months and consequently the vaccination output during the rest of the year was very poor.[23]

Under the new system, a temporary vaccinator was recruited locally from each local panchayat (population about 2,500) for one month in winter, during which they visited each house for vaccination and carried out an 'active search' for cases. A smaller number of senior vaccinators supervised their work. Simple recording forms replaced the household registers. Although the programme in each district could have been completed in one month, 'in view of the difficulty involved in training and in order to ensure adequate supervision, only one quarter of the district was taken up each month'.[24]

Despite limiting vaccination to the four winter months, the new mass vaccination strategy 'has produced better results in terms of high primary and total vaccination coverage'.[25] Although in 1971 the programme was still expanding, Appendix 4 shows the large increase in vaccinations carried out, from 2,823,098 in 1970–71 to 6,162,478 in 1971–72. The 1971 second quarter report to SEARO estimated an overall coverage of 74 per cent of the total population in the fifty districts in the programme, although the figure varied between areas.[26] In both Sagarmatha and Rapti zones primary vaccination coverage was less than 65 per cent in two districts.[27] To help with the change a new staff manual was produced in Nepali, and annual refresher training instituted to keep staff up to date. The WHO assisted in running the courses and in providing the necessary daily subsistence allowances to the participants which in the past had often been an issue. The arrangement was formalised in an exchange of letters between the government and WHO and became an addendum to the plan. This finance was additional to the annual requests from the government to WHO for support for equipment and supplies as the programme expanded as scheduled into new zones and districts. At the end of September 1971 SEARO's Regional Director, Guneratne, proposed that the 'misnomer' of the name of the revised plan of operation signed in November 1966 – Smallpox Eradication and Control of Other Communicable Diseases – be changed to Smallpox Eradication Programme, since the WHO Public Health Officer assigned to the project 'has been directing exclusively smallpox eradication activities'.[28]

Large quantities of vaccine were needed to meet the vaccination targets in Nepal's expanding programme. The WHO smallpox unit in Geneva was supporting countries to produce their own vaccine in sufficient quantity and to meet stricter international standards. In the South-East Asia Region, Burma (Myanmar) became self-sufficient in 1969 and Indonesia in 1970.[29] Nepal's plan outlined WHO's commitment to supply vaccine for 1967–69, increasing from 900,000 doses in 1967 to two million doses in 1969.[30] In January 1970, Dr Colin Kaplan from the UK visited to explore the feasibility of Nepal producing its own freeze-dried vaccine but concluded that it would be 'difficult to justify'.[31] The WHO continued to arrange Nepal's vaccine supply. Most came from the USSR, which was the largest contributor of vaccine to the global programme and between 1958 and 1979 donated more than 1,400 million doses.[32] With the USA now supporting the global programme, Cold War vaccine politics evident in the 1963–64 epidemic in Nepal faded. In 1971, New Zealand gave Nepal 250,000 doses following a visit by the King and Queen.[33] On 4 May, Arita in Geneva notified SEARO that the testing of the vaccine 'was finalized with satisfactory results' and that the New Zealand government would despatch the vaccine to SEARO to be forwarded to Nepal.[34]

Following the reorganisation of the vaccination programme, Nepal required even larger amounts of vaccine. Documents from Nepal at times referred to ampoules of vaccine and at others to doses. Sathianathan requested an additional 38,500 ampoules for November 1971 and 40,000 for January 1972 to cover programme needs until July 1972.[35] A week later HQ notified SEARO and copied to Sathianathan that on 4 October 575,000 doses were despatched from HQ to Nepal, which completed 1971 requirements. Most vaccine was supplied in ampoules; each was regarded as sufficient to vaccinate twenty to twenty-five people, but with the increasing use of bifurcated needles the number could increase by four to five times.[36] Although the global programme eventually had sufficient vaccine, at times reserve supplies were 'perilously low'.[37] Co-ordinating vaccine supply for the global programme from Geneva was complicated and time-consuming. In January 1972 a mix-up with Nepal's supply occurred. One million doses were to be sent directly to Nepal from Moscow via India, but the delivery was cleared through customs in India. Fortunately, the vaccine was held in cold storage a few miles from New Delhi and on 8 February was flown to Nepal.[38]

On reaching Nepal, vaccine was stored and then distributed to the increasing number of zones and districts involved in the SEP. Freeze-dried vaccine stored below 10°C (50°F) could be expected to remain fully potent for at least two years. In October 1972, Sathianathan asked for samples from a batch of vaccine with an expiry date of June 1972 to be tested for potency and if possible a new expiry date.[39] Proper storage remained an issue for Nepal. Refrigerator supply was part of WHO's commitment to the SEP, but project staff reports continued to note the variable state of the refrigerators that were or were not working, that needed repairs or where finance was lacking to buy kerosene or where the kerosene was of poor quality. The situation improved following the training of a technician, K. B. Shrestha, in Calcutta on a WHO fellowship.[40] The 1972 fourth quarter report noted that 'Refrigerators are functioning well in most areas. The project refrigerator technician has recently toured the eastern zones to service and repair the three or mal-functioning units.'[41]

Of greater maintenance concern were the programme's increasing number of vehicles. Joining the project in 1972 as a second WHO operations or technical officer was Jay Friedman, a former Peace Corps volunteer who had worked as an operations officer in the West and Central Africa smallpox programme.[42] Part of his responsibilities were 'many of the administrative details of the project concerning vaccine, supplies, and, most importantly, the vehicles of the project which are now in a rather sorry state and continually in need of repairs'.[43] In his third quarter report he noted that the 'complete lack of repair facilities in the terai necessitates all but the simplest repairs to be done in Kathmandu or India' but 'the SEP workshop is still very slow in repairing vehicles'.[44] A vehicle manual was introduced to try and improve the situation. Once a vehicle was repaired, it might easily break down again in the difficult terrain. 'After being overhauled in July, the Janakpur Zone Land Rover broke down once more in August.'[45] The other operations officer, Roy Mason, was stationed in Butwal (Lumbini zone) in the Tarai, and wrote that 'even in the dry season there are many creeks to cross'.[46]

The WHO staff posted to Nepal – and even more so when they were out in the field – were very aware of Nepal's obstacles. For programme personnel in New Delhi or Geneva, it was sometimes hard to believe. Henderson earlier had acknowledged the need to be on the ground to understand what was happening and related the use of district supervisors to the communication challenges. Head of the SEARO Smallpox Eradication Unit was Dr Nicole Grasset, a French epidemiologist, who had been working as a Red Cross adviser in Africa. Bhattacharya considers her 'inspirational role as a manager and negotiator is generally overlooked in existing historical studies'.[47] Grasset joined SEARO in 1971 and her early communications displayed her unfamiliarity with Nepal. Her written communications with Sathianathan appeared quite formal and she expressed disbelief and concern about various aspects. In June, she was unhappy at the reliance on the district supervisors for confirming suspect cases and was keen that this was undertaken by more senior staff in the area if SEP HQ staff could not go out.[48] A month earlier, Sathianathan had requested a large number of spare parts for vehicles, but Grasset thought that these were less the problem than proper maintenance and prompt repairs.[49] Two new Land Rovers had arrived but had defective pistons. The replacement parts were sent but she asked: 'Is the delay due to not finding qualified mechanics to replace the pistons?' That might be a reasonable question, but Nepal lacked appropriate mechanics whether qualified or not. She found it hard to 'easily justify' requests for annual increases in subsidies or another operational officer if staff mobility was in question. Grasset did, nevertheless, mention the possibility of using a helicopter in an emergency. Over the next few years, she visited Nepal on various occasions.

At the 1972 inter-country seminar in New Delhi, also attended by Dr M. P. Shrestha who was the medical officer in charge of Gandaki zonal hospital in Pokhara, project chief Shrestha (P. N.) spoke about the development of reporting in Nepal and how the SEP 'had to develop its own reporting system from its own staff in the district'.[50] Smallpox patients 'usually do not seek medical help' and so health institutions 'do not play any significant role in the reporting of smallpox cases'. Furthermore, in some areas people hid cases to avoid discovery and some 'often also refuse to cooperate in the surveillance and containment measures taken by the

SEP staff'.[51] A breakdown of the fourteen outbreaks of smallpox in Nepal in 1971 showed that four notifications were by a panchayat, four by vaccinators, one from a hospital, two from health posts, one from a pharmacy, one by an assistant supervisor and one from field investigations.[52]

During 1970 and the first half of 1971, the SEP focused on its staff immediately investigating all reports of suspect cases and then putting into place effective containment action. Only a few reports came from areas outside the project. Information about the confirmed outbreak was 'promptly' sent telegraphically to national and zonal SEP headquarters and then 'generally' was followed by staff (including WHO staff) going to the outbreak area and helping district staff organise the containment. Four containment teams were trained and posted to different locations, but 'Due to certain financial and administrative problems, these teams did not function effectively and in time became non-operational due to resignations, etc.'[53]

After July 1971 and the limiting of the vaccination programme to the four winter months, increased emphasis could be put on surveillance and the active search for cases by all district personnel. Under the new system

> When the senior vaccinator visits a panchayat, he makes enquir[i]es of suspect cases of rash with fever from the Pradhan Panch, other panchayat leaders, school teachers if any, health institutions if any, and malaria units if any. He also visits other places and people from whom information may be available and also looks for cases in as many houses as possible. He seeks the cooperation of panchayat leaders for prompt reporting of suspect cases to district SEP office. All reports of suspect cases are immediately investigated by the district supervisor.[54]

During 1971–72 there were 486 such reports of which most were chickenpox or measles.[55] Details about actual smallpox cases were telegraphed immediately to national headquarters, while suspect case information was collated monthly. National HQ in turn sent weekly reports to WHO HQ in Geneva, while monthly and quarterly reports went to SEARO.

Further modifications were added. From mid-1972 a scab specimen from each outbreak was sent for laboratory examination.[56] In addition to telegraphic reporting of all outbreaks by district SEP offices, weekly postal and later telegraphic reporting of smallpox cases (including nil reports) was introduced. No reporting targets were indicated, but 'Except in occasional circumstances, this system worked satisfactorily.'[57] In September 1972, four surveillance teams were formed. These, Shrestha noted, would not face 'the previous financial and administrative problems' that had thwarted the earlier teams.[58] They were based in Kathmandu, but their main function was to improve and strengthen district activities. As soon as national HQ received a report, it sent a team to the outbreak area who would help district staff in the epidemiological investigations and containing the outbreak.

Both Mason and Friedman supplied regular field notes that went to SEARO. With the improved and increased amount of reporting, the files for the project in Nepal become much more extensive; they also, however, often give the impression that WHO staff are running the project as only their voices are recorded. Friedman has also written an unpublished account of a trip he made with Dr Benu Karki who joined the project in December 1972. They were to investigate an outbreak in Doti district in western Nepal in March 1973. The account reveals further layers within WHO even in a relatively small country such as Nepal and the different treatment and needs of foreign and local staff. Importantly, it also endorses the effective role of a district supervisor.[59] In view of the area's remoteness and difficulty to access from Kathmandu, Sathianathan 'persuaded his boss, the WHO Representative Dr. Peter Kim' to charter a plane for the outward journey. On arrival, Friedman as 'an honoured foreign guest' was given a horse to ride for the '3 hour trek to the east up a steep hill', while 'my Nepali colleagues had to walk'. All, however, would then be on foot for the day-and-a-half walk to the outbreak area, although an extra porter to carry 'essential supplies needed for a long trek, including a case of beer' was engaged. They found that a serious shortage of food existed as the wider area had had a bad harvest and British planes were dropping food supplies to the scattered villages. A thorough investigation of the outbreak found that

> All people susceptible to smallpox in Jurali and surrounding villages had been vaccinated. Since there had been no new cases for 18 days

and the source of infection had been determined, we decided there was nothing more for us to do. The containment was very well done, which was noteworthy since this was the district staff's first experience with a smallpox out-break.[60]

The following day Friedman and Karki stopped at a small health post in Silikot village where they 'were very pleased to see the smallpox recognition poster with a picture of a mother and child pinned up on the wall in this very remote place.'[61]

Karki was unmarried and spent much of his time travelling throughout Nepal and often on foot. One of his hardest and most 'frustrating' tasks was finding somewhere to stay for the night.[62] On one occasion in Arghakhanchi district he began looking from 4 o'clock in the afternoon. It was winter. At every house he was told that there were only women in the house and so his request was declined. Two hours later, he and his porter found themselves at the entrance of a forest and had to retreat the same way they had come. By now it was about 7 o'clock and quite dark. A man called them. He said that he had seen them earlier but knew that nobody would give them lodging and that they would have to return. He took them back to his house and offered them a hot meal and somewhere to stay for the night. The next morning, they continued their field visit 'with due thanks to him. This was just one of many such events.'

At the 1972 seminar, Grasset provided a regional assessment of the programme. She talked of the countries that had become smallpox free 'in spite of the many difficulties', and this gave her hope for those where the disease was still endemic – India, Pakistan, Bangladesh (formerly East Pakistan) and Nepal.[63] War in 1971 led to the creation of Bangladesh as an independent nation but also to the displacement of millions of people.[64] Many were housed in refugee camps where smallpox was prevalent. Within these endemic countries, Grasset noted, large areas were free or 'appear to be nearing the point of interruption of transmission'. Within India, 80 per cent of cases were from a northern belt.[65] In Nepal, only two of the fourteen zones experienced outbreaks in 1972; two-thirds of active cases were in Kailali district in the west. 'Thus at the present time the vast majority of the country seems to enjoy a smallpox free state.'[66] This meant that 'We no longer have to *fight* on a vast battlefield but can now concentrate our efforts to restricted areas.'[67]

Staff could identify and work on priority areas and were now able to produce maps and charts showing districts, blocks and other units. She cautioned, however, that 'In the large areas which we have noted as being smallpox free or where the incidence is at a low level, all efforts should be made so as to maintain the smallpox free status or achieve such a status as soon as possible.'[68] 'The failures as you will see are not due to lack of vaccine, to lack of funds or to lack of manpower, but are for the most part due to lack of training, lack of organization, lack of inter-district coordination and lack of supervision.'[69] Improvements in all these aspects in Nepal were reaping benefits. From July 1972 all smallpox cases were traced directly or indirectly to importations.

1973–75: From non-endemic to 'Target Zero'

In October 1972 the cover of the WHO magazine *World Health* referred to the programme's aim of nil incidence as 'Target Zero'. While 1972 was marked by both progress and setbacks, the geographical extent of smallpox-infected areas worldwide was decreasing. The 'final stage' was to begin.[70] Accounts about the period from Nepal being classified as 'non-endemic' in March 1973 and its last case in April 1975 all focus on the situation in India. At the end of 1973, smallpox was endemic in only four countries worldwide – Bangladesh, Ethiopia, India and Pakistan. Except for one case from Bangladesh in 1973, all importations into Nepal between 1973 and 1975 were from India.[71] While smallpox in 1973 had spread in many parts of the Asian sub-continent and became re-established in previously smallpox-free areas, Nepal, as the *WER* noted, and the Indian state of Orissa were 'notable exceptions'.[72] Both had been able to detect the outbreaks in time, contain them to prevent further spread and the development of secondary cases, and document them as 'being directly or indirectly due to importations from known endemic areas'. Shrestha considered reporting to be 'sufficiently complete since 1973'.[73] Maintaining Nepal's non-endemic status, however, was touch and go at times.

While the main concern in this period was India, importations into Mugu district in May 1973 generated considerable and high-level concern in another direction. This mountainous area in Karnali zone was an area usually thought to be more than one incubation period away from India for transmission of the virus but was close to the border with the TAR.[74] With the SEP's focus on the Tarai, Mugu had only become part of the programme during the year. How had smallpox reached the area? Social anthropologist Melvyn Goldstein noted the lack of access to 'modern' medical facilities in his report about Limi panchayat in adjacent Humla district and that 'inoculations' (vaccinations) were not popular.[75]

Nepal notified Geneva of seven cases of smallpox and one death in the district for the week of 13–19 May.[76] In New Delhi, Grasset responded in the only example in the Nepal files of the way many accounts depict WHO as operating. Grasset sent two telegrams on 22 May. One went to Kathmandu to the WR Nepal – with a copy by pouch to Sathianathan – saying that SEARO had approved US$15,000 for 'immediately chartering helicopter to investigate outbreaks Tibetan border … Inform soonest Nepalese zones districts involved and further details necessary for cross notification Chinese authorities.'[77] In 1972, WHO had recognised the government of the People's Republic of China as having the sole right to represent mainland China. The second telegram was to Geneva for Henderson informing him of the situation and action.[78] Although the cases were in Nepal and Nepal's SEP staff would investigate, a further telegram on 29 May added 'presume only WHO smallpox staff involved in travel'.[79] The two-page telegram to Grasset from Kathmandu was far more informative about the outbreaks and illustrated the increasing sophistication of the reporting system in Nepal.[80] Importantly, it documented how district level surveillance and containment was already in action in the area – it had not required the national HQ or WHO staff to mobilise. The source of the outbreaks was Nainital district in Uttar Pradesh where both men – the index cases – had separately worked as labourers. They then separately travelled back from India into Nepal directly through the hills rather than the more usual route through the Tarai. The outbreaks in Nepal were in two different panchayats and both were notified to the SEP office in Jumla on 7 May 'and containment action initiated' on 10 May. On 14 May a 'mass vaccination programme' in Mugu district began for the first time and was due to be completed on 14 June.

This activity illustrated that different communication networks were operating. The Mugu incident was an example of WHO operatives working separately from the programme's national staff, although in a small unit staff would know. Another aspect was the contrasting formality in the written correspondence between, for example, Grasset and Sathianathan or Shrestha, and informality shown between Friedman and Grasset and Henderson who Friedman addressed by their first name, or in the case of Henderson as D. A., and often used hand-written aerogrammes.[81] Lower-level staff likely had their own networks, but except for one letter are not reflected in the written project archive. This letter also shows networks outside the project. The project refrigerator technician, K. B. Shrestha, had complained to WHO about what he thought was WHO failing to meet its obligations regarding supplies. In a typed letter of apology addressed to the Regional Director and copied to the Director-General in Geneva, Shrestha explained that he was maintaining and repairing 'all refrigerators of Small-pox Eradication Project and other Health Services under the Health Department through out the country except some gas leaked refrigerators due to lack of repairing equipments'.[82] Shrestha had learned about the agreement between WHO and the Government and the responsibility of each 'from the administrative asst. Mr. B. L. Shrestha of W. H. O. Representative to Nepal'.

Although occurring much deeper into Nepal, the outbreaks in Mugu district fitted a characteristic pattern for 1973 of 'diffuse importation from all areas of Uttar Pradesh and Bihar'.[83] This resulted in 305 cases, with secondary spread only occurring on eight occasions. In October this pattern came to end. During November and December, the number of importations began to increase, with 'active outbreaks' in six districts at the end of the year. In five the source was from Bihar with one from Uttar Pradesh.[84] For the first half of 1974 the main pattern was repeated importations from Bihar and north-eastern Uttar Pradesh into eastern Nepal and from western Uttar Pradesh into western Nepal.[85] In western Nepal increased vaccination activities were underway, although not everyone was enthusiastic. In another example illustrating the complexity of people's beliefs, Goldstein noted that villagers declined revaccination saying they had already been vaccinated 'and since they were not sick they would rather hold on to the medicine until they needed it'.[86]

Some local spread occurred in the infected districts but rarely beyond one generation of the virus. In June 1974 Sathianathan received a letter from Henderson who was both concerned and encouraged at the situation but 'puzzled by the comparatively few outbreaks which seem to occur as a result of spread from the infected villages'.[87] Referring to a thirty-five case outbreak where there had been a delay in discovery, 'It seems remarkable to me that rarely is there spread to other villages, nor do cases occur more than a few days after discovery and containment of the outbreak.' While he wanted Sathianathan to 'Hold the line, at all costs!', he thought that 'All of us would be most interested in learning more in regard to your obviously effective containment procedures – notably conducted by the local supervisors themselves ... I feel there is something here which might well help other programmes.' Here was acknowledgement from the head of the global programme that Nepal's success was being built on local structures and personnel.

Across the Indian border in 1974, Bihar reported 126,872 smallpox cases and Uttar Pradesh 36,959, but in Bihar the situation was made worse by a late monsoon leading to major food shortages and 'increasing the already brisk annual flow of migrants across the border with Nepal'.[88] In the border area formal and informal communication methods were used. When staff in Nepal traced an outbreak to a source outside the country, they sent the details of the district, block and any other information via the regional office to the Indian SEP personnel responsible for that area.[89] Likewise, the Nepal programme received such information from India. Some people coming across the border were nomadic. While they tended to be unvaccinated and often resisted vaccination, they used to move daily from one village to another. They were a 'frequent headache' to those working in the border area.[90] 'I remember', recalls Karki, 'one of our district supervisors mobilizing his staff, encircling a group of them early in the morning and vaccinating them forcefully.'

During 1974, 180 outbreaks occurred in Nepal with the three most affected districts being Morang, Jhapa and Mahottari, which became infected towards the end of 1973. Cases continued to be reported throughout 1974 and from Morang into 1975. As the year progressed, local spread concentrated in two areas, the Bagmati zone and Morang district, and 'outbreaks were generated at fourth and fifth remove'.[91] Except for two isolated outbreaks at the beginning of 1974, all the outbreaks in Bagmati zone were part of two lengthy chains, both starting in Kabhre Palanchok district. The first chain lasted from mid-February to mid-September and involved five panchayats. The other started in early February and lasted till early September, spreading to three panchayats. Only two districts in the zone were not affected. In the first chain, most cases were Newars. 'The problem throughout this chain was vaccination resistance with a consequent difficulty in completing containment.'[92] This was associated with spread to new localities. The second chain also involved Newars, but the authors of the report were keen to emphasise that the search for cases was 'no less efficient' even though the outbreak in Chaubas panchayat was undetected for 107 days. They explained that the outbreak burnt out after four cases in seventeen days, then was undetected for ninety days, only coming to light when its two seeded outbreaks were being investigated in early September. The practice of friends and relatives visiting affected households 'played a major part in the transmission that occurred'.[93]

Geneva had become anxious at the deteriorating situation in Nepal which in 1974 had reported the country's highest annual total since notifications began in 1961 of 1,549 cases in twenty-eight districts (Appendix 1). In a memorandum to Grasset, Henderson wrote 'Is Nepal going to become our Achilles heel in 1975? I hope not but I'm worried.'[94] He acknowledged that Sathianathan and David Bassett, an American who had joined the project temporarily as a technical officer in 1974, were among 'the most competent advisers we have'.[95] From afar, as he read about the account of an outbreak and delayed detection and reporting in an area that was part of an integrated health services project which was supposed to be functioning well, Henderson thought that 'it sounds like a very sloppy operation'. All this raised another 'knotty problem' for Henderson – whether to return Nepal to the list of endemic countries as 'They've had rather more internal spread for far longer periods than should be tolerated. While I'm sure this would cause considerable governmental consternation, I'm afraid we'll have to reach a decision on this one way or the other in the next 4 to 6 weeks.'[96] Whether the memorandum was passed on to Nepal is not known but it is not in existing Nepal files.

Bagmati zone became clear of the original importation by the end of the third quarter, but Morang continued to be a problem. Sixteen outbreaks (ninety-five cases) were reported in Nepal in 1975, of which fifteen occurred in Morang district. All but two resulted from local spread and all but two were people unvaccinated prior to exposure.[97] The last five outbreaks in Morang were managed differently. Previously, 'all other outbreaks had been flexible and somewhat ad hoc', but a 'more disciplined method' was now employed.[98] Each outbreak was investigated, lists prepared of all the houses in the village and 'a systematic vaccination programme' was carried out. Staff then adopted the Indian SEP method of containment and appointed 'houseguards' from among the villagers who were to prevent unvaccinated people entering the house or any infected person leaving.[99] Two national assessment teams supervised the houseguards. Formal house-to-house searches were also undertaken. This new method was considered effective in the context of these outbreaks, although whether in other areas it would have prevented spread 'is open to conjecture'.[100] In March 1975 a cash reward of Rs 100 (US$10) was offered to the public for reporting an outbreak of smallpox. 'How much the reward would have helped had it been introduced earlier is open to discussion', considered project chief Shrestha, 'but since it did generate a huge number of suspect case reports, perhaps its impact would have been significant.'[101] Any potential for dividing communities was not mentioned.

The last outbreak of smallpox in Nepal occurred in Armadaha panchayat in Morang district, an area that already had experienced other outbreaks.[102] Most of the cases in 1974 had occurred among the Sathar tribal group who originated from India, but in 1975 among the Raj Bhansi, an indigenous Nepali caste group. On 6 March 1975, twenty-six-year-old Choba Lal Raj Bhansi and his relative Sundar Lal Raj Bhansi (who became the only case in an outbreak in another village on 19 March) visited a household infected from an earlier outbreak in Chinta Tole village. On 21 March, Choba Lal developed a smallpox rash. He was discovered on 24 March by the guards from Chinta Tole and containment was immediately started, 'using (Indian) containment books for the first time'. The illness was severe and by day ten of the rash he 'was in danger of dying. He had lesions in his throat and had great difficulty in taking even fluids.' In a rare example in the documents about caring for someone with the disease, his family was instructed 'in the technique of patiently spoon-feeding him with water, and he finally made a good recovery'. On 6 April, Choba Lal's wife, Jahaje, and one-year old daughter developed a smallpox rash. They had both been vaccinated on 24 March, and their illnesses were very mild. Unfortunately, Jahaje was seven months pregnant. On 7 April she gave birth to a premature son who died after a few days. 'The premature onset of labour was, in all probability, caused by her illness, despite its mildness.' Champawatti, her daughter, had an 'uneventful recovery from smallpox but her vaccination site became infected and formed an inch wide ulcer on her arm'. 'Possibly' due to an accompanying septicaemia, she developed osteomyelitis in one leg and in December 1975 was treated surgically at Biratnagar hospital and only began to walk at the age of eighteen months. The account concluded that 'When last seen in April 1976 the family was happily recovered although Champawatti's leg is slightly deformed.'[103]

In late March 1975, WHO epidemiologist Monnier spent two weeks in Nepal assessing the programme.[104] Somewhat to his surprise, Monnier concluded that it had been effective and that Target Zero had been reached despite the large number of imported cases. He considered that advice, direction and implementation of the SEP had been 'utmost effective on both WHO and national sides', and that reporting and containment were 'quite effective' and 'effective' when measured by non-local spread and the number of weeks of 'epidemiological silence' after containment measures. It was also 'very surprising that near 100 per cent of the sources of infection have been detected'. Morang district 'perhaps is the only failure', which he thought was 'due more to circumstantial facts'. He identified a range of operational problems. The 'massive invasion' of imported cases from Bihar had stretched the small number of staff, who had to deal with considerable staff shortages and lack of transport. He thought that supervision was 'poor' at all levels – absent WHO staff, no national replacement and 'rather poor interest in the programme' from the district supervisor. These programme issues were combined with severe monsoon conditions which destroyed roads. While this isolated some outbreaks, in others the local teams could not get there allowing further spread. Lastly there were social factors of the Dasain holidays, followed by further holidays for King Birendra's coronation, and that the 'WHO Technical Officer was unable to renew his expired trekking permit for field travel until 1 March.' Nevertheless, in the month before his arrival Monnier noted that operations were 'highly improved'. Indian staff had detected some hidden outbreaks, contained these and notified the Nepali team; Friedman was able to reach Morang; a reward of Rs 100 had 'stimulated' reporting and 'close' coordination with malaria staff had also improved reporting of cases. Significantly, Tiwari, 'a very efficient district supervisor' was transferred to Morang on 10 March. On 24 May 1975, Nepal officially attained the status of having no more cases of smallpox – 'zeropox'.[105]

Eradication

The last case of smallpox in Nepal could not be the end of the programme until first country eradication (elimination) was deemed achieved and then the goal of global eradication. As the Government's annual report commented, 'The greatest danger to this goal at present is complacency.'[106] While the focus in Nepal was on the situation within its borders, that danger of complacency was relevant both worldwide (particularly because of easier and faster means of travel that could facilitate spread of the disease) and in those few countries where there still were cases. Nepal's first task was to maintain zero cases until country eradication was declared. The WHO Expert Committee on Smallpox Eradication had determined in 1971 that this would be a period of at least two years from the last case and that because of the ease of virus transmission it could only be applied to a continent.[107] As a small landlocked nation state, the situation in surrounding countries was of paramount importance. The greatest threat had been from India, but in May 1975 India also reached zero incidence and, wrote Shrestha, 'the reservoir of infection for Nepal finally dried up once and for all'.[108] In Bangladesh the last case was in October, while no cases from China were detected in Nepal after 1961.

In June 1975 a two-day, high-level seminar was held in Kathmandu, chaired by Dr Nagendra Dhoj (N. D.) Joshi, Director-General of the Department of Health, and attended by government and WHO personnel.[109] Its purpose was to discuss the smallpox 'Operational Guide'. The project had about 800 full time and 4,200 part time staff throughout the country.[110] Present at the seminar were headquarters and zonal personnel involved with the SEP and project chief and regional officers from the malaria programme who were to assist with surveillance activities. Also participating was Dr Rita Thapa, now Chief of the Integration Division of the Department of Health but still one of very few women at this senior level in the health administration. In areas where health services were integrated, surveillance was to be carried out by the junior auxiliary health workers and supervised by their usual supervisors.

After introducing the guide, 'All points', said Shrestha, 'were now open for discussion and possible revision'.[111] The meeting had two rapporteurs – G. M. Singh, the health educator in Narayani zone, and Friedman from WHO. Under the new system, the proposal was to introduce surveillance of all houses in all districts, whereas previously this was possible only in the integrated districts and in the Tarai where malaria staff were undertaking this activity. Districts would be assigned different priorities (1–4) according to the risk of importation. The seven-page summary of the seminar is one of few documents that illustrated the nationwide nature of the SEP. It also demonstrated Shrestha's skills in negotiating Nepali officialdom.[112] Participants drew on their knowledge and experiences in different parts of the country to cover a range of issues such as pay, staffing, number of people seen and district categories. They also discussed the public's responses. Dr Bhim Bahadur Pradhan, civil surgeon, Kosi zone, commented that 'in upper-class houses vaccinators were frequently stopped by servants and dogs etc.' and this impeded surveillance.[113] Dr K. M. Dixit, project Chief of the Nepal Malaria Eradication Organization (NMEO), added that this also happened to malaria staff. Thapa highlighted the value of 'passive surveillance' and making use of outside resources. She had recently given a talk on smallpox to the Nepal Women's Organization in Rajbiraj, the administrative centre of Saptari district (Sagarmatha zone) who were planning a family planning and maternal child health (FP/

MCH) project. She used the smallpox recognition card and thought 'the village women seemed very enthusiastic'.[114] Shrestha thought this point should be included in the guide and the seminar participants agreed.

In another discussion about a very practical point, Shrestha asked about the experience of the malaria programme with stencils which were placed on the houses that staff visited.[115] The regional malaria officer for Biratnagar, S. M. Shrestha, outlined the method but added that 'normally only 50%' could be found on the houses. Dixit thought stencils were not very useful while Hari Prasad Duwal, acting senior supervisor, Sagarmatha zone said stencillers could sign several months in advance if not properly supervised. Shrestha (P. N.) said the stencils would be written with *geru* (ochre), but Dixit replied that the malaria organisation had found that 'unsatisfactory' and were now using pencils for stencilling. Shrestha indicated the smallpox programme would therefore use pencils, although added that this would not be visible sufficiently for the reward slogan and that *khari* (European nettle wood – *Celtis australis*) might be better. Dr B. R. Baidya, civil surgeon, Gandaki zone, raised the issue of the very low literacy rate in the hills and the appropriateness of writing. Shrestha brought the discussion to a close by saying that the reward slogan could be written by the 'best local method in each district' to which the participants again agreed.

From 15 July 1975, project staff throughout the country introduced the new operational guidelines which continued to undergo revisions. The reward for the first public informer reporting information that led to the discovery of an outbreak was increased to Rs1,000 (US$100) and generated a lot of suspect cases. Information bulletins 'reminding people of their duty to report cases' plus the offer of the reward went out three times a day on Radio Nepal.[116] Lantern slides were a popular method of health education and were regularly shown in Nepal's few cinemas. Posters, in Nepali, were distributed throughout the country, but project staff acknowledged that Nepal's literacy level was still no higher than around ten per cent and that the slogans painted on houses 'may therefore be of limited value'.[117]

Public education and the new guidelines aimed to establish and maintain surveillance. In the following two years only one 'dead' outbreak of four cases was uncovered. This was in Kailali district and had occurred more than two years previously.[118] By early 1976 the only country reporting cases was Ethiopia. In Nepal, as well as routine surveillance, special searches in vulnerable areas were also undertaken. One was a pock mark survey of Tibetan refugees, who mostly still lived in organised camps.[119] Of the forty-three people (out of 2,350) found with pock marks, six were infected in Nepal but none was known to the SEP because the infections occurred in places before they were part of the programme and, in general, were outside the camps. Had the infection occurred in a camp, thought Shrestha, further spread would have been likely but as there were no cases in the camps infection from Tibet was considered unlikely. Routine assessment of the surveillance activities was also carried out through the use of a 'subjective questionnaire' administered by district supervisors in their own districts and by two national assessment teams formed early in 1976 with financial assistance from UNICEF. Its main objective was to find out the level of people's knowledge about surveillance and the reward.[120] By July 1976, all eighteen Tarai districts (except the inner districts of Chitaun and Dang) had been assessed, involving 323 panchayats, 29 markets and 21,888 people or houses. Results were variable with generally better levels of awareness in eastern districts than those in the west, leading Shrestha to conclude that 'there is plenty of scope for improvement'. Importantly, no cases of smallpox had been detected.

While the level of surveillance was being maintained and intensifying with the use of large numbers of malaria workers, vaccination also needed to continue although this was now at a lower rate. From 1975 it was carried out in only one-third of the country each year. Vaccinations decreased from 5,694,195 in 1975–76 to 2,029,033 in 1976/77 (Appendix 4).[121] Supplies of vaccine were still needed. In September 1975 SEARO director Guneratne requested a donation of 35,000 ampoules from 'the Government of India to His Majesty's Government of Nepal' as 'excellent potent and heat stable vaccine is produced in the four production centres'.[122] Like Nepal, India also had no more cases and 'excellent' progress had been made in Bangladesh, but 'neighbouring countries must continue vaccination for two more years'.

With increasing optimism about the progress of the SEP in Nepal and even before the last case, the activities of senior national and

WHO staff were being directed elsewhere. In August/September 1974 Sathianathan was in Geneva where he undertook refresher training in country health programming.[123] He was then involved 'to a great extent' in project formulations of various health projects in Nepal until his departure in April 1976. Shrestha continued his duties as Chief of the SEP, but in March 1976 was also appointed as Deputy Chief of the FP/MCH project.[124]

As time passed with no further cases, attention turned to preparing for the certification of eradication. On 4 August 1976 Dr David Robinson from the UK arrived for a month as a short-term consultant for writing up the SEP's documentation for the international commission which would make the decision.[125] He would then return for six weeks in April–May 1977 just before and during the commission's visit scheduled for April. Dr K. B. Shrestha joined the project in September as his counterpart medical officer. After Sathianathan's departure, Friedman was the WHO's most experienced staff member with the project with supervision from New Delhi by Dr L. N. (Lev) Khodakevich. In November 1976, a consultative group headed by the Secretary of the International Commission, Professor Jan Kostrzewski (Medical Division, Polish Academy of Science, Warsaw, Poland) reviewed the programme and assessed 'its preparedness' for the visit of the commission.[126] Other members of the group were SEARO's country representative, Dr A. R. (Ray) Mills, Dr K. B. Shrestha, Friedman, Khodakevich and another SEARO medical officer Dr N. A. (Nick) Ward. By using the word 'his', the outline indicated these were Kostrzewski's recommendations. Surveillance was to be intensified 'in every panchayat in every district' using the SEP integrated health workers and malaria staff and that this was to be followed immediately by an independent assessment. Civil administration was also to be involved both before and during the final certification; activities were to be documented fully and that there should be a 'major propaganda drive' during the whole process.[127] A 'Special Addendum' to the operational guidelines was prepared and 'is to be followed by all staff, until the commission has made known its findings'.[128] The following February, Khodakevich again visited and reported that almost all Kostrzewski's proposals had been or were being implemented and that surveillance had been intensified in all categories of districts.[129] Letters from the Minister of Health were also sent to each pradhan panch and from the Director General to hospitals, health centres and health posts requesting they also organise surveillance for smallpox.

Khodakevich's report indicated that a commission would visit Nepal from 5–13 April with a prior briefing meeting for the countries involved in New Delhi at the regional office on 4 April. As well as Nepal, it was also visiting India and Bhutan to certify eradication. On 13 April the Commission would be in Kathmandu and 'will participate in celebration of the new year, which will, hopefully, [be] the first year of smallpox free status'. The report, however, gave no hint of an earlier 'delicate problem' concerning the venue of the announcement. Both Mills and Friedman considered that the announcement should be made in Kathmandu and not New Delhi. 'Dr Shrestha [P. N.] feels, and I am sure the Health Secretary and other more senior officials would agree', wrote Mills in a letter to Ward at SEARO on 21 January, 'that the announcement should be made in Kathmandu. Dr Shrestha even seems reluctant to travel to New Delhi for the final discussions of 20–23 April.'[130] The visit to Nepal was initially planned for 13–20 April, the 13th being the Nepali New Year and as a holiday was another problem. Mills then proposed 'from a political and diplomatic point of view' some options, concluding with 'Jay and I both agree that an announcement in New Delhi of Nepal's eradication would be as though Nepal was, once again being considered as part of India.'

Joining Kostrzewski was Dr Takashi Kitamura, Chief, Division of Poxviruses, National Institute of Health, Tokyo, Japan and Dr Donald Mackay, Ross Institute, London School of Hygiene and Tropical Medicine, England. At the briefing meeting, Shrestha presented to the commissions of both India and Nepal a paper on the activities of 'the smallpox eradication programme in Nepal from its inception in 1962 up to the present', which was followed by discussions of the programme.[131] Later, at the first meeting of the Commission for Nepal, 'a tentative schedule for work and travel was proposed and accepted'. On 5 April it travelled to Kathmandu and held meetings with the Minister of Health, Pitambar Dhoj Khati, the Secretary of Health, Mr Manmohan Lal Singh, and the Director General of Health Services, Joshi. In the national Smallpox Eradication office, they met with project staff, with Thapa, Director of Community Health and Integration, and Dixit, Chief of Malaria.

Over the next week the commission visited twenty-five of the seventy-five districts. It was divided into two teams, with one visiting districts in western Nepal and the other to the east. Shrestha (P. N.) and Robinson joined Mackay's western team and Friedman and K. B. Shrestha joined Kitamura for the eastern team. The teams did not have long, but each attempted

> to visit different terrains and population groups within its area, in order to see the eradication programme functioning under diverse but representative conditions. During this fieldwork, the Commission paid visits to zonal and district smallpox offices, malaria units, health posts, bazars, schools and villages in an attempt to determine the sensitivity of the surveillance system and to discover whether there was any possibility or evidence of smallpox transmission continuing in Nepal since the last known case in April 1975.[132]

On 12 April the commission met to have final discussions with project staff in Kathmandu. Unable to find any evidence of the presence of smallpox, it therefore concluded that the surveillance system in Nepal was 'sufficiently sensitive' to have detected any evidence in the past two years and that therefore the requirements for smallpox eradication 'as established by the WHO Expert Committee on Smallpox Eradication (1971)' had been 'fully met; thus the eradication of smallpox in Nepal is considered to have been achieved'.[133] Among its other recommendations, the Commission appreciated 'the degree and expertise in epidemiological surveillance and containment achieved by workers' in the SEP and hoped that when the SEP concluded 'this expertise will be utilized to the benefit of other programmes dealing with control of communicable disease'.[134]

The following day, the Commission declared that smallpox had been eradicated from Nepal. At the celebrations in Kathmandu at City Hall, the Prime Minister, Dr Tulsi Giri, the Minister for Health, Khati, and Secretary of Health, Singh, all spoke of the achievement. Each identified a particular aspect of the programme that highlighted different perspectives and agendas for those involved and that there were multiple stories to Nepal's eradication of smallpox. Giri acknowledged and thanked WHO for its 'valuable co-operation', but eradicating smallpox was Nepal's achievement led by King Birendra Bir Bikram Shah Dev and his wish that 'Ending hunger and disease is one of the chief aims of the economic development of the country.'[135] He noted that 'In comparison with other sectors, it is necessary to put in more sacrifices and work in the field of health. It is essential to understand the significance of this point and behave and perform accordingly.' Both he and the other speakers finished with the salutations *Jaya Desh! Jaya Naresh!* (Hail country! Hail King!).

Khati turned his attention to the development of health services. More specifically, he talked of His Majesty's Government's 'historical struggle' against smallpox for the past '15 years' and the importance of community participation and the panchayats.[136] By referring to fifteen years he was looking further back than the 1967 start of the SEP to the pilot project. 'The success we have achieved is due to all the health workers, Panchas, members of the Class Organisations, social workers as also to the World Health Organisation' and 'the timely cooperation from all sectors'.[137] He also mentioned that the King in addressing the Eighth All Nepal Medical Conference of the Nepal Medical Association stressed the need for basic health services to be made available 'for every Nepalese living in all corners of the country' and to stress prevention of diseases rather than cure. 'I want to let you know that His Majesty's Govt. is making ceaseless efforts to make available both preventive and curative services according to its financial capacity.' Despite the declaration, people should not be complacent, and they would be continuing 'for some years its programme of surveillance and primary vaccination. It will be the responsibility of all of us to arrange for the vaccination of all new-born babies.'

Singh took another perspective and talked of how eradication of the disease ended the 'heart-wrenching separations' of parents from their children dying from smallpox.[138] The world found a 'useful ally' in WHO 'who decided to throw in its weight and resources behind the complete eradication of small-pox'. Pointedly, he added, 'Needless to say, the WH.O. contributions to the eradication of the disease were more than matched by our own national resources. But for the deep concern we felt for the eradication for this disease all this money would not have come to be spent.' He thanked all for their hard work over years and said that the Prime Minister would be giving out commendation certificates as a 'small token of appreciation'. Activities would continue with surveillance and vaccinations 'and for much longer time in the expanded immunization activities to which the Government is strongly committed'. His speech was also a reminder that smallpox for many Nepalis from all sections in society was experienced as a clinical disease. He talked of a 'deep surge of peace and satisfaction'. 'The pleasing sights of children playing about with abandon and gaiety will now replace the frightful sights of children being struck down, felled and on most occasions, mortally wounded by the disease.'

Conclusion

Eradication of smallpox from Nepal after 1970 occurred in three phases. Achieving non-endemic status in 1973 built on the steady expansion of the SEP nationwide after 1967. Throughout implementation of the global health programme, Nepal received the vaccine it needed, and storage and distribution challenges were worked through. While from the WHO perspective the change in strategy from mass vaccination to surveillance and containment was the key factor that made worldwide success possible, in Nepal the initial change in strategy was made in 1971 and was for vaccination to take place annually for one month during the winter. This aligned with people's long-time preference as to when to vaccinate. Importantly, limiting the vaccination period freed up district personnel to focus on looking for cases during the rest of the year. Communication within the country was improving, but even if headquarters personnel investigated cases and outbreaks, the programme's effective decentralised structure was key to its success.

Reporting continued to improve. Between 1973 and the last case of smallpox in Nepal in 1975, the SEP turned much of its attention towards its southern border since any cases were being traced to outside the country. At times it was touch and go as to whether there was local spread. The outbreak in Mugu district was a reminder to WHO that the disease could reach anywhere in the country. The regional office's top–down response of rushing to investigate was not typical of the way the SEP in Nepal operated. Concerned that the source of the outbreak might be over Nepal's northern border in the TAR, WHO staff were helicoptered into the remote area but only to find that containment was well in hand and that the cases could be tracked back to India.

After 1975 the challenge for the programme in Nepal was to maintain the status of zero cases, although the elimination of smallpox from India and elsewhere in the Himalayan area in 1975 made this easier. For global eradication of the disease to be accepted, rigorous assessment was needed. Nepal could not be complacent. Intensive preparations for the international commission's visit demonstrated that the certification process was externally driven, although Nepali and WHO staff familiar with the country were part of the assessment team. These WHO staff also knew that Nepal having achieved so much would not take kindly to having the success announced in India, and they worked behind the scenes to ensure that it took place in Nepal. The celebration speeches in Kathmandu on 13 April 1977 highlighted key features: that it was Nepal's success; that the SEP was part of wider development in Nepal; that success was due to the support of many; and that while the WHO provided key support much of the cost was borne by Nepal. The eradication of smallpox from Nepal was an extraordinary achievement, and it was also the country's first nationwide healthcare programme. Those involved could justly feel a sense of triumph. The most poignant comment, however, was the reminder that for most Nepalis smallpox was not about a vaccination or about surveillance and containment but was a clinical disease that only a few years earlier was widespread in their country and brought considerable pain and suffering in their lives.

Notes

1 SEA/WHO, File 828, Box 210, Personal letter from Henderson to Dr A. Oles, Medical Officer, SEARO, 15 December 1970 (dictated by Henderson but signed by Arita).
2 *Ibid.*
3 Fenner et al., *Smallpox and Its Eradication*, p. 524; SEA/WHO, File 828, Box 210, Henderson to Oles, 15 December 1970.
4 *WER*, 48:11 (March 16, 1973), Table 1: Provisional number of cases by week (including suspected and imported cases) – Reports received by 13 March 1973, Smallpox surveillance – 1973, p. 127. See also SME/77.1, Shrestha, Robinson and Friedman, *The Nepal Smallpox Eradication Programme*, p. 12. This report (p. 28) refers to July 1973 as Nepal being declared non-endemic.

5 SEA/WHO, File NEP_SME_001JKT5, Box 215, Quarterly field report, second quarter 1975.
6 SEA/WHO, File 658, Box 220, SEA/Smallpox/79, 4 August 1977, Eradication of smallpox in Nepal: Report of the International Assessment Commission, 6–13 April 1977, p. 2.
7 Fenner et al., *Smallpox and Its Eradication*, p. 526.
8 SEA/WHO, File 827, Box 211, A. Monnier, Assessment of Nepal eradication programme, 26 March to 12 April 1975, p. 4.
9 Fenner et al., *Smallpox and Its Eradication*, pp. 524, 635. See also Vivek Neelakantan, 'Eradicating smallpox in Indonesia: The archipelagic challenge', *Health and History*, 12:1 (2010), 61–87.
10 WHO/SE/71.30, Inter-regional seminar on surveillance and assessment in smallpox eradication, World Health House, New Delhi, India, November 30–December 5, 1970, p. 2.
11 Ciro A. de Quadros, 'Experiences with smallpox eradication in Ethiopia', *Vaccine*, 29S (2011), D30–5.
12 WHO/SE/71.30, Inter-regional seminar 1970, D. A. Henderson, Summary – Status of the global programme, p. 7.
13 Bhattacharya, *Expunging Variola*, pp. 168–9.
14 WHO/SE/71.30, Inter-regional seminar 1970, A. Oles, Review of the status of smallpox in the South-East Asia Region, p. 17.
15 *Ibid.*, p. 18.
16 WHO/SE/71.30, Inter-regional seminar 1970, P. N. Shrestha, Importation of smallpox cases into Nepal, p. 2.
17 Dr Purushottam Narayan Shrestha. https://prabook.com/web/dr_purushottam_narayan.shrestha/956605 (accessed 18 October 2019).
18 *Ibid.*
19 Information about the Maldives from www.searo.who.int/maldives/about/previousWR/en/ (accessed 5 April 2017).
20 Email communication to author, Hema Dassanayake and Shiv Kumar Varma, 21 and 22 June 2021.
21 SEA/Smallpox/75 27 October 1976, M. Sathianathan, WHO Medical Officer, Smallpox Eradication Nepal: Assignment report, October 1970–April 1976, WHO project NEP SME 1, p. 2.
22 *Ibid.*
23 SE/WP/72.12, Inter-country seminar 1972, Shrestha, Present status and future plans for the smallpox eradication programme in Nepal, p. 2.
24 *Ibid.*
25 *Ibid.*
26 SEA/WHO, File NEP_SME_001JKT4, Box 215, Quarterly report – Nepal 9, second quarter 1971, Annex 1.

27 *Ibid.*, p. 3.
28 *Ibid.*, Regional Director (signed N. C. Grasset) to WHO Representative, Kathmandu, 30 September 1971.
29 Fenner et al., *Smallpox and Its Eradication*, p. 469.
30 Plan of operation 1967, p. 13.
31 SEA/Vaccine/34, Dr C. Kaplan, WHO Short-term Consultant, Assignment report on production of freeze-dried smallpox vaccine, Nepal (WHO project: SEARO 38), 1 April 1970.
32 Fenner et al., *Smallpox and Its Eradication*, p. 469.
33 SEA/WHO, File NEP_SME_001JKT4, Box 215, Regional Director, SEARO to Chief SE/HQ, 28 April 1971; ANZ, AAFB 632 W2883 144/31 R1845774, Sera and Vaccines – Smallpox Vaccine, 1969–1974, Department of Health, Gift of smallpox vaccine to Nepal.
34 SEA/WHO, File 828, Box 210, I. Arita, SE/HQ to Regional Director, SEARO SE, 4 May 1971.
35 *Ibid.*, Regional Director to Chief SE/HQ, 22 October 1971.
36 Fenner et al., *Smallpox and Its Eradication*, p. 472. For how variable this could be in the field, see SE/68.7, I. D. Ladyni, WHO Inter-Country Smallpox Adviser, 'Studies of smallpox vaccination by bifurcated needles in Kenya' https://apps.who.int/iris/handle/10665/67972 (accessed 25 September 2019).
37 Fenner et al., *Smallpox and Its Eradication*, p. 468.
38 SEA/WHO, File NEP_SME_001JKT4, Box 215, Chief SE to Regional Director, SEARO SE, 29 October 1971; also, 11 January, 4 and 10 February 1972.
39 *Ibid.*, Regional Director SEARO to Chief SE HQ, 6 October 1972.
40 SEA/WHO, File 658, Box 220, SEA/Smallpox/50 20 January 1972, R. Wasito, WHO Medical Officer, Assignment report on Smallpox Eradication and Control of other Communicable Diseases, Nepal (WHO project: Nepal 9), 8 January 1968–31 October 1972.
41 SEA/WHO, File NEP_SME_001JKT4, Box 215, Tour notes, fourth quarter 1972, Jay S. Friedman, Technical Officer.
42 Diane Drew (Interviewer), CDC, Nurse and Jay Friedman (Interviewee), CDC, Operations Officer, 'FRIEDMAN, JAY', *The Global Health Chronicles* https://globalhealthchronicles.org/items/show/3505 (accessed 14 June 2020). In Nepal, Friedman referred to himself as a technical officer. The titles 'operations officer' and 'technical officer' are often used interchangeably in the Nepal documents and are used as cited in the source.
43 SEA/WHO, File NEP_SME_001JKT4, Box 215, J. S. Copland to Friedman, 14 February 1972. Copland, normally based in Geneva, was in New Delhi for a month; Unit head Grasset was away in Indonesia.
44 SEA/WHO, File NEP_SME_001JKT4, Box 215, Tour notes, third quarter 1972, Jay S. Friedman, Technical Officer.

45 *Ibid.*
46 *Ibid.*, Field notes, fourth quarter 1972, R. Mason, Operations Officer.
47 Bhattacharya, *Expunging* Variola, p. 168.
48 SEA/WHO, File NEP_SME_001JKT4, Box 215, Grasset to Sathianathan, 7 June 1971.
49 *Ibid.*, 18 May 1971.
50 SE/WP/72.13, Inter-country seminar 1972, Shrestha, Development of reporting system in Nepal, p. 2.
51 *Ibid.*
52 SEA/WHO, File 438, Box 211, Annex 1 Smallpox outbreaks in 1971, Nepal fourth quarter 1?.12.71, Nepal: Case notification up to 1973. The precise date is obscured.
53 SE/WP/72.13, Inter-country seminar 1972, Shrestha, Development of reporting system in Nepal, p. 2.
54 *Ibid.*, pp. 3–4.
55 *Ibid.*, p. 3.
56 SME/77.1, Shrestha, Robinson and Friedman, 'Nepal Smallpox Eradication Programme', p. 81.
57 WHO/SE/78.107, Shrestha, Smallpox eradication in Nepal, p. 5.
58 SE/WP/72.13, Inter-country seminar 1972, Shrestha, Development of reporting system in Nepal, p. 5.
59 Jay Friedman, 'Trekking for smallpox in Nepal'. www.zero-pox.info/narratives/friedman_nepal.pdf.
60 *Ibid.*
61 *Ibid.*
62 Dr Benu Karki, email communication with author, 8 September 2021.
63 SE/WP/72.8, Inter-country seminar 1972, N. C. Grasset, Smallpox eradication in Asia, p. 3.
64 See Bhattacharya, *Expunging Variola*.
65 SE/WP/72.8, Inter-country seminar 1972, Grasset, Smallpox eradication in Asia, p. 4.
66 *Ibid.*
67 *Ibid.*, p. 5.
68 *Ibid.*, p. 6.
69 *Ibid.*, p. 47.
70 Fenner et al., *Smallpox and Its Eradication*, p. 528.
71 WER, 48:26 (29 June 1973), p. 264.
72 WER, 48:32 (10 August 1973), p. 317.
73 WHO/SE/78.107, Shrestha, Smallpox eradication in Nepal, p. 5.
74 SME/77.1, Shrestha, Robinson and Friedman, 'Nepal Smallpox Eradication Programme', p. 28.
75 Melvyn C. Goldstein, 'A report on Limi Panchayat, Humla District, Karnali Zone 1974', *Contributions to Nepalese Studies*, 2:2 (1975), 99.

76 *WER*, 48:21 (25 May 1973), p. 228.
77 SEA/WHO, File 828, Box 210, Grasset to World Health Kathmandu, 22 May 1973.
78 *Ibid.*, Grasset to Unisante Geneva, 22 May 1973.
79 *Ibid.*, Grasset to World Health Kathmandu, 29 (original dated 26 but crossed out) May 1973.
80 *Ibid.*, 29 May (a note on 30 May added that they had immediately telephoned Dr Mahendra Singh of the Indian SEP).
81 Friedman comments that smallpox workers on the whole were informal with each other. While addressing most other Nepali doctors as 'Dr', after a couple of years in Nepal he began calling Shrestha 'Puru', while Karki who he worked closely with was always 'Benu'. Email to author, 20 July 2021.
82 SEA/WHO, File 828, Box 210, 18 December 1973.
83 SME/77.1, Shrestha, Robinson and Friedman, 'Nepal Smallpox Eradication Programme', p. 28.
84 *Ibid.*
85 *Ibid.*, p. 34.
86 Goldstein, 'A report on Limi Panchayat', p. 99.
87 SEA/WHO, File 828, Box 210, Henderson to Sathianathan, copied to Grasset, 5 June 1974.
88 SME/77.1, Shrestha, Robinson and Friedman, 'Nepal Smallpox Eradication Programme', p. 34.
89 *Ibid.*, p. 83.
90 Dr Benu Karki, email communication to author, 8 September 2021.
91 SME/77.1, Shrestha, Robinson and Friedman, 'Nepal Smallpox Eradication Programme', p. 34.
92 *Ibid.*, p. 41.
93 *Ibid.*, p. 47.
94 SEA/WHO, File 828, Box 210, SME to Regional Director, SEARO SPX, 27 December 1974.
95 SEARO had posted Mason on a temporary assignment to Bihar. Bassett worked with the Nepal SEP June 1974 to February 1975. Email to author, 13 June 2021.
96 SEA/WHO, File 828, Box 210, SME to Regional Director, SEARO SPX, 27 December 1974.
97 SME/77.1, Shrestha, Robinson and Friedman, 'Nepal Smallpox Eradication Programme', p. 47.
98 *Ibid.*, p. 84.
99 The term 'watchguard' was also used.
100 SME/77.1, Shrestha, Robinson and Friedman, 'Nepal Smallpox Eradication Programme', p. 85.

101 WHO/SE/78.107, Shrestha, Smallpox Eradication in Nepal, p. 4.
102 SME/77.1, Shrestha, Robinson and Friedman, 'Nepal Smallpox Eradication Programme', p. 52.
103 *Ibid.*
104 SEA/WHO, File 658, Box 220, A. Monnier, Assessment of Nepal Eradication Programme, from 26 March to 12 April 1975, p. 4; further visit 1–6 June 1975.
105 SEA/WHO, File NEP_SME_001JKT5, Box 215, Quarterly field report, second quarter 1975.
106 *Ibid.*, His Majesty's Government of Nepal, Ministry of Health, Department of Health Services, Smallpox Eradication Project, Kalimati, Kathmandu, annual report, fiscal year 2031/32 (1974/75), p. 5.
107 WHO Expert Committee on Smallpox Eradication & World Health Organization (1972). WHO Expert Committee on Smallpox Eradication [meeting held in Geneva from 22 to 29 November 1971]: second report, p. 6. https://apps.who.int/iris/handle/10665/40960.
108 WHO/SE/78.107, Shrestha, Smallpox eradication in Nepal, p. 10.
109 SEA/WHO, File 658, Box 220, Smallpox eradication seminar, Kathmandu, Nepal Asadh 2–3, 2032/16–17 June 1975.
110 SEP/HMG, annual report 1974/75, p. 10.
111 SEA/WHO, File 658, Box 220, Smallpox eradication seminar 1975, p. 1, File 658.
112 He was less encouraging of SEP staff.
113 SEA/WHO, File 658, Box 220, Smallpox eradication seminar 1975, p. 3.
114 *Ibid.*, p. 4.
115 *Ibid.*, pp. 4–5; Arnold Boulter, WHO Technical Officer, Health Laboratory Services, conversation with author, Waitati, 21 August 2023.
116 SME/77.1, Shrestha, Robinson and Friedman, 'Nepal Smallpox Eradication Programme', p. 86.
117 *Ibid.*, pp. 86–7. Sathianathan had requested a copy of the latest reward poster that was being used in India. SEA/WHO, File 658, Box 220, L. B. Brilliant to Sathianathan, 11 September 1975.
118 SME/77.1, Shrestha, Robinson and Friedman, 'Nepal Smallpox Eradication Programme', p. 69.
119 SEA/WHO, File 658, Box 220, P. N. Shrestha, Pock mark survey of Tibetan refugees in Nepal, 1976.
120 SEA/WHO, File 658, Box 220, P. N. Shrestha, Assessment of smallpox surveillance in Nepal.
121 WHO/SE/78.107, Shrestha, Smallpox eradication in Nepal, pp. 3–4.

Success 251

122 SEA/WHO, File NEP_SME_001JKT4, Box 215, 18 September 1975.
123 SEA/Smallpox/75, Sathianathan, Assignment report 1976, p. 2.
124 SEA/WHO, File 658, Box 220, Quarterly field report, first quarter 1976, 26 March 1976.
125 *Ibid.*, Quarterly field report, third quarter 1976, 20 September 1976. Bassett left Nepal 14 August 1976. As WHO inter-regional staff, he had spent much of the previous year on assignments in Bangladesh and Ethiopia. Email to author, 13 June 2021.
126 SEA/WHO, File 658, Box 220, Outline proposals for activities of the Smallpox Eradication Programme for the four months prior to the visit of the International Commission to certify smallpox eradication, April 1977.
127 *Ibid.*
128 SEA/WHO, File 658, Box 220, Nepal Smallpox Eradication Project operational guidelines, special addendum in preparation for International Commission.
129 *Ibid.*, Tour notes of Dr L. N. Khodakevich, WHO medical officer, Smallpox Unit, Nepal 26 February–1 March 1977.
130 *Ibid.*, Letter from A. R. Mills, WR to Nepal, to N. A. Ward, SPX, New Delhi, 21 January 1977. Friedman also wrote separately on the same day to Ward, considering it would be a 'disaster' to do otherwise.
131 *Ibid.*, SEA/Smallpox/79 4 August 1977 Restricted, Eradication of smallpox in Nepal, Report of the International Smallpox Assessment Commission, 6–13 April 1977, p. 2.
132 *Ibid.*, p. 1.
133 *Ibid.*
134 *Ibid.*, p. 2.
135 SEA/WHO, File 658, Box 220, Speech by His Excellency the Rt. Honourable Prime-Minister Shree Dr Tulsi Giri on the occasion of declaration of eradication of small-pox from Nepal, City Hall, 13 April 1977, unofficial translation.
136 *Ibid.*, Speech by [Honb'le] Minister for Health Mr Pitambar Dhwoj Khati on the occasion of declaration of eradication of small-pox.
137 Class organisations were non-political and based on groupings such as peasants and women. They operated parallel to the panchayat structure. See Leo E. Rose, 'Nepal's experiment with "Traditional Democracy"', *Pacific Affairs*, 36:1 (1963), 16–31.
138 SEA/WHO, File 658, Box 220, Observations made by M. L. Singh, Secretary, Ministry of Health, H.M.G. on the occasion of declaration of eradication of small-pox in Nepal by International Commission on Small-pox.

Conclusion

Implementing a global health programme – and making it work

On the fortieth anniversary of the end of the smallpox programme the WHO Director-General, Dr Tedros Adhanom Ghebreyesus, called for the world now facing a new threat to work together and draw on what had been learned from implementing the successful smallpox programme.[1] He spoke of the importance of 'basic public health' tools used successfully: disease surveillance, case reporting, contact tracing and mass communication campaigns to inform affected populations. Valuable skills and knowledge in these areas developed over the course of the smallpox programme, but often are overshadowed in accounts that glorify central control, institutions and centrally placed actors that have dominated the narrative.[2] The eradication of smallpox continues to be portrayed widely as a 'dramatic tale of technological and organizational triumph'.[3] The 'extraordinary achievement' of the WHO-led global smallpox programme after 'so long a history', celebrated the authors of the official history published in 1988, was possible 'when countries throughout the world collaborated in a common aim, making use of the structures of an international organization and acting under its auspices'.[4] The website of WHO reaffirms that smallpox eradication 'remains among the most notable and profound public health successes in history' while that of the CDC proclaims that 'Many people consider smallpox eradication to be the biggest achievement in international public health.'[5]

Smallpox is the only human disease to have been eradicated and achieving the programme's goal of zero cases was an enormous achievement for those implementing the programme. Many people felt a sense of pride at being part. Nevertheless, the lessons from the smallpox programme are mixed. Eradication remains a controversial concept. In 1980, WHO Director-General Dr Halfdan Mahler (1973–88) wrote that while important lessons could be learned 'the idea that we should single out other diseases for worldwide eradication campaigns is not among them'.[6] Mahler highlighted the uniqueness of smallpox, but such campaigns sat uncomfortably with the aspirations of integrated primary healthcare. In 1974, as the smallpox programme entered the final stages, the WHA passed a Resolution formally establishing an Expanded Programme of Immunization (EPI). Documents from WHO from the early years of EPI 'continually reaffirm' that immunisation should be part of and not separate from primary healthcare.[7]

The achievement, however, *was* taken as a lesson and has been highly influential in showing the feasibility of disease eradication as a public health goal.[8] Success with smallpox raised the possibility for similar achievements with other diseases. Within a few months of smallpox eradication being declared, 'the first of many conferences' was held to consider what disease should be the next target.[9] As the authors of the official history acknowledged and duly urged caution, the programme provided 'illuminating evidence of the need for caution in deciding upon other eradication programmes'.[10] It was not to be used as a template and noted that 'the difficulty of its achievement should not be underestimated'.[11] Global project leader Henderson later recalled that at the time 'our staff did not speculate about the possibility of eradicating another disease. From personal experience, they knew that smallpox eradication had barely succeeded.'[12]

Success with smallpox also showed that implementation was possible even in countries that offered enormous challenges that are usually presented as reasons for why something does not work or work as well as planned. If the eradication strategy was to reach its goal, those involved in its implementation had to find a way to overcome challenges. In a much-cited article, US historian Paul Greenough has written about American physician-epidemiologists working in South Asia during the latter stages of the programme and argued that even if perhaps justifiable in an eradication campaign 'coercion' and 'intimidation' are not appropriate where the objective is control rather than eradication.[13] Unfavourable past experiences with vaccination can leave a legacy for future programmes. In 2019 the WHO identified vaccine hesitancy as one of the ten threats to global health.[14] Vaccine hesitancy – the reluctance or refusal to vaccinate despite the availability of vaccines – threatened to reverse progress made in tackling vaccine-preventable diseases.

Implementing a Global Health Programme: Smallpox and Nepal presents an alternative to the standard narrative of how eradication was achieved. It is a study of smallpox in the small Himalayan nation state of Nepal, and how the disease that once ravaged one of the world's least developed countries was eradicated as part of the WHO's global smallpox programme – but differently. Its value, therefore, extends beyond medical history and Nepal to policymakers today grappling with major health challenges.[15] Biomedical research continues to dominate global health – and definitions of what constitutes global health may differ, but 'doing' global health has become an important part of this now established field of research, study, and practice.[16] The book places the country and its people at the centre. Nepal was one of the last group of countries to achieve eradication. As the many major obstacles to implementing the programme in Nepal became apparent, an underlying question emerged – why was it successful? Why was the Smallpox Eradication Project (SEP) not only Nepal's first nationwide healthcare programme but also successful in reaching its target of zero cases when the difficulties seemed overwhelmingly against it? Often not asked or studied, why something works remains as relevant a question today for implementing health programmes successfully as it was for Nepal and smallpox in the 1960s and 1970s. Like the overall global programme, success should not be assumed because it happened.

Any smallpox programme had important factors in its favour such as the disease only involved human to human transmission of the virus and appropriate, affordable vaccine existed. For the programme to succeed, people needed to be vaccinated, but few Nepalis were able to access vaccination prior to the WHA's declaration in 1959 of the goal to eradicate the disease worldwide. Over time the global programme moved away from mass vaccination to focus on a surveillance and containment strategy. This required active monitoring and appropriate responses to any cases to prevent spread, but Nepal had an extremely limited trained workforce and services. Implementing the programme in Nepal needed a different approach to overcome the very considerable challenges of the country's physical and human environment and make it work.

Nepal's success was built on a decentralised operational system established within Nepal which adapted to the country's conditions. It was also one of the cheapest programmes. Shrestha as project chief (1969–77) and Sathianathan (1970–76) his WHO counterpart gave the programme direction and stability at a time of ongoing change in Nepal. Few others in such senior positions had their level and continuity of involvement. A decentralised operational strategy, however, was already being implemented when they were appointed. Project headquarters was in Kathmandu, but district supervisors, whose significant role the monumental official history of the global programme acknowledged, became the 'vital element' in Nepal's success. Nowhere else in the chapter conclusions drawn from different national programmes or in the wider literature is such a decentralised strategy referred to as a reason for success. It took time to achieve, but zone by zone and district by district the project expanded year by year as scheduled in the 1967 plan until in 1972–73 it incorporated the whole country. Organising around the 'district' was not a new concept as Nepalis had long lived with local government where, for example, taxes were collected in an area rather than by a central authority in Kathmandu. The smallpox programme was most successful where there were effective district supervisors who could be relied upon. Only through such decentralisation in practice could problems such as areas being cut off during monsoon flooding or poor communications be worked around. Despite some improvements, most of Nepal could be reached only on foot and reports could still take two to four weeks to reach the project headquarters from distant parts of the country. Central staff had to be able to rely on and trust staff in the field and had to be able to defend the system to regional and central WHO. Gradually, nationwide reporting and epidemiological knowledge of the disease throughout the country increased. Although at a government level the project was independent and not integrated into the country's basic health services that gave it flexibility, it aligned with national development policies and aspirations. Importantly, with political changes and the ascendancy of the monarchy, the programme had the support of the King.

The book highlights the importance of local context and uses a longer and wider lens than the programme archive to view the disease's presence in Nepal and people's responses. People's stories are at the forefront. Neither national nor international authorities had any accurate idea about the prevalence of smallpox in Nepal until the mid-1960s as statistics were lacking, but through their daily lives Nepalis knew that this feared disease was widespread and that many died, especially children. People with pockmarks were a visible reminder of those who survived. Nepalis developed their own practical, cultural, and religious responses. Mass vaccination was retained throughout but in 1971 was adapted to a time-limited annual campaign that aligned with people's longstanding preference for vaccination in winter. The book has drawn on different voices to tell multiple and different stories from the local to the global – and the many levels between – and has argued that these are integral to understanding Nepal's experiences with smallpox and the global programme. Nepal's story becomes visible and Nepali people can claim their history and their part in global smallpox history.

Using the approach of an historical case study of a small nation state's experiences might appear counter-intuitive for thinking of global relevance but this method allowed for in-depth exploration of the complexities of the programme, the many perspectives and the multiple levels of engagement and negotiation involved in its implementation. Accounts also revealed different perceptions of Nepal's achievement and tensions between 'global' (and donor) priorities and those of the national government. With the passage of time, it becomes easy to overlook that success was not guaranteed. The WHO worked with nation states, but Nepal was not a priority for policymakers and planners at a global level who considered that progress in Nepal would depend on progress in the wider region – particularly India which had the most cases of the disease worldwide. Nepal began to engage with global smallpox policy through its membership of the South-East Asia Regional Office of WHO from 1953 which led to the introduction of a joint Government/WHO pilot control project in the Kathmandu Valley in 1962. Although this was viewed negatively in the official history, this pilot nevertheless provided the foundation from which the intensified programme in Nepal developed after 1967.

While smallpox has remained popular in a range of literature and this book provides evidence to think about the global narrative and its ongoing refashioning, eradication of the disease was a global public health initiative of the member states of the WHA. From this perspective, it is necessary to look beyond newer historical narratives of the influence of Cold War politics or a timeline dominated by US involvement and embed the implementation of these national programmes into their local context. Each chapter in the book has a particular focus with its own conclusions, but here I want to draw together themes from throughout that were not only key aspects in Nepal but also have wider relevance for planning and implementation.

More than prevention

Smallpox had a long history in Nepal. The full title of the WHO 'Handbook for Smallpox Eradication Programmes in Endemic Areas' implied that people involved with the intensified programme would be working in places where the disease was still present.[17] Although much of the world was free, in 1967 smallpox was still widespread in many countries. The manual contained clinical information about the disease, but this was provided to assist staff with diagnosis rather than care of a person suffering from having smallpox. The extensive archive from the global smallpox programme that has survived and is digitised depicts, especially in the final stages, increasing knowledge about the disease and how it spread in a community. It shows how the strategy of surveillance and containment worked. How to look after someone with smallpox was not included. Such details are similarly rare in the programme archive for Nepal, even in the pilot project, or in other accounts at the time of the 1963 epidemic when there were many cases. The mention in the 1977 report of the country's last case of the disease of how to assist feeding for someone with smallpox is surprising.[18]

The common theme in the two stories at the start of this book, however, is the anguish that smallpox caused in people's lives whether they lived in a crowded town or a remote mountain village. Smallpox occurred throughout much of Nepal in the 1960s but although serious was only one of the many communicable disease challenges confronting the country's predominantly rural population. Nationwide health services did not exist and those that were provided were patchy and fragmented. As Shrestha later noted, health services were not the source of notifications for programme staff as people with smallpox were looked after in the domestic environment of their home.[19] For people with the disease and their families their experience of smallpox was intensely personal and one they might not survive. Good nursing care – usually by a child's mother – was extremely important. When I talked with people, memories were still vivid of the care they were given while they were sick or – if they were the carer – of the demands it involved. I was also surprised by the number of people I met from all walks of life and all sections of society who said that they had had smallpox when they were young. The control and later eradication of smallpox was to the people of Nepal, therefore, not only about prevention. It was also about a very real disease that was present in their lives. At the 1977 celebrations for the country's smallpox eradication success Secretary of Health Singh acknowledged parents' heartbreak.[20]

Vaccine and vaccination

People's experiences of smallpox and the presence of the disease in the community influenced their ideas and actions, including vaccination. The existence of cheap and effective vaccine worldwide contributed to making smallpox an appropriate target for a worldwide eradication strategy as low-income countries struggled with limited resources for health services. Much of the cost of the global programme fell to the individual state. Also, promoting acceptance of vaccination was not helped when people knew of others who had been vaccinated but still got the disease. The global intensified programme after 1967 used the newer freeze-dried vaccine, which was more stable in the warmer temperatures of countries where the disease was still endemic. In Nepal, freeze-dried vaccine was also used in the earlier pilot project. The new bifurcated needle had the benefit of reducing vaccine wastage which extended the number of vaccinations from the quantity of vaccine supplied. Although concern about the quality of the vaccine was an important factor in the programme after 1967, the issue was well recognised. During the 1963 epidemic Nepali officials in Kathmandu asked Dr Edward Crippen at USAID for 'Dry-Vac' rather than the liquid form available from India.[21]

In Nepal, belief in a goddess who could cause or protect a person from smallpox could not be assumed to equate with opposition to an intervention to prevent the disease. Most people continued to believe in the goddess and were vaccinated. Beliefs and culture are often viewed negatively in the literature when they come into contact with a programme such as the global smallpox programme, but they can also be harnessed in support. The timing of when or when not to vaccinate was important in Nepal and influenced people's willingness or unwillingness to be vaccinated. Gardner, the newly imposed British Resident, found this in 1816 as did US Peace Corps volunteers Messerschmidt and Morrison in 1964. The training period for the pilot project was shortened to take advantage of people's preference for vaccination in the colder winter months. Later, the major change in vaccination strategy in 1971 to time-limited annual mass vaccination in winter similarly aligned with people's ideas and practices. Despite the shorter period, vaccinations increased.

In the official history, issues around people's responses to vaccination focus on beliefs but this can be too narrow. While beliefs influenced people's actions regarding vaccination, they were nevertheless part of a spectrum of factors that included vaccine, vaccination methods and practical issues such as access. Despite the introduction of vaccination into Nepal in 1816, its spread was limited and so remained unavailable to most Nepalis. In the 1950s and early 1960s the government expanded vaccination services, but people talked about vaccinators coming into their community when they out working in the fields or of not going to villages further away from a road or a central location. Sometimes the factors influencing vaccination were separate but often they were linked. People's preferences for vaccination in winter could reflect lack of activity in the fields at that time of year but also that in the cold temperatures infected vaccination sites were less likely to occur.

Earlier vaccination methods, as the WHO Expert Committee on Smallpox acknowledged in 1964, could be traumatic.[22] The later bifurcated needle was more acceptable.

Environment

Nepal's topography is rugged and many areas often difficult to access. The WHO official history contains the only published account of Nepal's programme and confirms that global policy-makers and programme planners focused on India and that they considered Nepal an epidemiological extension of activities in India's northern plains and cities. Their attention, therefore, was directed to southern Nepal and the long and largely open border region of the Tarai. While the later stages of Nepal's programme in the 1970s were influenced heavily by the situation in neighbouring countries and the importation of cases into Nepal, a decade earlier smallpox was widespread throughout much of the country and no area could be excluded from the possibility of the disease appearing. Indeed, Shrestha made this point in his comments on the draft for the official history about Nepal's programme.[23] International experts assumed wrongly that the hills and mountains to the north were beyond the transmission of the virus. The 1963 epidemic in the Mt Everest region – which they were not aware of – showed that it could and how. The densely populated capital Kathmandu, where smallpox was endemic, acted as a central transmission point. Tourism was beginning to develop, and foreign climbing expeditions arrived in Kathmandu to recruit local staff to carry expedition supplies to the mountain. Two weeks later the first case of smallpox appeared. In the final efforts of the global programme in Ethiopia, operatives were chasing the virus into remote areas of the central highlands.[24] That it did not happen in Nepal perhaps also contained the element of luck.

The writing of smallpox eradication history is full of accounts and pictures that vividly portray the many challenges faced by those working to implement the WHO-led programme around the world. Nepal's limited infrastructure compounded the practical challenges presented by its terrain and climate. Although roads began to be built as part of Nepal's development policy, communication in

Nepal throughout the years of the smallpox programme often was easier if people crossed from Nepal into India and travelled in India before returning across the border to another area in Nepal. In the hills and mountains most travel and delivery of messages throughout the smallpox eradication programme was on foot and was therefore slow. Only near the end was it possible to send a report of a case of smallpox telegraphically to Kathmandu. These challenges became much worse during the summer monsoon period when rain and flooding made travel treacherous and rivers impassable; cloudy weather meant it was unsafe to fly in the mountains. As Henderson found from distant Geneva or Grasset in New Delhi, often it was hard to comprehend the magnitude of the difficulties on the ground in Nepal.

Logistics

Good logistics was important for the success of the smallpox programme, whether thinking globally or within each nation state. Not only did there need to be a suitable vaccine but also supplies needed securing and transporting to places where and when they were needed. Nepal did not produce its own vaccine and so relied on external sources. As the programme expanded into more and more of Nepal's seventy-five districts, hundreds of thousands of doses from different countries were supplied through the WHO and arrived in Kathmandu for distribution into the districts and then beyond to workers in the field. Air transport was expensive and, apart from some use by foreigners and towards the end, played little part in the global programme in Nepal after 1967. Motor vehicles were used in the few areas with roads, but Nepal lacked mechanics to maintain and repair them and so they were often out of action. As in their everyday lives, most programme workers walked. Awareness of the importance of logistics was not new. A major issue in 1816 was how to get the vaccine from Bengal in northern India to Kathmandu in the heat of summer through the malarial Tarai region. In 1963 vaccine was flown into the Mt Everest region for Sir Edmund Hillary's group, but in the Lamjung area Morrison walked for two days to Pokhara before being able to fly to Kathmandu to secure supplies.

Another equally important logistics concern was storage. Initially the country lacked the ability to provide the required refrigeration to maintain the vaccine's potency. This was particularly important with the earlier liquid vaccine. Some countries got around the issue by the frequent despatch of supplies within the timeframe calculated to maintain the efficacy of the vaccine. Such a system relied on a country having the communication infrastructure to enable that to happen which Nepal did not have. People's preferences for vaccination in winter was a bonus. Freeze-dried vaccine improved the situation but still required appropriate storage. Refrigeration, however, was another unfamiliar technology in Nepal, and the country lacked people who could maintain and repair the refrigerators. As the programme expanded more were needed; reports frequently commented on problems such as refrigerators not working or a district lacking kerosene to operate them. Very few areas had electricity. Support from WHO through a fellowship for a Nepali technician to train in India to learn how to maintain the refrigerators was central to improving the situation in the later part of the programme.

Training

Nepal was one of the most under-developed countries in the world in the middle of the twentieth century. It was less a question that services and infrastructure were not operating well, but rather that they did not exist and that most of the population even if they wanted to, could not access 'modern' health services. By the 1960s, Nepal's extremely low literacy rate was improving but most people's education was at primary school level. The government planned widespread development and modernisation to be financed through foreign aid, but the country had few trained health workers or other personnel for any of the many areas of expertise required. Throughout the years of WHO involvement with the smallpox programme in Nepal, WHO staff were aware that Nepal's needs were considerable; overseas fellowships filled some gaps, but other in-country training was vital. In some countries, foreigners were brought in to assist the smallpox programme. Although in 1963 and early 1964 foreigners in Nepal responded to local people's requests for help, and obtained and gave vaccinations, smallpox control and eradication was a government programme; the archives make it clear that the government strictly limited the number of WHO or other foreigners who could be involved.

A key aim of the HMG/WHO pilot project (1962–65) was to build up a core of expertise in Nepal to then enable the project to expand beyond the Kathmandu Valley. Reports from visiting WHO staff and short-term consultants usually acknowledged that vaccinator technique was satisfactory but were critical of most other aspects. In 1965, organisers of the local vaccination initiative in Morang and Sunsari districts in the Tarai trained vaccinators who were drawn from educated members of the community such as teachers. Under the programme after 1967, appropriate training and supervision of local staff was vital if the expansion was to progress and succeed. Mass vaccination remained important, with the last districts only being brought into the programme in 1972–73. Large numbers of people were needed at each stage. By this time, however, the focus of programme implementation was on the increasing importance of reporting suspected cases and instituting surveillance and containment measures. Extra WHO support to provide annual staff training was approved and became a regular addendum to the SEP's plan of operation. Senior level training was held in Kathmandu, was mostly in English and drew on foreign expertise for example in epidemiology, but vaccinator training was carried out in the districts where training was in Nepali and carried out by local personnel. The success of this training and prevention of local spread was acknowledged in Geneva by Henderson.

Implementing a global health programme – looking forwards

In their history of WHO, Cueto, Brown and Fee conclude that success with smallpox began with a 'bilateral program linked to a conventional model of development, but SEP's staff gained relative autonomy and overcame the tradition of multilateral agencies being subservient to political powers as they increasingly exercised legitimate international authority'.[25] The programme's experiences in Nepal provide a different narrative that emphasises local aspirations and agency. According to the country's Prime Minister in

1977, the SEP was Nepal's achievement, led by the King and carried out with WHO's 'valuable co-operation'.[26] One month after the Kathmandu celebrations, the Minister of Health spoke at the seventh plenary meeting of the Thirtieth World Health Assembly in Geneva. Khati referred to Nepal's 'long association' with WHO in the South-East Asia Region and 'the tremendous benefits' of emphasising the prevention of diseases rather than their cure.

> For it is our knowledge that, if we can prevent disease itself, we shall not be called upon to invest more on the curative side of medicine. It is in this light that we view the recent declaration of my country as being free from smallpox. In the eradication of smallpox, immunization has played a significant role. It is through the investment on the preventive side of medicine that I think the eradication of smallpox has been made possible.[27]

Involvement at a global and regional level was important as it demonstrated Nepal's commitment to the international community; it also brought some much-needed resources into Nepal as the success of the global programme depended on its implementation within a country. Nepal's second delegate, Director-General of Health Services Dr N. D. Joshi, attended a range of other meetings. One was about the progress of an Expanded Program on Immunization (EPI) initiated in 1974. Joshi spoke of being 'proud' that Nepal was free of smallpox and that

> Nepal was seeking to embark on an expanded programme of immunization but, without self-reliance for vaccine production, the targets would not be met. As one of the sponsors of the draft resolution on the regional production of vaccines his delegation hoped for its adoption and early implementation and for WHO's full commitment to the regional production of vaccines.[28]

In 1977 Nepal introduced a very limited EPI in three districts with DPT vaccination (for diphtheria, pertussis [whooping cough] and tetanus) and BCG (for tuberculosis).[29]

In 1988 the member countries of the WHA voted to undertake the eradication of polio; the WHO, together with Rotary International, UNICEF and CDC launched the Global Polio Eradication Initiative with the goal of eradicating polio by the year 2000. In 2014, WHO declared Nepal polio-free after maintaining polio-free status for three consecutive years. As the years have passed and smallpox remains the only human disease to have been eradicated to date, the

Conclusion 265

certainty of achieving such a global goal becomes much less certain and the element of luck – as Henderson acknowledged for smallpox – more apposite. Among the wider population, the smallpox story was itself slipping into the past. Other diseases became more important or indeed always were more important. In 2001, fears of bioterrorism after the 9/11 attacks, rekindled interest in smallpox, especially in the USA, which began to stockpile smallpox vaccine. The centenary of the 1918 influenza pandemic, however, reawakened memories of what could happen on a global scale with the outbreak of a disease for which there was no cure. The emergence of COVID-19 and the events that followed were a stark reminder for the world.

Nepal's different story with the global smallpox programme was written about in the official history but there it has remained. Historians have a role to play in writing about global health and its history that is broader and more inclusive, but this book has the added value of historical accounts written from different perspectives that are scarcely visible from a 'global' perspective. Having lived in a small village in the mountains of Nepal led me to appreciating the importance of 'history from below', of thinking 'outside-in' and how talking to real people 'disrupted' narratives. That was why I began this book in the remote mountain valleys of the Mt Everest region and in the hill town of Kirtipur with Nepali people's experiences of the disease. As much as the eradication of smallpox was a public health programme, the disease of smallpox was about life and death to the people of Nepal. The fact that Nepal was not very important or interesting from a global perspective (and so for the authors of the official history) has no bearing on the possible value and interest of a national history or people's stories. When I replied to the woman who asked me what I was going to do with her story, I did not realise that Nepal had such an important story to tell.

Notes

1 WHO, 'WHO Director-General's opening remarks at the media briefing on COVID-19 – 8 May 2020'.
2 William Muraskin, 'The power of individuals and the dependency of nations in global eradication and immunisation campaigns', in Christine Holmberg, Stuart Blume and Paul Greenough (eds), *The*

Politics of Vaccination: A Global History (Manchester: Manchester University Press, 2017), pp. 321–36.
3 Anne-Emanuelle Birn, 'Small(pox) success?', *Ciencia & Saude Coletiva*, 16:2 (2011), 592.
4 Fenner et al., *Smallpox and Its Eradication*, p. 1346.
5 WHO, Smallpox. www.who.int/health-topics/smallpox#tab=tab_1; CDC, History of Smallpox. www.cdc.gov/smallpox/history/history. html (accessed 30 January 2024).
6 Birn, 'Small(pox) success?', 592.
7 Stuart Blume, Jagrati Jani and Sidsel Roalkvam, 'Saving children's lives: Perspectives on immunisation', in Sidsel Roalkvam, Desmond McNeill and Stuart Blume (eds), *Protecting the World's Children: Immunisation Policies and Practices* (Oxford: Oxford University Press, 2013), p. 9.
8 *Ibid.*
9 D. A. Henderson, 'The global eradication of smallpox: Historical perspective and future prospects', in Sanjoy Bhattacharya and Sharon Messenger (eds), *The Global Eradication of Smallpox* (New Delhi: Orient BlackSwan, 2010), p. 34.
10 Fenner et al., *Smallpox and Its Eradication*, p. 1369.
11 *Ibid.*, p. 1367.
12 Henderson, *Smallpox: The Death of a Disease*, p. 302.
13 Paul Greenough, 'Intimidation, coercion and resistance in the final stages of the South Asian Smallpox Eradication Campaign, 1973–1975', *Social Science & Medicine*, 41:5 (1995), 633–45.
14 WHO, 'Ten threats to global health in 2019' www.who.int/news-room/spotlight/ten-threats-to-global-health-in-2019 (accessed 11 January 2023).
15 Sanjoy Bhattacharya, Alexander Medcalf, and Aliko Ahmed, 'Humanities, criticality and transparency: Global health histories and the foundations of inter-sectoral partnerships for the democratisation of knowledge', *Humanities and Social Sciences Communications*, 7:1 (2020), 1–11.
16 Johanna Hanefield and Hanna-Tina Fischer, 'Global health: Definitions, principles, and drivers', in Robin Haring (ed.), *Handbook of Global Health* (Cham: Springer, 2021), p. 9. DOI.org/10.1007/978-3-030-45009-0
17 World Health Organization, SE/67.5 Rev. 1, Handbook for Smallpox Eradication Programmes in Endemic Countries, July 1967.
18 SME/77.1, Shrestha, Robinson and Friedman, *The Nepal Smallpox Eradication Programme*, p. 52.

19 SE/WP/72.13, Inter-country seminar 1972, Shrestha, Development of reporting system in Nepal, p. 2.
20 SEA/WHO, File 658, Box 220, Observations made by M. L. Singh, Secretary, Ministry of Health, H.M.G. on the occasion of Declaration of Eradication of Small-pox in Nepal by International Commission on Small-pox.
21 Crippen, 'Smallpox, Nepal 1963 … Prelude to Eradication?', p. 4.
22 WHO Expert Committee on Smallpox: First report, p. 31.
23 SEA/WHO, File 1239, Box 666, Attached comments, Acting WPCR Nepal to Regional Director, SEARO, 29 November 1984.
24 de Quadros, 'Experiences with smallpox eradication in Ethiopia', D30-5.
25 Cueto, Brown and Fee, *The World Health Organization*, p. 145.
26 SEA/WHO, File 658, Box 220, Speech by His Excellency the Rt. Honourable Prime-minister Shree Dr. Tulsi Giri on the occasion of Declaration of Eradication of Small-pox from Nepal, City Hall, 13 April 1977, unofficial translation.
27 World Health Assembly, 30. (1977). Thirtieth World Health Assembly, Geneva, 2–19 May 1977: part II: verbatim records of plenary meetings: summary records and reports of committees, p. 208. https://apps.who.int/iris/handle/10665/86037
28 WHA 30, part II: verbatim records of plenary meetings: summary records and reports of committees, p. 250.
29 Dixit, *Nepal's Quest for Health* (2014), p. 78.

Appendix 1

Smallpox cases reported by year, 1961–75

Year	Number of smallpox cases	Number of districts reporting cases	Number of districts in the SEP
1961	5	–	0
1962	–	–	0
1963	1105	3	3
1964	135	3	3
1965	70	3	3
1966	164	–	3
1967	110	–	3
1968	249	8	15
1969	163	7	29
1970	76	1	41
1971	215	6	50
1972	399	9	58
1973	277	18	75
1974	1549	28	75
1975	95	2	75

Source: WHO/SE/78.107, P. N. Shrestha, Smallpox eradication in Nepal, p. 5; *WER*.

Appendix 2

Selected health and socio-economic indicators, 1951–76

	1952–54[1]	1961[1]	1971[1]	1976[2]
Population	8,256,625	9,412,996	11,555,983	
% rural	97.1	96.4	96	
% urban	2.9	3.6	4	
Kathmandu Valley	410,995	459,990	618,991	
No. villages				28,780
No. towns over 5,000 people	10	16	16	
% under 15 years	38.4	39.9	40.4	
Median age (years)	21.0	23.2	22.8	
Annual rate of population growth (%)				2.52 (1974–75)
Crude birth rate/1000*	40.0 (1951–61)	41.0 (1961–71)	42.0	44.7 (1974–75)
Crude death rate/1000*	27.0 (1953–61)		21.4 (1961–71)	19.5 (1974–5)
Infant mortality rate/1000*	255 (1954)	193 (1961–71)	172	132.5
Life at birth expectancy (years)*	25.6 m 25.7 f	30.2 m 33.0 f	42.9 m 38.9 f (1961–71)	46.0 m 42.5 f (1974–75)
% Nepali mother tongue+	48.7	51.0	52.4	

(continued)

	1952–54[1]	1961[1]	1971[1]	1976[2]
Per capita annual income (approx.)				$90–100
Literacy rate (%)	4.3	8.9	14.3	
	7.8 m	16.4 m	24.7 m	
	0.7 f	1.8 f	3.7 f	
School enrolments:	(1950)[3]	(1961)[3]	(1973)	
Primary	8,505	182,533	301,439	
Secondary	1,680	21,115	215,993	
Schools:				
Primary and middle	310	1,237		
High	11	83		
Health institutions	(1956)[4]	(1966)[5]		
Hospitals	34	57		61
Beds	625	1,756		2,238
Other	24	98		434
aushadhalaya	63			82
Health workers	(early 1950s)			
Doctors	about 50	230		338
Other		387		2,246

* Population censuses were carried out in 1952–54 (considered the benchmark for modern scientific census in Nepal), 1961 and 1971. Although questions were included in the census, Nepal lacked a vital registration system; estimates vary in different studies.

+ The census asked for mother tongue and not ethnicity.

Sources: [1] ESCAP, *Population of Nepal*; [2] SME/77.1, Shrestha, Robinson and Friedman, 'The Nepal Smallpox Eradication Programme', pp. 96–8; [3] Wood, 'Educational planning in Nepal and its economic implications', p. 25; [4] Dixit, *The Quest for Health* (1999), pp. 51–2; [5] WHO/SEP, Yarom, Draft report on a visit to Nepal 1966, pp. 4–5.

Appendix 3

Financial inputs by the Government of Nepal and WHO, 1962–76 (US$)*

Year	Government of Nepal	WHO	Total
1962	2,447	–	2,447
1963	3,598	–	3,598
1964	4,702	–	4,702
1965	5,334	–	5,334
1966	6,000+	17,828	23,828+
1967	31,000+	68,875	99,875+
1968	53,615	100,590	154,205
1969	64,334	64,414	128,748
1970	82,400	[11]6,589	198,989
1971	121,071	122,404	243,475
1972	147,339	158,629	305,968
1973	165,000	166,554	331,554
1974	163,500	94,993	258,493
1975	158,262	160,346	318,608
1976	169,343	129,815	299,158
Total	1,177,945	1,201,037	2,378,982

*Excluding the cost of 160,000 vials of vaccine

+Estimated

Source: Fenner et al., *Smallpox and Its Eradication*, p. 795.

Appendix 4

Vaccinations carried out through the HMG/WHO smallpox programme

Year	Number of primary vaccinations	Total number of vaccinations
1962–63	–	218,025
1963–64	–	69,107
1964–65	–	160,796
1965–66	–	201,243
1966–67	–	643,699
1967–68	13,698	1,246,033
1968–69	282,613	2,195,942
1969–70	521,571	2,136,468
1970–71	503,462	2,823,098
1971–72	598,958	6,162,478
1972–73	992,860	6,516,395
1973–74	1,049,405	6,418,402
1974–75	367,470	6,187,676
1975–76	604,240	5,694,195
1976–77	269,768	2,029,033

Source: WHO/SE/78.107, P. N. Shrestha, Smallpox eradication in Nepal, p. 4.

Glossary

control reduction of disease incidence, prevalence, morbidity and mortality to a locally acceptable level as a result of deliberate efforts; continued intervention measures are required to maintain the reduction

elimination reduction to zero of the incidence of a specified disease in a defined geographical area as a result of deliberate efforts; continued intervention measures are required

endemic a disease present in a geographical area or population at a relatively high rate compared with other areas or populations

epidemic widespread occurrence of an infectious disease in a community at a particular time

eradication permanent reduction to zero of the worldwide incidence of an infection caused by a specific agent as a result of deliberate efforts; intervention measures are no longer needed

immunisation coverage estimated percentage of the population who have received a specific vaccine

inoculation a method (in health) of artificially inducing immunity to an infectious disease; often used interchangeably with both variolation and vaccination

surveillance and containment active searching to find cases, rigorous isolation of patients, and vaccination and surveillance of close contacts to contain outbreaks ('ring vaccination')

vaccination inoculation of uninfected persons with milder vaccinia; **mass vaccination** involves delivering immunisations to a large number of people at one or more locations in a short interval of time

variolation inoculation of uninfected persons with the fluid retrieved from the pustules of smallpox

Bibliography

Primary sources

Archive collections and libraries in Nepal, New Zealand, Switzerland, the UK and the USA

Nepal

Archives held at Khunde Hospital (KH)
  Annual Reports 1967–83
  Various files of correspondence – incomplete
  Boxes of assorted files and loose papers
Madan Puraskar Pustakalaya – Nepali language items on smallpox
Online: *Journal of Nepal Medical Association*, 1963–77 (incomplete)

New Zealand

Auckland War Memorial Museum/Tāmaki Paenga Hira
  MS-2010–1, Hillary, Sir Edmund, personal papers
Archives New Zealand/Te Rua Mahara o te Kāwanatanga, Head Office, Wellington (ANZ)
  ABHS 6949 W4628 NDI 64/14/2, Himalayan Climbing Expeditions & Schoolhouse Project
  EA W2824 18/13/13/14 /1, Economic and Technical Assistance to individual countries – Nepal – Sir Edmund Hillary's Himalayan Projects
  AAFB 632 W2883 144/31 R1845774, Sera and Vaccines – Smallpox Vaccine, 1969–74
University of Otago, Dunedin
  MS–1760, University of Otago, Department of Preventive and Social Medicine Records, Professor Cyril W. Dixon

Gill, M. B., 'The Sherpas: A survey of an isolated mountain community' (Department of Preventive and Social Medicine diss., 1961)
Weekly Epidemiological Record (WER)

United Kingdom

British Library, India Office Records (IOR), London
    R/5/37 and R/5/38, Letters to India 1816
    R/5, Kathmandu Residency records c1792–1872
    F/4/550/13379, Board of Control records 1784–1858
    L/PS/11, Political and secret annual files Nepal 1912–30
    L/PS/12, Political and secret (external) files 1931–50
    (These contain a few assorted files related to the British Residency/ Legation in
    Kathmandu and some annual reports)
    V/24/4346, Reports on vaccination in the Punjab 1910–26
The National Archives (TNA), Kew
    FO 371/22175, Nepal: annual report 1937
    FO 766/27, Transfer of files to the Indian Embassy
    BW 129/5, Nepal: British Council activities, annual reports
School of Oriental and African Studies (SOAS), University of London
    Regions Beyond Missionary Union publications, 1903–52
    Box 452, Conference of British missionary societies
Online: Digital Himalaya (University of Cambridge) www.digitalhimalaya.com/

Switzerland

World Health Organization (WHO), Geneva
    Smallpox Eradication Archives (SEA/WHO)
        WHO HQ correspondence and papers
        WHO SEARO correspondence and papers
        WHO photographic collection
    Library
    'A report on health and health administration in Nepal 1969', Directorate of Health Services, Ministry of Health, Kathmandu
    Journal of Nepal Medical Association, 1963–77
    World Health
Online: World Health Organization www.who.int/
WHO IRIS https://apps.who.int/iris/

Bibliography

USA

Divinity library of Yale University library, New Haven, Connecticut
United Mission to Nepal archives (UMN) Record Group No. 212
International Nepal Fellowship archives (INF) Record Group No. 214
Online: Centers for Disease Control and Prevention (CDC) www.cdc.gov/smallpox/symptoms/index.html
Global Health Chronicles, CDC (Jay Friedman) https://globalhealthchronicles.org/items/show/3505
Regmi Research Series https://ecommons.cornell.edu/handle/1813/57329
Target Zero – Smallpox Eradication Archives www.zero-pox.info/

Official publications

Basu, R. N., Z. Jezek and N. A. Ward, *The Eradication of Smallpox from India* (New Delhi: World Health Organization, South-East Asia Regional Office, 1979).

Economic and Social Commission for Asia and the Pacific (ESCAP), *Population of Nepal*, Country Monograph Series No. 6 (Bangkok: United Nations, 1980).

Fenner, F., D. A. Henderson, I. Arita, Z. Jezek and I. D. Ladnyi, *Smallpox and its Eradication* (Geneva: World Health Organization, 1988).

World Health Organization, *The First Ten Years of the World Health Organization* (Geneva: World Health Organization, 1958).

World Health Organization, *The Second Ten Years of the World Health Organization, 1958–1967* (Geneva: World Health Organization, 1968).

World Health Organization, *The Third Ten Years of the World Health Organization, 1968–1977* (Geneva: World Health Organization, 2008).

World Health Organization, Regional Office for South-East Asia, *Twenty Years in South-East Asia, 1948–1967* (New Delhi: World Health Organization, Regional Office for South-East Asia, 1967).

World Health Organization, Regional Office for South-East Asia, *A Decade of Health Development in South-East Asia, 1968–1977* (New Delhi: World Health Organization, Regional Office for South-East Asia, 1978).

World Health Organization, Regional Office for South-East Asia, *Collaboration in Health Development in South-East Asia, 1948–1988: Fortieth Anniversary Volume* (New Delhi: World Health Organization, Regional Office for South-East Asia, 1992).

Private papers

I am very grateful for being able to consult documents from the personal papers of:

Dr Edward Crippen (courtesy of his family and Don Messerschmidt)
Dr Donald A. (Don) Messerschmidt

Interviews and written correspondence

Formal and informal interviews, conversations and written communication have taken place throughout the research and writing of this book and have been documented. In many cases this information was gathered or provided on multiple occasions and linked me with other people. This is noted in the chapter notes. I am very grateful to the following people:
  Kiran Bajracharya, pharmacist, introduced me to his Newar community
  Professor Hemang Dixit, consultant paediatrician, educationalist and author
  Jay Friedman, WHO Technical Officer, SEP 1972–77
  The Hillary family
  Dr Philip Houghton, Himalayan Schoolhouse Expedition, 1963
  Dr Benu Bahadur Karki, Medical Officer SEP from 1972, periodically in charge
  Dr Donald Messerschmidt and Bruce Morrison, Peace Corps volunteers, Lamjung area in 1963–64
  Dr Pratyoush Onta, historian, Research Director, Martin Chautari, Kathmandu
  Major Peter Pitt, surgeon, British Military Hospital, Dharan, 1966–68
  Dr Kami Temba Sherpa, Medical Officer, Khunde Hospital and Himalayan Trust
  Dr Lhakpa Norbu Sherpa, first Sherpa to be awarded a PhD, cultural authority
  Dr Rita Thapa, Director, Maternal and Child Health, for short period in charge SEP
I would like to acknowledge and thank my anonymous interviewees in Kathmandu, Khumbu and Kirtipur for their stories about their experiences with smallpox and my interpreters for their additional information.

Publications by those involved

Arita, Isao, *The Smallpox Eradication Saga: An Insider's View* (Hyderabad: Orient BlackSwan, 2010).
———, *Smallpox Eradication: Target Zero* (Japan: Mainichi Press, 1979).

Brilliant, L. B., *The Management of Smallpox Eradication in India: A Case Study and Analysis* (Ann Arbor, MI: University of Michigan Press, 1985).
Cockburn, W. Charles, 'Progress in international smallpox eradication', *American Journal of Public Health*, 56:10 (1966), 1628–33.
de Quadros, Ciro A., 'Experiences with smallpox eradication in Ethiopia', *Vaccine* 29S (2011), D30–5.
Dixon, C. W., *Smallpox* (London: J. & A. Churchill, 1962).
———, 'Smallpox in Tripolitania, 1946: An epidemiological and clinical study of 500 cases, including trials of penicillin treatment', *Journal of Hygiene*, 46:4 (1948), 351–77. DOI:10.1017/s0022172400036536.
Fenner, Frank, *Nature, Nurture and Chance: The Lives of Frank and Charles Fenner* (Canberra: ANU E Press, 2006).
———, 'Smallpox in Southeast Asia', *Crossroads: An Interdisciplinary Journal of Southeast Asian Studies*, 3:2/3 (1987), 34–48.
Fenner, F., A. J. Hall and W. R. Dowdle, 'What is eradication?', in W. R. Dowdle and D. R. Hopkins (eds), *The Eradication of Infectious Diseases* (Chichester: John Wiley & Sons, 1998), pp. 3–17.
Foege, William H., *House on Fire: The Fight to Eradicate Smallpox* (Berkeley, CA: University of California Press and Milbank Memorial Fund, 2011).
Frederiksen, Harald, Nemesio Torres Muñoz and Alfredio Jauregui Molina, 'Smallpox eradication', *Public Health Reports*, 74:9 (1959), 771–8.
Frederiksen, Harald and James P. Sheehy, 'Smallpox control by mass vaccination with dried vaccine', *Public Health Reports*, 72:2 (1957), 163–72.
Henderson, D. A., 'Epidemiology in the global eradication of smallpox', *International Journal of Epidemiology*, 1:1 (1972), 25–30.
———, 'Frank Fenner (1914–2010): A guiding light of the campaign to eradicate smallpox', obituary, *Nature*, 469:7328 (6 January 2011), 35.
———, 'The global eradication of smallpox: Historical perspective and future prospects', in Sanjoy Bhattacharya and Sharon Messenger (eds), *The Global Eradication of Smallpox* (New Delhi: Orient BlackSwan, 2010), pp. 7–35.
———, 'Principles and lessons from the smallpox eradication programme', *Bulletin of the World Health Organization*, 65:4 (1987), 535–46.
———, *Smallpox: The Death of a Disease: The Inside Story of Eradicating a Worldwide Killer* (New York: Prometheus Books, 2009).
Henderson, D. A. and Petra Klepac, 'Lessons from the eradication of smallpox: An interview with D. A. Henderson', *Philosophical Transactions of the Royal Society*, B 368:20130113 (2013), 4.
Hopkins, Donald R., *Princes and Peasants: Smallpox in History* (Chicago, IL: University of Chicago Press, 1983). The 2nd (2002) edition was published as *The Greatest Killer: Smallpox in History*.
Karki, B. B., 'A review of global smallpox eradication', *Journal of Nepal Medical Association (JNMA)*, 13:1–2 (1975), 18–24.
Marennikova, S. S. (ed.), *How It Was: The Global Smallpox Eradication Program in Reminiscences of Its Participants* (Novosibirsk: CERIS, 2018).

Schnur, Alan, 'Innovation as an integral part of smallpox eradication: A fieldworker's perspective', in Sanjoy Bhattacharya and Sharon Messenger (eds), *The Global Eradication of Smallpox* (New Delhi: Orient BlackSwan, 2010), pp. 106–50.
Shrestha, P. N., 'History of smallpox', *JNMA*, 10:2 (1972), 107–11.
Singh, Satnam, 'Some aspects of the epidemiology of smallpox in Nepal', *Indian Journal of Public Health*, 14:4 (1970), 129–35.

Other

Miscellaneous newspaper cuttings
United States Operations Mission to Nepal, *Glimpses of Progress in Nepal 1952–1961* (Kathmandu: United States Information Service, 1961).

Secondary sources

Adhikari, Jagannath and David Seddon, *Pokhara: Biography of a Town* (Kathmandu: Mandala Book Point, 2002).
Agrawal, Hem Narayan, *The Administrative System of Nepal: From Tradition to Modernity* (New Delhi: Vikas, 1976).
Amrith, Sunil S., *Decolonizing International Health: India and Southeast Asia, 1930–65* (Basingstoke: Palgrave Macmillan, 2006).
Arnold, David, *Colonizing the Body: State Medicine and Epidemic Disease in Nineteenth-Century India* (Berkeley, CA, and London: University of California Press, 1993).
——, 'Social crisis and epidemic disease in the famines of nineteenth-century India', *Social History of Medicine*, 6:3 (1993), 385–404.
Baldwin, Peter, *Contagion and the State in Europe, 1830–1930* (Cambridge: Cambridge University Press, 1999).
Banister, Judith and Shyam Thapa, *The Population Dynamics of Nepal* (Honolulu, HI: East-West Center, 1981).
Bartlett, M. S., 'Measles periodicity and community size', *Journal of the Royal Statistical Society. Series A (General)*, 120:1 (1957), 48–70.
Bashford, Alison, 'The history of public health during colonialism', in Harald Kristian (Kris) Heggenhougen and Stella Quah (eds), *International Encyclopedia of Public Health* (Amsterdam: Elsevier/Academic Press, 2008), pp. 398–404.
——, *Imperial Hygiene: A Critical History of Colonialism, Nationalism and Public Health* (Basingstoke: Palgrave Macmillan, 2004).
Bastos, Christina, 'Borrowing, adapting, and learning the practices of smallpox: Notes from colonial Goa', *Bulletin of the History of Medicine*, 83:1 (2009), 141–63.
Baylac-Paouly, Baptiste, 'Confronting and emergency: The vaccination campaign against meningitis in Brazil (1974–1975)', *Social History of Medicine*, 34:2 (2021), 632–49.

Benenson, Abram S. (ed.), *Control of Communicable Diseases in Man*, 12th edn (Washington, DC: American Public Health Association, 1975).

Bennett, Michael, *War Against Smallpox: Edward Jenner and the Global Spread of Vaccination* (Cambridge: Cambridge University Press, 2020).

Bhattacharya, Sanjoy, *Expunging Variola: The Control and Eradication of Smallpox in India 1947–1977* (New Delhi: Orient Longman, 2006).

———, 'Global and local histories of medicine: Interpretative challenges and future possibilities', in Mark Jackson (ed.), *A Global History of Medicine* (Oxford: Oxford University Press, 2018), pp. 243–62.

———, 'International health and the limits of its global influence: Bhutan and the worldwide Smallpox Eradication Programme', *Medical History*, 57:4 (2013), 461–86.

———, 'Re-devising Jennerian vaccines? European technologies, Indian innovation and the control of smallpox in South Asia, 1850–1950', *Social Scientist*, 26:11/12 (1998), 27–66.

———, 'Uncertain advances: A review of the final phases of the Smallpox Eradication Program in India, 1960–1980', *American Journal of Public Health*, 94:11 (2004), 1875–83.

———, 'WHO-led or WHO-managed? Re-assessing the Smallpox Eradication Program in India, 1960–1980', in Alison Bashford (ed.), *Medicine at the Border: Disease, Globalization and Security, 1850 to the Present* (Basingstoke and New York: Palgrave Macmillan, 2006), pp. 60–75.

Bhattacharya, Sanjoy and Carlos Eduardo D'Avila Pereira Campani, 'Re-assessing the foundations: Worldwide smallpox eradication, 1957–67', *Medical History*, 64:1 (2020), 71–93.

Bhattacharya, Sanjoy, Mark Harrison and Michael Worboys, *Fractured States: Smallpox, Public Health and Vaccination Policy in British India 1800–1947* (New Delhi: Orient Longman, 2005).

Bhattacharya, Sanjoy, Alexander Medcalf and Aliko Ahmed, 'Humanities, criticality and transparency: global health histories and the foundations of inter-sectoral partnerships for the democratisation of knowledge', *Humanities and Social Sciences Communications*, 7:1 (2020), 1–11.

Bhattacharya, Sanjoy and Sharon Messenger (eds), *The Global Eradication of Smallpox* (New Delhi: Orient BlackSwan, 2010).

Birn, Anne-Emanuelle, 'Small(pox) success?', *Ciencia & Saude Coletiva*, 16:2 (2011), 592.

———, 'The stages of international (global) health: Histories of success or successes of history?', *Global Public Health*, 4:1 (2009), 50–68.

Blume, Stuart, *Immunization: How Vaccines Became Controversial* (London: Reaktion Books, 2017).

Blume, Stuart, Jagrati Jani and Sidsel Roalkvam, 'Saving children's lives: Perspectives on immunisation', in Sidsel Roalkvam, Desmond McNeill and Stuart Blume (eds), *Protecting the World's Children: Immunisation policies and practices* (Oxford: Oxford University Press, 2013), pp. 1–30.

Brimnes, Niels, 'Fallacy, sacrilege, betrayal and conspiracy: The cultural construction of opposition to immunization in India', in Christine Holmberg, Stuart Blume and Paul Greenough (eds), *The Politics of Vaccination: A Global History* (Manchester: Manchester University Press, 2017), pp. 51–76.

———, 'Variolation, vaccination and popular resistance in early colonial South India', *Medical History*, 48:2 (2004), 199–228.

Brockington, Fraser, *World Health* (Harmondsworth and Baltimore, MD: Penguin, 1958).

Chen, Lu, 'China in the Worldwide Eradication of Smallpox, 1900–1985: Recovering and Democratizing Histories of International Health', PhD Diss., University of York, 2021.

Closser, Svea, *Chasing Polio in Pakistan: Why the World's Largest Public Health Initiative May Fail* (Nashville, TN: Vanderbilt University Press, 2010).

Crosby, Alfred W., 'Smallpox', in Kenneth F. Kiple (ed.), *The Cambridge World History of Human Disease* (Cambridge: Cambridge University Press, 1993), pp. 1008–13 http://dx.doi.org/10.1017/CHOL9780521332866.190

Cueto, Marcos, Theodore M. Brown and Elizabeth Fee, *The World Health Organization: A History* (Cambridge: Cambridge University Press, 2019).

Dixit, Hemang, *Fifty Years of NMA* (Kathmandu: Nepal Medical Association, 2001).

———, *My 2 Innings*, 2nd edn (Kathmandu: Makalu Publication House, 2009).

———, 'National health – the task ahead', *JNMA*, 10:1 (1972), 45–50.

———, *The Quest for Health: The Health Services of Nepal* (Kathmandu, Nepal: Educational Enterprise, 1995, 2nd edn 1999). The 3rd (2005) and 4th (2014) editions were published as *Nepal's Quest for Health* (Kathmandu: Educational Publishing House).

Dowdle, Walter R., 'The principles of disease elimination and eradication', *Bulletin of the World Health Organization*, 76:Suppl. 2 (1998), 22–5.

Dunn, Frederick L., 'Medical-geographical observations in Central Nepal', *Milbank Memorial Fund Quarterly*, 40:2 (1962), 125–48.

Enkin, M. W. and A. R. Jadad, 'Using anecdotal information in evidence-based health care: Heresy or necessity?' *Annals of Oncology*, 9 (1998), 963–96.

Ferrari, Fabrizio M., *Religion, Devotion and Medicine in North India: The Healing Power of Śītalā* (London: Bloomsbury, 2015).

Fisher, James F., *At Home in the World: Globalization and the Peace Corps in Nepal* (Bangkok: Orchid Press, 2013).

Fraser, Stuart M. F., 'Leicester and smallpox: The Leicester method', *Medical History*, 24:3 (1980), 315–32.

Frechette, Ann, *Tibetans in Nepal: The Dynamics of International Assistance among a Community in Exile* (New York: Berghahn Books, 2002).

Frèrot, Mathilde, Annick Lefebvre, Simon Aho, Patrick Callier, Karine Astruc and Ludwig Serge Aho Glèlè, 'What is epidemiology? Changing definitions of epidemiology 1978–2017', *PLoSONE*, 13:12 (2018), e0208442.

Fujikura, Tatsuro, 'Technologies of improvement, locations of culture: American discourses of democracy and "community development" in Nepal', *Studies in Nepali History and Society*, 1:2 (1996), 271–311.

Gill, Michael, *Mountaineering Midsummer: Climbing in Four Continents* (London: Hodder & Stoughton, 1969).

Gimlette, G. H. D., *Nepal and the Nepalese* (London: H. F. & G. Witherby, 1928).

Goldstein, Melvyn C., 'A report on Limi Panchayat, Humla District, Karnali Zone 1974', *Contributions to Nepalese Studies*, 2:2 (1975), 89–101.

Greenough, Paul, 'Intimidation, coercion and resistance in the final stages of the South Asian Smallpox Eradication Campaign, 1973–1975', *Social Science & Medicine*, 41:5 (1995), 633–45.

———, 'The uneasy politics of epidemic aid: The CDC's mission to Cold War East Pakistan, 1958', in Christine Holmberg, Stuart Blume and Paul Greenough (eds), *The Politics of Vaccination: A Global History* (Manchester: Manchester University Press, 2017), pp. 19–50.

Hanefield, Johanna and Hanna-Tina Fischer, 'Global health: Definitions, principles, and drivers', in Robin Haring (ed.), *Handbook of Global Health* (Cham: Springer, 2021), doi.org/10.1007/978-3-030-45009-0_1

Harper, Ian, *Development and Public Health in the Himalaya: Reflections on Healing in Contemporary Nepal* (London and New York: Routledge, 2014).

———, 'Mediating therapeutic uncertainty: A mission hospital in Nepal', in Mark Harrison, Margaret Jones and Helen Sweet (eds), *From Western Medicine to Global Medicine: The Hospital Beyond the West* (New Delhi: Orient BlackSwan, 2009), pp. 303–29.

Harrison, Mark, 'A global perspective: Reframing the history of health, medicine, and disease', *Bulletin of the History of Medicine*, 89:4 (2015), 639–89.

Hasrat, Bikrama Jit, *History of Nepal as Told by Its Own and Contemporary Chroniclers* (Hoshiarpur, Punjab: V. V. Research Institute, 1970).

Hays, J. N., *The Burdens of Disease: Epidemics and Human Response in Western History*, rev. edn (New Brunswick, NJ: Rutgers University Press, 2009).

Heydon, Susan, 'Death of the king: The introduction of vaccination into Nepal in 1816', *Medical History*, 63:1 (2019), 24–43.

———, 'Medicines, travellers and the introduction and spread of "modern" medicine in the Mt Everest region of Nepal', *Medical History*, 55:4 (2011), 503–21.

———, 'Missions, visitors and international aid', *Studies in Nepali History and Society*, 24:1 (2019), 73–104.

———, *Modern Medicine and International Aid: Khunde Hospital, Nepal, 1966–1998* (New Delhi: Orient BlackSwan, 2009).

———, 'Which medicine? Medicine-taking and changing Sherpa lives', *Himalaya*, 34:2 (2015), 38–50.

Hillary, Edmund, *High Adventure* (London: Readers Book Club, 1957).

———, Sir Edmund, *Schoolhouse in the Clouds* (London: Hodder & Stoughton, 1964).

Hillary, Louise, *A Yak for Christmas* (Garden City, NY: Doubleday, 1969).

Hindman, Heather, 'The everyday life of American development in Nepal', *Studies in Nepali History and Society*, 7:1 (2002), 99–136.

Hitchcock, John T., 'Some effects of recent change in rural Nepal', *Human Organization*, 22:1 (1963), 75–82.

Hodges, Sarah, 'The global menace', *Social History of Medicine*, 25:3 (2012), 719–28.

Holmberg, Christine, Stuart Blume and Paul Greenough (eds), *The Politics of Vaccination: A Global History* (Manchester: Manchester University Press, 2017).

Izzard, Ralph, *An Innocent on Everest* (New York: E. P. Dutton, 1954).

Jackson, Mark, 'One world, one health? Towards a global history of medicine', in Mark Jackson (ed.), *A Global History of Medicine* (Oxford: Oxford University Press, 2018), pp. 1–18.

Jannetta, Ann, *The Vaccinators: Smallpox, Medical Knowledge, and the 'Opening' of Japan* (Stanford, CA: Stanford University Press, 2007).

Johnson, Ryan and Amna Khalid (eds), *Public Health in the British Empire: Intermediaries, Subordinates, and the Practice of Public Health, 1850–1960* (New York and London: Routledge, 2012).

Justice, Judith, *Policies, Plans & People: Foreign Aid and Health Development* (Kathmandu: Mandala, in association with University of California Press, 1989).

Justice, Judithanne, 'The invisible worker: The role of the peon in Nepal's health service', *Social Science & Medicine*, 17:14 (1983), 967–70.

Khan, Yasmin, *The Raj at War: A People's History of India's Second World War* (London: Vintage, 2016).

Kirkpatrick, Colonel, *An Account of the Kingdom of Nepaul Being the Substance of Observations Made during a Mission to That Country in the Year 1793* (New Delhi: Manjusri Publishing House, 1969 [1811]).

Koplan, J. P., T. C. Bond, M. H. Merson, K. S. Reddy, M. H. Rodriguez, N. K. Sewankambo, J. N. Wasserheit and Consortium of Universities for Global Health Executive Board, 'Towards a common definition of global health', *The Lancet*, 373:9679 (2009), 1993–5.

Kotar, S. L. and J. E. Gessler, *Smallpox: A History* (Jefferson, NC: McFarland, 2013).

Kramer, Paul A., 'Region in global history', in Douglas Northrop (ed.), *A Companion to World History* (Oxford: Blackwell, 2012), pp. 201–12.

Landon, Perceval, *Nepal*, 2 vols (New Delhi: Asian Educational Services, 1993 [1928]).
Larson, Heidi J., Caitlin Jarrett, Elisabeth Eckersberger, David M. D. Smith and Pauline Paterson, 'Understanding vaccine hesitancy and vaccines and vaccination from a global perspective: A systematic review of published literature, 2007–2012', *Vaccine*, 32:19 (2014), 2150–9.
Latham, Michael E., *Modernization as Ideology: American Social Science and 'Nation Building' in the Kennedy Era* (Chapel Hill, NC: University of North Carolina Press, 2000).
Liechty, Mark, Pratyoush Onta and Lokranjan Parajuli, 'Introduction: Cultural politics in the long 1950s', *Studies in Nepali History and Society*, 24:1 (2019), 1–14.
Liechty, Mark, *What Went Right: Sustainability versus Dependence in Nepal's Hydropower Development* (Cambridge: Cambridge University Press, 2022).
Lienhard, Siegfried, *Songs of Nepal: An Anthology of Nevar Folksongs and Hymns* (Delhi: Motilal Banarsidass, 1992).
Liu, Chieng-Ling, 'Relocating Pastorian medicine: Accommodation and acclimatization of Pastorian practices against smallpox at the Pasteur Institute of Chengdu, China, 1908–1927', *Science in Context*, 30:1 (2017), 33–59.
Lock, Margaret and Vinh-Kim Nguyen, *An Anthropology of Biomedicine* (Chichester: Blackwell, 2010).
Macekura, Stephen J. and Erez Manela (eds), *The Development Century: A Global History* (Cambridge: Cambridge University Press, 2018). DOI:10.1017/9781108678940
Macfarlane, Alan, 'Death, disease and curing in a Himalayan village', in Christoph von Fürer-Haimendorf (ed.), *Asian Highland Societies in Anthropological Perspective* (New Delhi: Sterling, 1981), pp. 79–129.
McKay, Alex, '"An excellent measure": The battle against smallpox in Tibet, 1904–47', *Tibet Journal*, 30/31:4/1 (2005–06), 119–30.
Manela, Erez, 'A pox on your narrative: Writing disease control into Cold War history', *Diplomatic History*, 34:2 (2010), 299–323.
———, 'Smallpox and the globalization of development', in Stephen J. Macekura and Erez Manela (eds), *The Development Century: A Global History* (Cambridge: Cambridge University Press, 2018), pp. 83–103.
Marasini, Babu Ram, 'Health and hospital development in Nepal: Past and present', *JNMA*, 42:149 (2003), 306–11.
Martin, Chautari, *Early Developments in Telephones and Electricity in Nepal*, Research Brief 26 (Kathmandu: Martin Chautari, 2019).
Messerschmidt, Don, 'The scourge of smallpox: Nepal 1964', *ECS Nepal*, 73 (January 2008) www.ecs.com.np/feature_detailed.php?f_id=76.
Mierow, Dorothy, *Thirty Years in Pokhara* (Kathmandu: Pilgrims Book House, 1997).
Mihaly, Eugene Bramer, *Foreign Aid and Politics in Nepal: A Case Study*, 2nd edn (Lalitpur: Himal Books, 2002).
Millar, W. S., 'Some aspects, mainly medical, of the Gurkha recruiting season, 1955', *Journal of the Royal Army Medical Corps*, 103:3 (1957), 147–54.

Mills, Anne, 'Vertical vs horizontal health programmes in Africa: Idealism, pragmatism, resources and efficiency', *Social Science & Medicine*, 17:24 (1983), 1971–81.

Mills, Anne, J. Patrick Vaughan, Duane L. Smith and Iraj Tabibzadeh, *Health System Decentralization: Concepts, Issues and Country Experience* (Geneva: World Health Organization, 1990).

Millward, Gareth, *Vaccinating Britain: Mass Vaccination and the Public since the Second World War* (Manchester: Manchester University Press, 2019).

Minsky, Lauren, 'Pursuing protection from disease: The making of smallpox prophylactic practice in colonial Punjab', *Bulletin of the History of Medicine*, 83:1 (2009), 164–90.

Moore, Alfred and Jack Stilgoe, 'Experts and anecdotes: The role of "anecdotal evidence" in public scientific controversies', *Science, Technology, & Human Values*, 34:5 (2009), 654–77.

Moore, George and Berwyn Moore, 'Experience of a US Public Health Officer: 1950s Nepal', *Public Health Reports*, 120:5 (2005), 463–6.

Muraskin, William, 'The power of individuals and the dependency of nations in global eradication and immunisation campaigns', in Christine Holmberg, Stuart Blume and Paul Greenough (eds), *The Politics of Vaccination: A Global History* (Manchester: Manchester University Press, 2017), pp. 321–36.

Murdoch, Lydia, 'Carrying the pox: The use of children and ideals of childhood in early British and imperial campaigns against smallpox', *Journal of Social History*, 48:3 (2015), 511–35.

Nano, Atsuko, 'Inoculators, the indigenous obstacle to vaccination in colonial Burma', *Journal of Burma Studies*, 14 (2010), 91–114.

Neelakantan, Vivek, 'Eradicating smallpox in Indonesia: The archipelagic challenge', *Health and History*, 12:1 (2010), 61–87.

Nicholas, Ralph W., 'The goddess Sitala and epidemic smallpox in Bengal', *Journal of Asian Studies*, 41:1 (1981); 21–44.

Nichter, Mark, *Global Health: Why Cultural Perceptions, Social Representations, and Biopolitics Matter* (Tucson, AZ: University of Arizona Press, 2008).

Oduntan, Oluwatoyin Babatunde, 'Culture and colonial medicine: Smallpox in Abeokuta, Western Nigeria', *Social History of Medicine*, 30:1 (2017), 48–70.

Ogden, Horace G., *CDC and The Smallpox Crusade* (Washington, DC: US Department of Health and Human Services, Center for Disease Control, 1987).

Ohja, Durga P., 'History of land settlement in Nepal Tarai', *Contributions to Nepalese Studies*, 11:1 (1983), 21–44.

Oldfield, Henry Ambrose, *Sketches from Nipal*, 2 vols (London: W. H. Allen, 1880).

O'Leary, Zina, *Researching Real-World Problems: A Guide to Methods of Inquiry* (London: SAGE Publications, 2005).

Packard, Randall, *A History of Global Health: Interventions into the Lives of Other Peoples* (Baltimore, MD: Johns Hopkins University Press, 2016).
——, 'Visions of postwar health and development and their impact on public health interventions in the developing world', in Frederick Cooper and Randall Packard (eds), *International Development and the Social Sciences: Essays on the History and Politics of Knowledge* (Berkeley, CA: University of California Press, 1997), pp. 93–115.
Pandey, M. R., I. L. Acharya and A. Moyeed, 'Clinical survey of small pox', *JNMA*, 2:1 (1964), 8–11.
Peace Corps, *The Peace Corps' Contributions to the Global Smallpox Eradication Program* (Washington, DC: Office of Strategic Information, Research, and Planning (OSIRP), 2016), https://s3.amazonaws.com/files.peacecorps.gov/../Peace_Corps_Global_Smallpox.pdf
Penschow, Jennifer D., *Battling Smallpox before Vaccination: Inoculation in Eighteenth Century Germany*, Clio Medica Series (Leiden: Brill, 2022).
Pigg, Stacy Leigh, 'Inventing social categories through place: Social representations and development in Nepal', *Comparative Studies in Society & History*, 34:3 (1992), 491–513.
——, 'The credible and the credulous: The question of "villagers' beliefs" in Nepal', *Cultural Anthropology*, 11:2 (1996), 160–201.
——, 'Unintended consequences: The ideological impact of development in Nepal', *Comparative Studies of South Asia, Africa and the Middle East*, 13:1/2 (1993), 45–58.
Pitt, Peter, *The Scalpel and the Kukri: A Surgeon & his Family's Adventures among the Gurkhas* (Chippenham, UK: Peter Pitt, 2005).
——, *Surgeon in Nepal* (London: John Murray, 1970).
Porter, Dorothy, 'How did social medicine evolve, and where is it heading?', *PLoS Med*, 3:10 (2006), e399.
Prasai, Bhisma Raj, *Afu Lai Farkera Hereko* (Looking Back at Oneself) (Kathmandu: Ghost Writing Nepal, 2017).
Rahul, Ram, *The Himalaya as a Frontier* (New Delhi: Vikas Publishing House, 1978).
Raj, Yogesh, 'Management of the relief and reconstruction after the Great Earthquake of 1934', *Studies in Nepali History and Society*, 20:2 (2015), 375–422.
Raj, Yogesh, Deepak Aryal and Shamik Mishra, 'Documents related to the early hospitals in Nepal', *Studies in Nepali History and Society*, 21:2 (2016), 347–400.
Reinhardt, Bob R., *The End of a Global Pox: America and the Eradication of Smallpox in the Cold War Era* (Chapel Hill, NC: The University of North Carolina Press, 2015).
Roberts, Gilbert, 'Health and medicine', in James Ramsey Ullman, *Americans on Everest* (Philadelphia, PA: J. B. Lippincott, 1964), pp. 343–50.

Roberts, Jonathan David, 'Participating in eradication: how Guinea worm redefined eradication, and eradication redefined Guinea work, 1985–2022', *Medical History*, 67:2 (2023), 148–71.

Roalkvam, Sidsel, Desmond McNeill and Stuart Blume (eds), *Protecting the World's Children: Immunisation Policies and Practices* (Oxford: Oxford University Press, 2013).

Robertson, Thomas B., 'DDT and the Cold War jungle: American environmental and social engineering in the Rapti valley of Nepal', *Journal of American History*, 104:4 (2018), 904–30.

———, '"Front Line of the Cold War": The US and Point Four Development Programs in Cold War Nepal 1950–1953', *Studies in Nepali History and Society*, 24:1 (2019), 41–72.

Rose, Leo E., 'Nepal's experiment with "traditional democracy"', *Pacific Affairs*, 36:1 (1963), 16–31.

———, *Nepal: Strategy for Survival* (Berkeley, CA: University of California Press/Kathmandu: Mandala Book Point, 1971).

Saavedra, Monica, 'Politics and Health at the WHO Regional Office for South East Asia: The Case of Portuguese India, 1949–61', *Medical History*, 61:3 (2017), 380–400.

Sharma, Sudhindra, 'Trickle to torrent to irrelevance? Six decades of foreign aid in Nepal', in Dipak Gyawali, Michael Thompson and Marco Verweij (eds), *Aid, Technology and Development: The Lessons from Nepal* (London and New York: Routledge, 2017), pp. 54–74.

Sherpa, Lhakpa Norbu (ed.), *Khumjung Secondary School: Celebrating 50 Years of Education 1961–2011* (Lalitpur: Golden Jubilee Celebration Committee, 2011).

Shrestha, Hari Prasad and Prami Shrestha, 'Tourism in Nepal: A historical perspective and present trend of development', *Himalayan Journal of Sociology & Anthropology*, 5 (2012), 54–75.

Skerry, Christa A., Kerry Moran and Kay M. Calavan, *Four Decades of Development: The History of U.S. Assistance to Nepal 1951–1991* (Kathmandu: United States Agency for International Development, 1991).

Slusser, Mary, 'Nepali sculptures: New discoveries', in P. Lal (ed.), *Aspects of Indian Art: Papers Presented in a Symposium at the Los Angeles County Museum of Art, October, 1970* (Leiden: Brill, 1972), pp. 93–104.

Sobocinska, Agnieszka, 'New histories of foreign aid', *History Australia*, 17:4 (2020), 595–610. DOI: 10.1080/14490854.2020.1838932

Stepan, Nancy, *Eradication: Ridding the World of Diseases Forever?* (Ithaca, NY: Cornell University Press, 2011).

Stiller, Ludwig F., *Nepal: Growth of a Nation* (Kathmandu: Human Resources Development Research Center, 1999 [1993]).

———, *The Silent Cry: The People of Nepal: 1816–1839* (Kathmandu: Sahayogi Prakashan, 1976).

Stiller, Ludwig F. and Ram Prakash Yadav, *Planning for People* (Kathmandu: Human Resources Development Research Center, 1993).

Streefland, Pieter, 'The frontier of modern western medicine in Nepal', *Social Science & Medicine*, 20:11 (1985), 1151–9.
Streefland, Pieter, A. M. R. Chowdhury and Pilar Ramoz-Jimenez, 'Patterns of vaccination acceptance', *Social Science & Medicine*, 49:12 (1999), 1705–16.
Subedi, Madhusudan Sharma, *Medical Anthropology of Nepal* (Kathmandu: Udaya Books, 2001).
——, *State, Society and Health in Nepal* (London and New York: Routledge, 2018).
Survey of India. *Records of the Survey of India 8, Exploration in Tibet and Neighbouring Regions, Part 2: 1879–1892* (Dehra Dun: Survey of India, 1915).
Suzuki, Akihito, 'Smallpox and the epidemiological heritage of modern Japan: Towards a total history', *Medical History*, 55:3 (2011), 313–18.
Svalheim, Peter (trans. Katherine M. Parent), *Power for Nepal: Odd Hoftun & the History of Hydropower Development* (Kathmandu: Martin Chautari, 2015).
Taylor, Carl E., 'A medical survey of the Kali Gandak and Pokhara valleys of Central Nepal', *Geographical Review*, 41:3 (1951), 421–37.
Tenzing Norgay (as told to) James Ramsey Ullman, *Man of Everest: The Autobiography of Tenzing* (London: The Reprint Society, 1956).
Tokunaga, Atsushi, 'Experiences of medical survey in Central Nepal', *Journal of the Indian Medical Association*, 29:6 (1957), 221–4.
Tucker, Jonathan B., *Scourge: The Once and Future Threat of Smallpox* (New York: Grove Press, 2001).
Tworek, Heidi J. S., 'Communicable disease: Information, health, and globalization in the interwar period', *American Historical Review*, 124:3 (2019), 813–42.
Ullman, James Ramsey, *Americans on Everest* (Philadelphia, PA: J. B. Lippincott, 1964).
Vaidya, B. N. and H. V. Gurubacharya, 'On smallpox', *JNMA* 4:4 (1966), 339–43.
van Spengen, Wim, *Tibetan Border Worlds: A Geohistorical Analysis of Trade and Traders* (London: Kegan Paul International, 2000).
Vargha, Dora, 'Vaccination and the communist state: Polio in Eastern Europe', in Christine Holmberg, Stuart Blume and Paul Greenough (eds), *The Politics of Vaccination: A Global History* (Manchester: Manchester University Press, 2017), pp. 77–98.
Wadley, Susan S., 'Sitala: The cool one', *Asian Folklore Studies*, 39:1 (1980), 33–62.
Walloch, Karen L., *The Antivaccine Heresy: Jacobson v. Massachusetts and the Troubled History of Compulsory Vaccination in the United States* (Rochester, NY; Woodbridge, Suffolk: Boydell & Brewer, 2015).
Ward, Michael, 'In eastern Nepal', *The Lancet*, 263:2 (1952), 238–9.

Wehrle, P. F., J. Posch, K. H. Richter and D. A. Henderson, 'An airborne outbreak of smallpox in a German hospital and its significance with respect to other recent outbreaks in Europe', *Bulletin of the World Health Organization*, 43:5 (1970), 669–79.

Whelpton, John, *A History of Nepal* (Cambridge: Cambridge University Press, 2005).

———, 'A reading guide to Nepalese history', *Himalaya*, 25:1 (2005), Article 5.

Wickett, John and Peter Carrasco, 'Logistics in smallpox: The legacy', *Vaccine* 29S (2011), D131–4.

Willard, Nedd, 'The anger of a goddess', *World Health* (October 1972), 18–21.

Williams, Gareth, *Angel of Death: The Story of Smallpox* (Basingstoke: Palgrave Macmillan, 2010).

Worth, Robert M. and Narayan K. Shah, *Nepal Health Survey 1965–1966* (Honolulu, HI: University of Hawaii Press, 1969).

Wright, Daniel, *History of Nepal* (New Delhi: Rupa & Co, 2007 [1877]).

Yin, Robert K., *Case Study Research and Applications: Design and Methods*, 6th edn (Thousand Oaks, CA: SAGE Publications, 2018).

Zangbu, Ngawang Tenzin (as told by), *Stories and Customs of the Sherpas*, ed. Frances Klatzel (Kathmandu: Mera Publications, 2000).

Index

Adiga, Ram Bhadra 102, 125, 128, 153–4, 184
administrative system 70, 74, 85, 104, 133, 180–1, 194–6, 198, 201
  see also district; panchayat system; zone
Afghanistan 120, 187, 206, 218
air transport 37, 76, 105, 110–11, 151–2
American Mount Everest Expedition (AMEE) 1, 95
Arita, Isao 27, 152, 178, 223
Ayurvedic medicine 53, 72, 77, 102

Bangladesh (East Pakistan) 31, 228–9, 236
Bhaktapur 130
  Thimi 102–3
Bhattacharya, Sanjoy 10–11, 220, 225
Bhutan 35
Big Red Book *see* eradication history
Bihar 37, 107, 231–2, 235
Bir Hospital 72, 102, 169, 199
  infectious disease unit (Teku) 169
Biratnagar 46, 134
Brahmin 47, 111
  see also Nepal: society

Britain
  British Military Hospital (Dharan) 171
  post 1947 relations with Nepal 109
British Council 149
British India, relations with Nepal 55, 69–70, 73, 76
  war 1814–16 5, 69
British Residency (Kathmandu)
  see also individual people
  hospital 57–58
Buddhism 48, 59, 70, 154
Burghart, Richard 68
Burma (Myanmar) 223

Candau, Marcolino 83, 120, 122, 143, 187
case study 10, 12, 256
CDC 27, 29, 36, 207, 252, 264
Ceylon (Sri Lanka) 123, 146–7
China 120, 123, 149
  relations with Nepal 25, 69
Christian missions 73, 78–9, 108, 121
  Nepal Evangelistic Band (International Nepal Fellowship) 78, 211
  United Mission to Nepal (UMN) 78, 172
Cold War 6, 9, 11, 31, 81, 100, 106, 223

colonialism 5, 46, 70, 80
communicable diseases 5, 52, 82, 103, 181, 210, 258
  prevention 75, 111, 243, 264
communication 73, 76, 103, 119, 126, 131, 151–2, 179, 197–8, 206–7, 209, 231, 261
  see also air transport; radio; roads; telephone; walking
constitution 74
  of 1962 85, 104, 195
Crippen, Edward 99, 101, 103–6

decentralisation 9, 17, 181, 193–4, 201, 218
development (as ideology) 196, 204
  see also foreign aid
district 71, 85, 118, 194–8, 200
district smallpox supervisors 194–5, 198, 201, 225, 227, 232, 235
Dixit, Hemang 32–3, 71, 169
Dixon, Cyril 28–9, 46, 170
Dunn, Frederick 59

earthquake (of 1934) 72
East India Company
  see British India
education 75, 119, 152–3, 156, 238, 262
epidemics 50, 72, 93, 104, 177
  smallpox
    1816 49
    1963–64 1–2, 15, 93–113, 128–9, 260
epidemiologists 181, 253
  see also individual people
epidemiology 45, 181
eradication (concept) 3, 143, 146, 252
eradication history 11, 14, 24–5, 28–31, 252, 257, 260, 263

official (Big Red Book) 9, 24–8, 34–6, 125, 194–5, 218–9, 253, 260
polio (poliomyelitis) 264
role of historians 30
smallpox programme's ongoing history 7, 37–8, 257, 265
40th anniversary 7, 252
Ethiopia 229, 239, 260
Everest, Mt 1, 25, 52, 70, 94, 209

Fenner, Frank 26–8
First World War 74
Fisher, Michael 69
Foege, William 29
foreign aid 16, 75–6, 79–80, 82, 86, 120, 149, 158, 179, 196, 207
  see also individual country programmes
foreigners 1, 15, 36, 52, 71, 77–8, 80, 86, 93, 106, 109, 112, 227, 262
  see also visitors; technology
Friedman, Jay 36, 224, 227, 231, 240

Gardner, Edward 55
Gimlette, George 57
Giri, Tulsi 103, 242
Global Commission for the Certification of Smallpox Eradication 7, 25–6
global health 9, 24, 254, 257–8
  role of historians 265
Gurkhas 57, 70, 106, 109–10, 157, 171
Gurung 106, 109, 157

health system 5, 71–2, 77, 83, 106, 108, 120–1, 130, 134, 152, 174, 176–7, 179, 182–3, 207, 237, 243

Index

Department of Health Services 72, 105, 109, 128, 135, 181, 183, 196–7, 200, 202, 204
  1969 report 125, 168, 210
  five-year plans 77, 119
  hospitals 71, 78–9, 107
    see also individual hospitals; Christian missions
  staff 180
Henderson, Donald 12, 27, 37, 172, 177, 180, 187, 194–5, 207–8, 218, 220, 232–3, 253, 263
Hillary, Sir Edmund 4, 51, 96, 98–9, 151
Hinduism 48, 59, 70, 154
Houghton, Philip 96

immunisation *see* vaccination
  Expanded Programme on Immunization (EPI) 244, 253, 264
India 75, 95, 109, 120, 171, 182, 229, 236, 239
  aid to Nepal 79
  border with Nepal *see* Nepal: border with India
  Indian Soldiers Board 110, 121
  relations with Nepal 241
  smallpox *see* smallpox eradication
International Committee of the Red Cross 121
International Sanitary Regulations 100, 170

Japan 206

Kalimati 204
Kantavati 47
Karki, Benu Bahadur 28, 227–8, 232
Kathmandu 1, 59, 99, 101, 122, 176, 210, 227, 242

Kathmandu Valley 2, 50–1, 99, 118, 125, 151, 169
Khumbu 1, 50, 59, 94, 96
Khunde Hospital 67, 99, 152, 161, 211
Kirkpatrick, William 49
Kirtipur 2, 101, 159

Lal, Krishan Murari 182–4, 196
Lalitpur (Patan) 155
Lamjung 106, *see* epidemics: smallpox: 1963–64
Landon, Perceval 58, 72
logistics 16, 205, 261
logistics approach 145
long 1950s 73, 77

Mahler, Halfdan 28, 253
malaria 122, 130
  global eradication campaign in Nepal 77, 82–3, 129, 180, 204, 207, 237
Marennikova, Svetlana 30
Mason, Royston 36, 224
Messerschmidt, Donald 106, 109, 157
modern medicine 1
monarchy 67, 204
  royal coup 1960 85, 104
Morrison, Bruce 106, 110–11

National Planning Commission 75
Nepal 15, 24, 32, 70, 242
  border with India 69, 73, 107, 209, 220, 232
  climate 206, 235
  cultural diversity 70
  economic development 75, 180, 195–6, 202, 204
  foreign policy 69
  formation of modern state 68–9
  language 67–8
  physical geography 24, 120, 260
  society 49, 70, 72, 77, 157, 238, 244

294　Index

Nepal Health Survey (1965–66) 17, 169, 173–7
  smallpox 174
  vaccination 174
Nepal Medical Association (NMA) 83
  Biratnagar branch 119, 135
  see also Prasai, Bhisma Raj
  Journal of Nepal Medical Association 33, 102, 134
New Zealand 1, 28, 68, 96, 161, 223
  see also Dixon, Cyril; Hillary, Sir Edmund; Houghton, Philip
Newar 2, 47, 51, 53, 101, 154, 184, 233
newspapers 13, 71, 101, 104, 172, 186

Oldfield, Henry 57

Pakistan 208, 229
panchayat system 85, 109, 135, 182–3
panchayats 33, 106, 111, 133, 153, 181, 211, 243
Peace Corps 37, 106–9, 111
  see also Messerschmidt, Donald; Morrison, Bruce
Pitt, Major Peter 171
Pokhara 77, 107, 110, 120, 208
population 5, 50, 169, 180, 202, 210
  growth 70, 77
  migration 70, 209–10
porters 2, 52, 95, 110, 122
Prasai, Bhisma Raj 53, 134, 153
Preston, David 28
public health 8, 121, 181, 253
  quarantine 84
  tools 8, 252

radio
  Radio Nepal 119, 238
Ram, Hari 49
Rana, Maharaja Chandra Shamsher 58, 68, 72, 76
Rana, Maharaja Jang Bahadur 50, 70
Rana regime 67, 71, 74
  downfall of 74
Rapti valley 80, 130
refrigerators 120, 125, 146, 150, 205–6, 224, 231, 262
roads 1, 37, 76, 120, 131, 206, 208–9, 236, 260

Sagauli, Treaty of 55, 69
Sathianathan, M. 36, 201, 221, 223, 225, 227, 233, 240
Second World War 5, 31, 73, 79, 81, 123
Shah, Birendra, King of Nepal 236, 242
Shah, Girvan, King of Nepal 47, 51, 56
Shah, Mahendra, King of Nepal 25, 74, 195, 204
Shah, Prithvi Narayan, King of Nepal 68, 78
Shah, Rana Bahadur, King of Nepal 47
Shah, Tribhuvan, King of Nepal 74
Sherpa 70, 95, 161, 176
Sherpa, Ang Jangbu 97
Sherpa, Kami Temba 70
Sherpa, Lhakpa Norbu 1, 95–6
Shrestha, K. B. 205, 224, 231
Shrestha, Purushottam Narayan 7, 26, 28, 195, 197, 199, 220–1, 234, 240
Sikkim 35
Singh, Satnam 33, 169, 171, 180, 202, 209
Singha Durbar 13, 125, 129
  Ministry of Foreign Affairs 203

Sitala 47, 59, 154, 157
smallpox 120, 171, 253
  control 53, 119, 122, 143–4, 254
  disease 4, 18, 45, 169, 171, 235, 243, 257
  epidemiology 50, 52, 145, 202
  pock mark surveys 239
  record-keeping 14, 209
  reporting 14, 31, 50, 101, 109, 170, 197, 208, 220, 225–7, 229, 238
  worldwide spread 4
  see also vaccination
smallpox eradication 11, 26, 120, 123–4, 133, 148, 153, 194, 243, 257–8
  global goal 6, 121–5, 144, 178, 196, 236
  intensified programme 6, 16, 163, 168, 177–8, 180, 208, 223
  Target Zero 229, 233–5
smallpox in Nepal 4, 13–14, 31, 45, 49–51, 93, 112, 169–70, 218, 225, 232–4
  beliefs 52, 96–7, 157–8, 184, 210, 259
  care in the home 2, 4, 46–7, 257
  cases 1961 120–1
  see also Tibetans (in Nepal)
  epidemiology 48, 52, 77, 95–6, 103, 109, 124, 208–9, 220, 260
  healers 47, 102
  importations Mugu district 1973 229–30
  requests for help 104, 109
  rituals 101
smallpox programme in Nepal 6–7, 10–12, 17, 73, 86, 118, 121, 144, 151, 158, 160, 168, 180–2, 187, 195–6, 200, 204, 229, 232, 234, 242–5, 254–5
  Government of Nepal/WHO Smallpox Control Pilot Project 16, 102, 124–33
  local initiative 1965 16, 118, 134–7, 153, 183
  revised plan of operation 1966 133, 151, 179, 181–2, 184, 209
  Smallpox Eradication Project (SEP) 17, 169, 184, 186, 193, 197, 200, 202, 204, 221
  additional funding from WHO 187, 203, 222
  assessment and evaluation 199, 211, 219
  staff 197–8, 225, 233, 263
  training 198, 201, 222, 263
  staff 152
  vehicle maintenance 206, 224–5
smallpox success in Nepal 218–9, 221, 236, 254–6, 264
  1975–77 236–9
  International Commission for the Assessment of Smallpox Eradication in Nepal 240–2
  declaration of eradication 241
  Kathmandu celebration 242–4
Soviet Union (USSR) 6, 178
  vaccine 123, 205
success 10, 12, 24, 27, 252–4
surveillance and containment 7, 18, 195, 208, 218, 220, 226–7, 235, 243, 263
Swayambhunath 47, 101

Tarai 32, 69, 76–7, 107, 169, 197, 208–9, 239
taxation 70–1
technology 6, 75, 196

Tedros, Adhanom Ghebreyesus 7, 252
telephone 76, 151
Thailand 120, 147
Thapa, Bhimsen 56
Thapa, Rita 154, 237
Tibet Autonomous Region (TAR) of China 1, 120
Tibetans (in Nepal) 57, 69–70, 100, 107, 239
Tiwari, Hira Prasad 201, 236
tourism 104
  see also visitors
traders 69, 109

United Nations (UN) 5, 82
United Nations Children's Fund (UNICEF) 147, 186, 239
United Nations Educational, Scientific and Cultural Organization (UNESCO) 30
United States Agency for International Development (USAID) 99, 103, 148
United States of America (USA) 5, 31
  aid programme 80, 106
  relations with Nepal 79
United States Operations Mission (USOM) 80, 83
  Moore, George 59
Uttar Pradesh 30, 37, 58, 107, 231–2

vaccination 1, 9, 16, 70, 84, 123, 143, 149, 258
  behaviour 16, 144–5, 253, 259
  bifurcated needles 105, 205, 260
  mass vaccination 3, 145–6, 153, 202, 218, 222, 263
  vaccination in Nepal 5, 57, 108, 112, 131, 133, 176
  1816 introduction 5, 55
  beliefs 97–8

  compulsory 102–3
  post 1951 59, 119, 130, 135, 147–8, 171–2, 186, 211
  other vaccines 161
  requests for vaccination 98, 109
  vaccination behaviour 3, 97, 111, 128–9, 153–6, 159, 184, 219, 221, 232
  acceptance 4, 97, 110, 147, 177
  refusal 97, 99, 231
  vaccine supply 56, 58, 72, 84, 93, 104–5, 126, 130, 136, 147, 186, 205, 207, 211, 223–4, 239, 264
variolation 53–4, 58, 98, 110, 159, 184
vertical programme 144, 179, 253
visitors 13, 59, 68, 79, 122
  climbing expeditions 70, 95

walking 1, 52, 95, 110, 122, 151, 206, 261
Wasito, R. 206
Whelpton, John 32, 196
WHO South-East Asia Regional Office (SEARO) 6, 28, 81–2, 118, 134, 136, 169, 178, 220
  Grasset, Nicole 225, 228
  Guneratne, V. T. Hevat 207, 222
  Mani, Chandra 81, 123, 179, 187, 203
  Regional Committee 6, 81, 84, 147
  regional personnel visiting Nepal 124–5, 127–8, 130, 152, 179, 182, 197, 199, 203, 219, 235
  workshop 1967 154, 160
women 154, 237
  carers 2–3, 51, 101, 258
  see also education
Wood, Hugh 149, 152

Index 297

World Health Assembly (WHA) 6, 27, 81, 118, 168, 178, 253
World Health Organization (WHO) 3, 5, 27, 81, 122, 152, 181, 187, 194, 206, 231, 253, 263
   Geneva HQ 177, 180, 194, 206
   in Nepal 81–2, 95–6, 203, 231
   smallpox conferences 146, 149, 219–21, 228

Weekly Epidemiological Record 100, 120–1, 170, 229
WHO expert committees on smallpox 132, 159, 236, 260
World Health magazine 34, 229
Wyeth Laboratories 95, 105

zone 85, 194, 197, 200, 206

www.ingramcontent.com/pod-product-compliance
Ingram Content Group UK Ltd.
Pitfield, Milton Keynes, MK11 3LW, UK
UKHW020943180225
455237UK00008B/104